Pediatric Cardiopulmonary Transplantation

Edited by

Kenneth L. Franco, MD

Associate Professor
Section of Cardiothoracic Surgery
Department of Surgery
School of Medicine
Yale University
New Haven, Connecticut

**Futura Publishing
Company, Inc.**
Armonk, New York

Library of Congress Cataloging-in-Publication Data

Pediatric cardiopulmonary transplantation / [edited] by Kenneth L.
   Franco
       p.   cm.
     Includes bibliographical references and index.
   ISBN 0-87993-397-6
     1. Heart—Transplantation.   2. Lungs—Transplantation.   3. Transplantation of
organs, tissues, etc. in children.
   I. Franco, Kenneth L.
     [DNLM: 1. Heart Transplantation—in infancy & childhood.   2. Lung
Transplantation—in infancy & childhood.   3. Heart-Lung Transplantation—in
infancy & childhood.   WG 169 P371 1997]
   RD598.35.T7P43   1997
   617.4′ 120592′ 083—dc21
   DNLM/DLC
   for Library of Congress   96-52001
                                                                           CIP

Published by
Futura Publishing Company, Inc.
135 Bedford Road
Armonk, New York 10504

LC#: 96-52001
ISBN#: 0-87993-397-6

Every effort has been made to ensure that the information in this book is up to date
and accurate at the time of publication. However, due to the constant developments in
medicine, neither the authors, nor the editor, nor the publisher can accept any legal or
any other responsibility for any errors or omissions that may occur.

Printed in the United States of America.

Printed on acid-free paper.

Contributors

Linda J. Addonizio, MD [1,7,8]
Associate Professor of Pediatrics
Medical Director, Pediatric Heart Transplant Program
College of Physicians and Surgeons of Columbia University
New York, New York

Ko Bando, MD [19]
Assistant Professor of Surgery
Division of Cardiothoracic Surgery
Indianapolis University Medical Center
Indianapolis, Indiana

Mark L. Barr, MD [17]
Associate Professor of Surgery
Co-Director, Cardiothoracic Transplantation
Director, Cardiothoracic Surgical Research
Division of Cardiothoracic Surgery
University of Southern California School of Medicine
Los Angeles, California

Stuart Berger, MD [10]
Chief of Pediatric Cardiology
Children's Hospital of Wisconsin
Milwaukee, Wisconsin

R. Morton Bolman, III, MD [13]
Professor and Chief
Division of Cardiothoracic Surgery
University of Minnesota
Minneapolis, Minnesota

Jonathan M. Chen, MD [7]
Department of Surgery
Division of Cardiothoracic Surgery
Columbia Presbyterian Medical Center
New York, New York

Numbers in brackets indicate chapters written or cowritten by the contributor.

Jean-Paul Couetil, MD [16]
Cardiothoracic Surgeon
Director, Heart and Lung Transplant Program
Department of Cardiothoracic Surgery
Broussais Hospital
Paris, France

Richard C. Daly, MD [12]
Associate Professor of Surgery
Consultant, Thoracic and Cardiovascular Surgery
Mayo Clinic
Rochester, Minnesota

Mark R. de Leval, MD, FRCS [9]
Consultant Cardiothoracic Surgeon
Great Ormond Street Hospital for Children
London, United Kingdom

Richard N. Eisen, MD [3]
Assistant Clinical Professor of Pathology
Yale University School of Medicine
Associate Attending Pathologist
Greenwich Hospital
Greenwich, Connecticut

Silviu Itescu, MD [1]
Assistant Professor of Pediatrics
Division of Autoimmune and Molecular Diseases
College of Physicians and Surgeons of Columbia University
New York, New York

Kenneth L. Franco, MD [15]
Associate Professor of Surgery
Division of Cardiothoracic Surgery
Yale University School of Medicine
New Haven, Connecticut

Michael D. Green, MD, MPH [2]
Associate Professor of Pediatrics and Surgery
Division of Pediatric Infectious Diseases
University of Pittsburgh School of Medicine
Children's Hospital of Pittsburgh
Pittsburgh, Pennsylvania

Bartley P. Griffith, MD [19]
Henry T. Bahnson Professor of Surgery
Chief, Division of Cardiothoracic Surgery
University of Pittsburgh Medical Center
Pittsburgh, Pennsylvania

Steven R. Gundry, MD [6]
Professor and Chief
Division of Cardiothoracic Surgery
Loma Linda University Medical Center
Loma Linda, California

Jeffrey D. Hosenpud, MD [10]
Professor and Chief
Division of Cardiovascular Medicine
Medical College of Wisconsin
Milwaukee, Wisconsin

Stuart W. Jamieson, MB, FRCS [11]
Professor and Chief
Division of Cardiothoracic Surgery
University of California Medical Center
San Diego, California

Valluvan Jeevanandam, MD [5]
Assistant Professor of Surgery
Surgical Director, Heart Transplant Program
Temple University Hospital
Philadelphia, Pennsylvania

David P. Kapelanski, MD, FACS [11]
Associate Clinical Professor of Surgery
Division of Cardiothoracic Surgery
University of California Medical Center
San Diego, California

Maryanne R. Kichuk, MD [1,7]
Assistant Professor of Pediatrics
Pediatric Cardiac Transplant Service
Division of Pediatric Cardiology
College of Physicians and Surgeons of Columbia University
New York, New York

Giovanni B. Luciani, MD [17]
Assistant Professor of Surgery
Division of Cardiovascular Surgery
University of Verona
Verona, Italy

George B. Mallory, Jr., MD [14]
Associate Professor of Pediatrics
Medical Director, Pediatric Lung Transplant Program
Washington University School of Medicine
St. Louis Children's Hospital
St. Louis, Missouri

Pankaj S. Mankad, MD, FRCS [9]
Consultant Cardiothoracic Surgeon
Royal Hospital for Sick Children
Edinburgh, Scotland

Christopher G.A. McGregor, MB, FRCS [12]
Professor of Surgery
Director, Cardiothoracic Transplant Program
Mayo Clinic
Rochester, Minnesota

Marian G. Michaels, MD, MPH [2]
Assistant Professor of Pediatrics and Surgery
Division of Pediatric Infectious Diseases
University of Pittsburgh School of Medicine
Children's Hospital of Pittsburgh
Pittsburgh, Pennsylvania

Robert E. Michler, MD [17]
Associate Professor of Surgery
Director, Heart Transplant Program
Division of Cardiothoracic Surgery
College of Physicians and Surgeons of Columbia University
New York, New York

D. Glenn Pennington, MD [4]
Professor and Chief
Division of Cardiothoracic Surgery
Bowman Gray School of Medicine
Winston-Salem, North Carolina

Mary S. Pohl, RN, BSN [20]
Clinical Trials Nurse
Division of Cardiothoracic Surgery
Barnes Hospital
St. Louis, Missouri

Sara J. Shumway, MD [13]
Professor of Surgery
Surgical Director, Heart Transplant Program
Division of Cardiothoracic Surgery
University of Minnesota
Minneapolis, Minnesota

Thomas L. Spray, MD [14, 20]
Professor and Chief
Division of Pediatric Cardiothoracic Surgery
University of Pennsylvania School of Medicine
Children's Hospital of Philadelphia
Philadelphia, Pennsylvania

Vaughn A. Starnes, MD [17]
Professor and Chief
Division of Cardiothoracic Surgery
University of Southern California School of Medicine
Children's Hospital of Los Angeles
Los Angeles, California

Mark T. Swartz, MD [4]
Director, Circulatory Support Program
Division of Cardiothoracic Surgery
St. Louis University
St. Louis, Missouri

Bruce F. Whitehead, MB, BS, FRCP [18]
Consultant Transplant Physician
Great Ormond Street Hospital for Children
London, United Kingdom

Foreword

Clinical cardiopulmonary transplantation has evolved dramatically since the first human heart transplant was performed by Dr. James Hardy in 1964. Of note, this was a xenograft procedure, and it is appropriate that it was, since the ultimate success of transplantation in helping large numbers of patients will depend upon the realization of successful xenografting. However, during the allograft era, which began for cardiac transplantation in 1967, there has been steady progress in terms of recipient selection, donor selection and management, surgical technique, postoperative management, and immunosuppression. The rapid progress in all of these areas has been associated with steady improvement in outcome, and widespread acceptance of transplantation has resulted. Because of the early successes in adult cardiac and, later, pulmonary transplantation, these methodologies have been introduced in the pediatric population. Because of concerns regarding growth and development, the influence of steroids, and the abilities of transplanted organs to grow, transplantation in the pediatric age group was relatively slow in coming. However, when faced with the inexorable progress of fatal illnesses and the established excellent results in the adult population, it became clear to the pediatric medical and surgical communities that transplantation was an appropriate alternative.

This volume deals with the transplantation of the heart, the lungs, and the heart-lung bloc in pediatric patients, examining the salient clinical problems as they are uniquely expressed in this age group. Much of what we have to learn regarding the further application of xenografting and the use of mechanical devices will be facilitated by the special perspective which pediatric transplantation affords.

John C. Baldwin, MD
Debakey/Bard Professor and Chairman
Department of Surgery
Baylor College of Medicine
Houston, Texas

Preface

Heart and lung transplantation remain effective therapeutic options for children with end-stage heart and lung disease, for which there is no medical treatment. Over the last ten years, a number of advances have occurred in the areas of immunosuppression, perioperative care, and surgical techniques. With increasing experience and improved results, more transplants will be needed, but the limiting factor will be the donor supply.

This book was written to document the current state of the art of pediatric thoracic organ transplantation. Many advances have occurred and are well summarized in the following chapters by authors who are recognized experts in their particular fields. They have written material in a comprehensive and clear manner. I hope that this book will help all who care for sick children with heart and lung disease.

I want to thank all of the contributors for their help in making this project a reality. This book took several years to complete, and would not have been possible if not for the support and dedication of Steve Korn and his publishing staff. This book is dedicated to all the children who will someday benefit from transplantation.

Kenneth L. Franco, MD
Editor

This book is dedicated to my wife, Jody, and son, Jonathan, for their support and understanding during the preparation of this work.

Contents

Chapter 1

Transplant Immunology and Pediatric Immunosuppression

Maryanne R. Kichuk, MD; Silviu Itescu, MD, Robert E. Michler, MD; Linda J. Addonizio, MD

Introduction

The immune system protects the body from various invaders by the identification of nonself from self. The immune response is a complex series of sometimes redundant initiations and terminations, often too confusing to follow and tedious to memorize, the result of which, years after studying the topic in medical school, is that its significance is regrettably forgotten. The importance of at least a rudimentary understanding of the immune system is essential to transplantation medicine. Without this, it is difficult to understand the workings of medications such as azathioprine and cyclosporin A(CsA), which are used in daily practice, and harder still to explain the necessity of such agents to anxious patients and their families.

Our goal in transplantation medicine is to manipulate the immune system in such a way as to induce immune tolerance: a condition of absent response to donor antigens with little effect on the immune response to unrelated antigens, and without the need for chronic immunosuppressive drugs. This is rather like having our cake and eating it, too. The perfect immune manipulation would produce a permanent state of tolerance to only donor antigens, leaving the remainder of the immune response intact against other potentially offensive and nonself antigens. As fledgling as our knowledge is, as imperfect as our efforts may be, we have been able to induce a state of pharmacologically engineered quasi-tolerance, which is, however, not without concomitant risks and dangers. It is this quasi-tolerant state which has allowed the success of organ transplantation, graft longevity, and the enhanced quality of life of the recipients.

In this chapter, we will simply review the basics of immunobiology, making note of their relativity to organ transplantation and rejection theory, and survey our current armamentarium of immunomanipulative therapeutics, including drug interactions and side effects.

From: Franco KL (ed). *Pediatric Cardiopulmonary Transplantation.* Armonk, NY: Futura Publishing Company, Inc.; © 1997.

Historical Background and the Recognition of Self

Medawar and Gibson, in their investigations during the 1940s and 1950s, used a mouse model that employed skin grafting from one site to another on the same mouse (autografts), or from genetically nonidentical individuals of the same species (allografts).[1] Invariably, rejection was the outcome in allograft transplantation and, as a result of this primary exposure, the recipient would evolve a specific immunologic memory for the donor, which on subsequent grafting would result in accelerated rejection.[2]

The existence of a complicated cell recognition system was suspected from the high incidence of rejection of allografted tissues. Further animal experimentation utilized skin grafting between individuals of the same inbred strain (syngeneic grafts), and between individuals from genetically disparate different species (xenografts). The success of the first case and the failure of the second seemed intuitively correct. Grafting between members of the same inbred strain should not result in rejection, because of the genetic homogeny of all the members. Transgressing species lines provided virtually limitless sites for nonself, nonspecies recognition and, therefore, resulted in rapid rejection. In addition, skin grafts performed on immunodeficient mice were not rejected.[3]

Exploration of the genetic basis for this process led to the discovery in mice of a group of related genes that exist within a particular chromosomal region and code for rapid graft rejection. The major histocompatability complex genes (MHC) code for glycoprotein molecules which are present on the surface of each cell and function as recognition sites for the determination of self from nonself. Two classes of molecules, called class I and class II, are encoded for by genes within the MHC region and each is slightly different from the other in structure and function, but both are involved in the process of rejection. The discovery of the MHC antigens allowed genetic matching of donor and recipient animals, and enhanced graft survival. It was hoped that the discovery of a similar system in humans could be applied practically to tissue grafting and organ transplantation. Initial studies in humans, performed using antibodies from pregnant women that reacted with leukocytes from different individuals, led to the identification of the human leukocyte antigen system (HLA). The genetic locus of the human MHC, encoding for the HLA group of proteins, is located on the short arm of the sixth chromosome. The human MHC system is extremely polymorphic, and is organized in a very similar manner to that of mice. It contains loci for class I, II, and III genes, as well as for certain cytokines.[4]

The class I HLA region of the human MHC complex contains six loci encoding for class I molecules. Three of these, HLA-A, -B, and -C are clinically important and are expressed on all nucleated cells. These three loci are highly polymorphic and contain at least 80 alleles. They are considered the classic antigens, since they form the major histocompatability barrier to allogeneic transplantation. The class II region contains approximately 14 loci, 7 of which encode for functionally important antigens. Genes located on these loci encode for α- or B-polypeptide subunits, which together, as an α-B-heterodimer, make up the complete class II molecule. Certain clusters of genes correspond to particular α- and B-peptide pairs, and three clinically relevant subregions have been described: HLA-DP; -DQ; and -DR. Each is highly polymorphic with from 10 to 30 alleles identified. Interspersed among the class I and class II loci are genes which encode for lymphokines, cytokines (including tumor necrosis factor-α [TNF-α]), collagen, and still others which may play a role in antigen processing and susceptibility to disease.[5,6]

The function of MHC (HLA) class I and II molecules is to bind peptide fragments of antigens, deliver them to the cell surface, and present them so that they can be recognized by T cells, thus initiating the immune response. The class I HLA molecule is made up of a membrane-bound glycoprotein heavy chain that is noncovalently connected to a β_2-microglobulin light chain. The heavy chain consists of two polymorphic (α_1 and α_2), and one nonpolymorphic (α_3) extracellular domains, as well as a transmembrane and an intracellular domain. High-resolution crystallography has illustrated that these molecules are complex heterodimeric protein structures made up of helices and β-pleated sheets that rest in three dimensions, the most external portion of which is a specific region of peptide binding and presentation. The class II HLA molecule is made up of four extracellular domains: α_1; α_2; β_1; β_2. Crystallographic pictures show two noncovalently connected halves formed by the alpha and beta domains, with a single helix and four strands making up the three-dimensional structure; the site for peptide binding is slightly different from that of the class I molecule.[7]

Class I HLA molecules are present on the surface of almost all nucleated cells. Class II molecules are present on specialized cells, termed antigen-presenting cells (APC), which are usually monocytes, macrophages, dendritic cells, and B cells. The class II molecules expressed on these cells serve to present foreign peptides to CD4+ helper T lymphocytes. Antigen-presenting cells also secrete cytokines, which further stimulate activation of T cells, and these include interleukin-1 and interleukin-6 (IL-1, IL-6), and tumor necrosis factor-α (TNF-α). Other cell types, such as vascular endothelium, can be induced to express HLA class II antigens after stimulation with δ-interferon, as may occur during the process of allograft rejection.[8]

Major histocompatability complex gene molecules shape the T cell repertoire of a particular individual during early ontogeny, by presenting a wide array of self-peptides, many of which are fragments of cell surface structures including other MHC molecules. Developing T lymphocytes must be educated to discriminate between self and nonself. During T cell development in the thymus, those cells having too strong (or conversely, too weak) an affinity for HLA and self-peptide are deleted. The remaining T cells having intermediate affinity are selected for maturation into peripheral T lymphocytes, presumably resulting in an immune responsiveness that is "just right." In a transplanted organ, the donor HLA molecule is perceived as foreign and its recognition by the recipient T cells initiates the ensuing immunologic cascade, termed the *alloresponse*. Because of the extreme nature of the polymorphism of HLA molecules and T cell receptor structures, maturation of T cells that are educated by recognition of self-peptides also provides a complement of T cells capable of interacting with exogenous antigens.[6,7] Recognition of the foreign HLA molecule may either occur directly by recipient CD4 or CD8 T cells, or indirectly, as peptides of the donor MHC class I or II molecules are presented by recipient APCs to recipient T cells. Both these scenarios are illustrated in Figures 1 and 2.

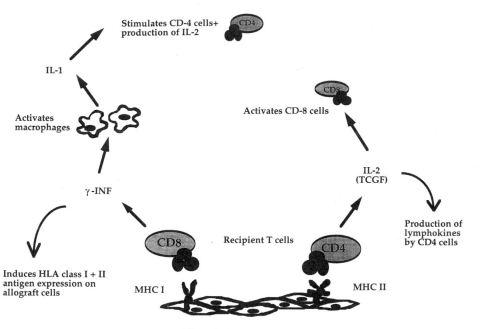

Figure 1. Direct alloresponse: both CD4 and CD8 recipient T cells can activate the direct alloresponse. Both cell types identify target major histocompatability complex (MHC) antigens by specific T cell receptors. CD4 cells are activated by donor MHC class II; CD8 cells interact with donor MHC class I antigens. Further production of lymphokines by these cells amplify the immune response.

The Heart of the Matter: The Immunologic Basis for Allograft Rejection

The steps that lead to immune recognition and initiation of the alloresponse are a chain reaction that begins with the encounter between an antigen (foreign protein) and a T cell.[5-10]

Direct recognition of the donor (or allo-) MHC molecule initiates a strong immune response. Lymphocytes that are capable of recognizing a particular alloantigen and inducing the direct alloresponse are present in circulation in numbers that are ten- to one-hundredfold greater than are lymphocytes, which recognize naturally occurring exogenous antigens. Both CD4 (helper) and CD8 (cytotoxic, suppressor) recipient T cells are capable of initiating the direct alloresponse. Both cell types identify target MHC antigens by specific T cell receptors. CD4 cells are activated by the specific antigenic reaction to the donor graft MHC class II complex, and once stimulated they produce large amounts of interleukin-2 (IL-2) and other lymphokines which accelerate the division of T cells and amplify the immune response. CD8 cells interact only with MHC class I antigen-bearing cells. They produce δ-interferon which activates macrophages

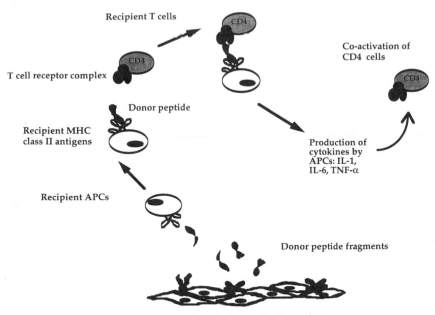

Figure 2. Indirect alloresponse: human leukocyte antigen (HLA) molecules shed by the donor organ provide a trigger for the indirect alloresponse. Donor antigens are scavenged by recipient antigen-presenting cells (APCs) and processed, then presented as peptides by recipient HLA class II antigens on the cell surface. The donor antigen-HLA complex can then interact with the T cell receptor on the surface of the CD4 cell, thus activating the cell and initiating an immune response against the specific major histocompatability complex (MHC) alloantigen.

and increases expression of allo-MHC proteins by the graft, thus amplifying the immune response. However, their primary importance is in killing target cells.[6,7,11]

In indirect antigen recognition, HLA molecules shed by the donor organ provide the trigger for the alloimmune response. Donor graft antigens are scavenged by recipient APCs, processed, and presented as peptides in the context of self (recipient) HLA. The HLA class II antigens bind the foreign peptide fragments intracellularly and form a complex which is translocated to the surface of the APC where it interacts with the T cell receptor on the surface of the CD4 cell. In this way, the CD4 cell is activated and an immune response is initiated against the specific MHC alloantigen. Concomitantly, the APC also secretes cytokines (IL-1, IL-6, and TNF-α) which coactivate the CD4 cells, thus propagating the alloimmune response. While the indirect response is the more usual or physiologic way for presentation of exogenous antigens to the immune system, it plays a secondary role to the vigorous direct alloresponse in the recognition and rejection of graft tissue.

The cytokines mentioned thus far have fairly specific functions. They are small soluble proteins that are produced by one cell, and act to alter the behavior of another cell. IL-1 is produced by macrophages and stimulates the helper T cell (CD4) response, inducing these cells to produce IL-2, or T cell growth factor (TCGF), which plays an important role in T cell proliferation, and also stimulates the production of other cytokines which modulate the effector functions of T cells, B cells, and macrophages. IL-2 stimulates CD4 cells to produce a cytotoxic T cell activating cytokine, directed toward the activation of CD8 cells. It also causes the release of δ-interferon from CD8 cytotoxic T cells, which induces the expression of HLA class I and II antigens on allograft cells which do not usually express these markers, thereby providing more targets for immunoreactivity, and potentiating the destructive capacity of T cells. If left untreated, this will serve to up-regulate the recipient immune system, and intensify the rejection process. IL-6 is produced by macrophages, and causes T and B cell growth and differentiation, and acute phase reaction. TNF-α, also called cachectin, is produced by natural killer cells (non-T, non-B lymphocytes) and macrophages, and causes local inflammation and endothelial activation. Cytokines produced as a result of routine infectious exposure in distant areas of the body, may also induce reactivity of the graft HLA system and have a "pro-rejection" effect. This theoretically supports the clinical practice of early detection and treatment of localized infections, such as sinusitis.[6,12]

Many of these T cell-derived cytokines function to activate B cells, resulting in cell growth and differentiation, and the production of membrane-bound or soluble antibodies or immunoglobulins (Ig). Membrane-bound antibodies serve as B cell receptors, and receptor diversity is provided by the variability of the Ig molecules. These membrane-bound immunoglobulins bind foreign antigens leading to activation of the B lymphocyte. The bound antigen is then internalized, processed, and transported to the B cell surface as a peptide bound by HLA molecules for presentation to T cells. In addition, B cell activation leads to secretion of soluble antibody with specificity for the particular inducing antigen. Secreted antibodies then coat the antigen (neutralization), enabling phagocytic cells that recognize the Fc portion of the Ig molecule to ingest the antigen (opsonization). Finally, soluble antibodies bound to antigen can directly trigger the complement cascade, enhancing opsonization and the destruction of the foreign antigen.[5,6,13]

Human Leukocyte Antigen Typing: Methodology and Relevance to Cardiac Transplantation

The prior details regarding the immunologic basis for rejection can now be applied to the more practical tasks of cardiac transplantation medicine. Current practice in cardiac transplantation is to base donor and recipient selection on ABO blood group compatibility. While survival of kidney and bone marrow allografts have correlated positively with the degree of HLA matching, the application of prospective HLA matching remains of controversial importance in cardiac transplantation. Historically, it has been taught that the prospective matching of heart donor and recipient is limited by the severe shortage of donor organs and myocardial preservation techniques which only ensure intact graft function with relatively short ischemic times.

Currently, there are three different methods used to type HLA antigens. The first method is that which is classically described using alloantisera. Most HLA typing in clinical practice is performed using the serologic method. Antibodies to a particular MHC molecule are added to T cells retrieved from an individual, and cause cytolysis of T cells specific for that HLA type. While it is a fairly rapid test, and can yield determination of both class I and class II antigens, serologic determination of HLA type has been shown to be inferior to genetic determination. Frequently, routine tissue typing at MHC class I loci is performed with serologic techniques and DNA genotyping is used for MHC class II loci. However, when only one class I antigen is reported at a given locus, it is assumed that the patient is homozygous when there may be a second allele that is untypeable by serologic determination.[8,14]

The second method utilizes T cells to detect class II MHC variability not determinable by serology. This in vitro detection method models in vivo graft rejection and is useful in screening for histoincompatibility between potential donors and recipients. This test is often referred to as a donor-specific cross-match. Donor T cells are cultured with irradiated recipient lymphocytes from an unrelated individual who is likely to be MHC disparate. The donor T cells are thus stimulated to proliferate and differentiate into effector cells; because the added lymphocytes are irradiated, they are unable to express a reciprocal response. The exuberant proliferation observed in these mixed lymphocyte cultures is the result of CD4 T cell recognition of MHC class II polymorphisms. The cytotoxic T cells that result are from CD8 cell recognition of MHC class I polymorphisms. If the donor T cells do not proliferate in response to recipient exposure, then it is likely that there are multiple common sites at the HLA-DR locus.[15]

Finally, direct structural analysis of genes present in an individual is the most reliable method of HLA determination. This can be done definitively by utilizing the polymerase chain reaction (PCR), which selectively replicates a particular stretch of genomic DNA. Once sufficient DNA is amplified from the gene in question, sequence analysis can be performed. This method has been effective in differentiation between serologically identical alleles, which in actuality are comprised of several closely related alleles, varying in expression by only one, or a few amino acids. A powerful alternative to PCR followed by sequencing is the PCR amplification with sequence specific primers (PCR-SSP). A completely matched primer will be more efficiently used in the PCR reaction than a primer with one or several mismatches, making typing specificity part of the amplification step. This shortens the amount of time necessary to yield an accurate tissue type, taking approximately 2 hours to complete. It is a rapid, inexpensive technique with high sensitivity, specificity, and reproducibility when compared with other PCR-based HLA class II typing techniques. Additionally, this typing methodology has a high degree of resolution; each primer pair defines two linked polymorphic sites which will facilitate identification and typing of heterozygous individuals.[16]

It is anticipated that, in the near future, routine HLA typing for all loci will employ DNA-based technology. Modern DNA typing methods permit determination of HLA type in a matter of hours; it is conceivable that donor HLA typing can be performed locally prior to organ harvesting, thus minimizing the risks associated with a long ischemic time. A recent study by DiSesa et al[9] retrospectively tested 47 cardiac transplant candidates against 1068 geographically accessible donors identified during a 1-year period by the United Network for Organ Sharing. When broad HLA specificities were used as the basis for donor-recipient matching, 94% of the 47 candidates had at least one donor with whom they shared four HLA antigens, suggesting that a significant degree of donor-recipient tissue matching may be achieved with the use of geographically accessible donors.[8,17]

Would HLA matching affect outcome? Retrospective analysis of HLA incompatibility and the incidence and severity of cardiac allograft rejection have produced conflicting results. These inconsistencies have been explained on the basis of patient heterogeneity, the use of variable immunosuppressive regimens, variation in HLA typing techniques, and the paucity of well-matched cardiac allografts.[8,16-24] Nonetheless, there is some clinical evidence that suggests that fortuitous, retrospectively identified HLA matching is associated with a reduced risk of rejection, improved graft survival, and patient outcome. Cocanougher et al[18] explored the relationship between HLA matching, allograft failure and recipient mortality as a result of graft coronary vasculopathy. Their findings suggest that patients with a high degree of HLA mismatch may have greater morbidity and mortality once coronary artery vasculopathy occurs.[20] However, another study by Zerbe et al, found that the severity of coronary artery luminal narrowing, as measured directly from epicardial coronary vessels obtained at retransplantation or autopsy, correlated with the incidence of rejection in the first 3 months after transplant, but not with the degree of HLA mismatch.[20] The lack of definitive evidence demonstrating a causal connection between graft vasculopathy and histoincompatibility raises the question of the immunologic etiology coronary artery disease (CAD). The majority of studies indicate that there is a beneficial effect of reduced HLA disparity between solid organ donors and recipients on graft longevity as measured by various parameters. The HLA-DR loci are particularly important in this regard, and, for example, a study by Wetzsteon et al has shown that reducing HLA-DR disparity between cardiac allograft recipients and their donors lower early acute rejection rates and improves graft survival.[13] One practical application of this knowledge is that patients with HLA-DR disparity may require more intense immunosuppression, and conversely, a good HLA-DR match may require less immunosuppression. In fact, a recent paper has shown that heart transplant recipients with at least one DR antigen could be more successfully weaned from long-term corticosteroid therapy than patients with no DR matches.[20] Retrospective tissue matching presents true clinical relevance, as it may be used to further individualize immunosuppressive therapy.

Allograft Rejection

Three types of rejection are seen in solid organ transplant recipients: hyperacute; acute; and chronic rejection.[24-28] These three phenomena are temporally separate, and have different immunologic etiologies. Hyperacute rejection is typically the result of humoral rejection and is mediated by preformed donor-specific antibodies in the recipient. It occurs minutes after vascular connections and reperfusion have been established in the donor organ, and donor-specific antibodies react with antigens on the graft vascular endothelium, stimulating the complement and clotting cascades. Complement activation results in endothelial activation, thrombosis, intravascular coagulation, edema, occlusion of graft vessels and ultimate loss of graft function. Death of the donor organ is imminent. Such grafts are not perfused, and quickly take on a white appearance. Pathologic specimens of hyperacute rejection show advanced graft destruction evidenced by fibrinoid necrosis of vessel walls, platelet and fibrin thrombus formation, mononuclear and neutrophil infiltration, and ischemic necrosis.

Alloreactive antibodies are detected by a prospective cross-match between donor lymphocytes and recipient serum, and a cross-match should always be performed in potentially sensitized recipients such as those who have received multiple transfusions. Currently, most centers screen serum from each prospective transplant recipient for the presence of preformed anti-HLA, panel reactive antibodies (PRA). These are detected by testing the recipient's serum reactivity against a panel of lymphocytes from a number of donors selected to represent all of the common HLA antigens. Since hyperacute rejection has been reported to be mediated by antidonor HLA antibodies of IgG, but not IgM, isotype, recipient serum is treated with dithiothreitol, a protease which inactivates antibodies of the IgM isotype and leaves IgG intact. The IgG fraction of serum is then tested against the lymphocyte panel. Depending upon the institutional standards, a PRA level of more than 10% may be considered positive and require a prospective donor-specific cross-match, since there is a higher likelihood that the recipient will have donor-specific anti-HLA antibodies.[30] It is often helpful to repeat PRA testing after any event which could potentially stimulate the immune system, such as a blood transfusion.

In addition to alloreactive antibodies, most humans have natural, preformed antibodies which react with antigens expressed by endothelial cells of disparate species. The most notable xenoantigen is the oligosaccharide moiety, galactose (α1–3) galactose, which is found as a constituent of many glycoproteins in all animals other than man and higher primates. These antibodies mediate hyperacute rejection of xenografts transplanted into humans, and at present remain the major barrier to successful clinical xenotransplantation.[26]

Acute rejection is the predominant and most familiar observed rejection response. It is primarily mediated by T cells ("cellular"), occurs within days, weeks, or months of transplant, and is initiated by either direct or indirect, CD4 and CD8 T cell recognition of donor graft HLA molecules.[27,28] Cellular rejection can be detected in routine endomyocardial biopsy specimens collected after cardiac transplantation, and is characterized by discrete perivascular or diffuse lymphocytic infiltrates detectable within the myocardium. With more advanced rejection, myocardial edema and cell necrosis are prominent features, and myocardiocytolysis is primarily mediated by CD8 ("killer") effector T cells which recognize class I MHC antigens. Billingham and associates established the first grading system for cardiac rejection nearly 20 years ago, and this system has been twice revised to accommodate the clinical subtleties associated with each classification.[29] Table 1 describes the microscopic appearance of each grade. As the severity of lymphocyte infiltration progresses, so does the degree of myocyte edema and necrosis. With advanced and prolonged rejection, myocyte damage may be irreversible and eminently result in graft loss.

While the significance of acute cellular rejection is undisputed, recent work has also

Table 1.

Grading of Rejection

Rejection Grade	Lymphocyte Infiltration	Myocyte Damage
0,NER	No evidence of rejection	None
1A	Focal perivascular but sparse infiltrate	None
1B	Sparse diffuse interstitial infiltrate	None
2	Solitary circumscribed focus of inflammatory cells	Some
3A	Obvious multifocal pattern of inflammatory infiltrate	Some
3B	Diffuse inflammatory process	Focal damage and edema
4	Aggressive polymorphous inflammatory infiltrate	Diffuse damage, hemorrhage, edema

identified antibody-mediated rejection as an important cause of acute vascular damage, myocyte injury, and graft loss.[30-33] Acute humoral or vascular rejection, described by Hammond, et al[31] and others, is characterized by deposition of IgG or IgM and complement (C3) in the coronary microvasculature. This form of rejection occurs in the first month after transplantation and can be detected by immunofluorescent staining of frozen tissue obtained at the time of endomyocardial biopsy. Humoral and cellular rejection can occur concomitantly; however, acute vascular rejection shows more severe left ventricular dysfunction and increased mortality, when compared with cellular or mixed cellular-humoral rejection. Early cases of vascular rejection may only be diagnosed by detecting vascular immune complexes; later cases may show diffuse endothelial swelling and interstitial edema. This may be manifested as severe ventricular hypertrophy and diastolic dysfunction soon after transplantation. True vasculitis is often seen in only relatively late lesions, however the presence of vascular immune complexes of Ig and complement is a consistent finding. It is important to note that routinely processed formalin-fixed, paraffin-embedded tissue specimens show a high percentage of vascular staining for Ig, due to labeling of passive Igs which are "fixed" in the vessels during processing. These passive immunoglobulins are washed away in preparation of frozen sections for immunofluorescent staining. Because of the high occurrence of vascular staining and the possibility of false-positive diagnoses of vascular rejection, formalin-fixed tissue specimens are not suitable for immunostaining.[33]

A recent study by Zales, et al[32] examined the incidence of humoral rejection, as measured by IgM and C3 deposition in the coronary microvasculature, and its relation to both short-term outcome and late follow-up of pediatric heart transplant recipients. One hundred and thirty-one biopsy specimens were obtained from 30 pediatric transplant recipients (mean age at time of transplant was 4.9 years, with a range of 2 days to 17 years). Deposition of IgM and C3 in the coronary microvasculature coexisted with cellular rejection in several specimens, however, the histologic features of vascular rejection were minimal in the mixed type. Deposition of IgM and C3 without cellular infiltrate was found in eight biopsies from four patients (13%); in three of these patients, the occurrence of isolated humoral rejection was within 3 weeks after transplantation. In two neonatal recipients, humoral rejection was associated with severe ventricular hypertrophy and diastolic dysfunction soon after transplantation. Long-term implications of humoral rejection were indeterminate, as only one patient demonstrating IgM and C3 deposition had angiographic evidence of coronary vasculopathy at 2 and 3 years after transplantation. CAD was later verified on autopsy.[32] In the study by Zales, et al[32] no relationship was found between pre-transplantation immunologic screening (PRA, or B cell cross-match) and the development of humoral rejection. However, Hammond, et al[32] and others have found an increased incidence of acute humoral vascular rejection in patients with a PRA greater than 5% or a positive donor-specific lymphocyte cross-match. In addition, both studies suggested that CAD develops in a subset of patients with persistent humoral rejection.

Chronic rejection occurs over months to years and is pathologically characterized by circumferential scaring of the coronary vessels associated with intimal proliferation, interstitial fibrosis, and luminal narrowing. This process has features which clearly differ from those of naturally occurring CAD; the lesions related to transplant are concentric, diffuse, and occur only in the donor vasculature. The etiology of this form of rejection is still in dispute, and proposed causes include repeated episodes of acute cellular rejection, hyperlipidemia, cytomegalovirus infection, and antidonor HLA or endothelial antibodies. The presence of specific antibodies against the donor endothelium has been reported by a number of centers to be associated with development of transplant atherosclerosis.[8,19,25,28,30,31] These antibodies may progressively increase with time after transplant, which could account for the indolent course and later presentation of this type of rejection. While the existence of antiendothelial antibodies directed against the donor graft has been demonstrated with varying prevalence, their significance at present remains unclear.

T cells of the CD4 (helper) family are likely to be of central importance initiating this process. By recognizing allo-MHC class II molecules, they begin a cytokine and growth factor-mediated cascade that promotes fibrous intimal hyperplasia and induces B cells to produce anti-HLA antibodies. Clinical detection of coronary graft vasculopathy has been limited by available imaging techniques. Coronary angiography often only demonstrates advanced disease; more promising in intravascular ultrasound, although large catheter size had prevented its use in infants and small children.

Approaches to Diminishing Recipient Immune Reactivity to the Allograft

The Induction of Specific Tolerance

The primary goal of transplantation medicine is to manipulate the immune system in such a way as to induce specific immune tolerance: a condition of absent response to donor antigens with little effect on the immune response to unrelated antigens, and without the need for chronic immunosuppressive drugs. While this goal remains elusive in human transplantation medicine, important insights have been gained from clinical studies in newborn humans and experimental animal models.[34-38]

Neonatal Immune Tolerance

There has been a fair amount of attention paid to the concept that neonates are conferred with an immunologic "grace period," based upon their immature and naive immune systems and, therefore, are better able to accept and sustain foreign transplanted tissues. This "window of opportunity" has been identified as the first 30 days after birth, and organs engrafted during this time are thought to elicit less aggressive activity from the still relatively immunosuppressed and uneducated newborn immune system. Organ transplantation occurring in recipients up to 3 months of age is, likewise, considered to have occurred during a privileged time.

In the neonate, both the humoral and cellular immune systems are suppressed. The fetus develops the capacity to produce immunoglobulin by the eighth to the tenth week of gestation, and synthesis begins by 20-weeks gestation. It is at about this time that maternal IgG crosses the placenta and appears in fetal circulation in titers high enough to suppress fetal immunoglobulin production. Naturally, this has a protective effect for the mother and for the fetus. It is also during the ninth or tenth weeks of gestation that T lymphocytes have completed differentiation in the thymus and are now in circulation as mature cells. By 12 weeks of gestation, the T cells are capable of responding to foreign antigens, but are held back by the presence of natural suppressor cells. Remember that B cells, which are abundant in the fetus, require further stimulation by T cell-derived lymphokines for further growth and differentiation. T cell function is suppressed in the fetus, therefore, little humoral immune reactivity occurs. It is supposed that this suppression state continues on into the newborn period, conferring the enhanced immune tolerance and greater graft acceptance. Theoretically, the net result of this is a requirement for less immunosuppression, and fewer episodes of rejection, and would also provide encouragement for xenograft transplantation in the newborn period. The reality is that the immunologic "window of opportunity" is still a disputable entity, and infants transplanted during this period do require significant immunosuppression, can suffer from rejection, and may go on to develop graft atherosclerosis. The remarkable adherence to a predetermined immunologic paradigm, programmed through generations of genetic planning, is in itself a proof of the fine tuning of the human immune system.[34,36]

Chimerism

Experimentation with allogeneic bone marrow chimeras has been ongoing since the 1950s, and was initiated by the early exploration for a treatment of lethal radiation exposure. Conceptually, it is simply a matter of "if you can't beat 'em, join 'em." Recipient species of mice are treated with high doses of whole-body irradiation to ablate all lymphoid cells, then infused with bone marrow from an allogeneic donor strain. When successful reconstitution of recipient mice was accomplished, the resulting chimeras were tolerant of both the donor and recipient antigens, as measured by in vitro testing or by in vivo transplantation. However, this approach was limited by the tendency for competent donor immune cells to attack the recipient, a phenomenon known as "graft-versus-host" reaction. The immunocompetent donor bone marrow placed in an immuno-ablated recipient leads to clinical features of acute and chronic graft-versus-host disease. In rodent models, these obstacles have been overcome by depleting the donor marrow of T cells using monoclonal antibodies prior to transplantation. This approach is associated with less successful marrow engraftment, possibly because donor T cells may attenuate residual immune defenses in the recipient, or supply some of the cytokines necessary for development of the donor marrow.

In widely disparate recipient-donor species, such as rodent/pig, allogeneic bone marrow chimeras are immunologically incompetent, even after bone marrow reconstitution. Possible explanations include incompatibilities between donor and recipient ligand-receptor pairs involved in T cell-dependent antigen reactivity, such as MHC-TCR, or accessory molecule interactions such as LFA3-CD2.[35-37]

Mixed Chimerism

One approach to this problem has been termed mixed bone marrow chimerism. Mixed chimeras are produced when the irradiated recipient is infused with a mixture of both donor and autologous (recipient) bone marrow. Successful engraftment results in a chimeric marrow, containing a mixture of both donor and recipient mature lymphoid cells. The reconstituted immune system is tolerant to both sets of antigens. MHC-dependent T cell immunocompetence is established, presumably because both peripheral and thymic APCs express recipient MHC and accessory molecules, and graft-versus-host disease does not occur, even when donor T cells are present in the marrow graft. Although this has been a successful model in rodent experiments, the application of mixed chimerism induction to humans and large animals may be limited by their inability to tolerate whole-body irradiation which ablates all marrow elements. Various nonmyeloablative regimens are currently being investigated and include a combination of high-dose thymic irradiation, low-dose whole-body irradiation, and infusion of anti-T cell antibodies. This work is promising and may eventually have clinical application, particularly in the field of xenotransplantation.[37,38]

Intrathymic Tolerance

Introduction of alloantigens into the adult thymus has induced tolerance to vascularized grafts in adult rodents. Animal experimentation in rats injected with donor alloantigens prior to transplantation has resulted in donor-specific post-transplant tolerance. Animals were concomitantly treated with murine monoclonal antibodies against rat cytotoxic/suppressor T cell subset, NK cells, and CD8 cells. In the clinical setting, pretreatment with donor antigens is a limiting factor, and further animal studies have been performed using simultaneous or post-transplant intrathymic inoculation of soluble antigens. Long-term donor-specific unresponsiveness has been induced in recipient animals challenged with second-set grafts greater than 100 days after inoculation and cardiac transplantation. These results suggest a promising strategy which may be used in human organ transplantation: the donor soluble antigen may be prepared after organ harvesting and may be administered by intrathymic injection at the time of, or immediately following transplantation.[38]

Nonspecific Immunosuppression

At present, immunomanipulative pharmacology is incapable of engendering specific immune tolerance, and we must rely upon nonspecific immunosuppression. Immunosuppression is the modulation of the immune system by pharmacologic agents, sufficiently suppressing the recipient's immune response to prevent graft rejection, while exerting limited effect on host defenses against infection. Our current armamentarium of immune suppressing drugs is fairly extensive and, in some cases, specifically directed toward a particular immunologic phenomenon. Infection still remains the greatest risk of immunosuppressive therapy and, in general, the more profound the immunosuppression, the greater the risk of infection. Prophylaxis against fungal, viral, and protozoal infections is recommended, especially during times of sustained enhanced immunosuppression, such as early after transplantation if induction therapy is used. Table 2 provides a ready reference for suggested pediatric regimens for most of the following medications.[6,9,39,40,41,42,43,44]

Table 2.

Immunosuppression

Medication (Generic, Brand)	Administration	Route	Interval	Comment	Toxicity
1 Cyclosporin A/CsA ·Sandimmune, Neoral	Initial	po	x 1 pre-transplant	Adjust CsA dose to renal/hepatic function. Titrate CsA dose to level: 400 ng/dl (whole blood) or 200 ng/dl (serum), early post-transplant. Neoral has enhanced GI absorption and bioavailability, however preparation may not be suitable for all patients.	Nephrotoxicity, hypocalcium, hypomagnesemia; hyperkalemia; vascular spasm, hypertension; tremor, headaches, amaurosis fugax, lowering of seizure threshold; hirsuitism, gingival hyperplasia, increased nasopharyngeal secretions, gallstones, PTLD.
	Maintenance	po	BID–TID	As above.	As above.
	Maintenance	iv	Slow-infusion divided BID–TID	IV dose is approximately 1/3 oral doses.	As above; notably hypertension may be severe and limited to the duration of infusion; anaphylactic reaction to diluent.
2 Azathioprine ·Imuran	Initial	po or iv	x1 pre-transplant	Same dose for oral and iv administration. Titrate to WBC count ≥ 4 thousand	Myelosuppression especially anemia, leukopenia; hepatitis, pancreatitis, PTLD
	Maintenance	po or iv	Q day	As above	As above
3 Prednisone ·Various Brands	Maintenance	po	BID	Higher doses given immediately after transplant, then tapered over ensuing months depending upon rejection history.	Diabetes, cushingoid habitus, increased appetite, gastritis, ulcers, growth retardation, osteoporosis, sodium retention.

#	Drug	Phase	Route	Schedule	Dose / Notes	Toxicities
4	Methylprednisolone • Solu-Medrol	Initial	iv	x1 in OR at	Single high dose.	Similar toxicities to Prednisone.
		Maintenance	iv	BID	May use higher doses immediately post-op. Maintenance steroids may be given i.v. if not tolerating po's. Solu-medrol dose = 5/4 Prednisone dose (mg).	As above.
5	FK-506/Tacrolimus • Prograf	Initial	iv	Post-Transplant, continuous infusion over 24 hrs	Adjust FK-506 dose to renal/hepatic function. Titrate FK-506 dose to desired level; therapeutic levels vary with assay and institution. Intravenous dose is half the oral dose.	Nephrotoxicity, hyperkalemia, hypomagnesemia, hyperuricemia; neurotoxicity including tremor, head aches, lowering of seizure threshold; diarrhea, nausea, vomiting; hyperglycemia; anaphylactic reaction; PTLD.
						As above.
6	Methotrexate • Various Brands	Post-transplant administration only.	po	Begin 2x/wk for 1 wk, then Q wk	Use for treatment of refractory rejection. Titrate to WBC count $\geq$ 4 thousand.	Myelosuppression especially anemia, leukopenia; may be given with leucovorin, a folic acid analog, to "rescue" the marrow and counteract some of the myelosuppressive effects.
7	Mycophenolate Mofetil • Cellcept	Maintenance	po	BID	Use in place of azathioprine; limited experience in children.	Nausea, vomiting, diarrhea; hepatotoxicity; less myelosuppression than azathioprine.

Note that dosages are often dependent upon institutional experience and desired drug levels. Many newer immunosuppressive agents have no standards for pediatric use.

All agents increase susceptibility to infection to varying degrees. Toxicities noted do not constitute a complete list. PTLD = post-transplant lymphoproliferative disease.

Drugs Which Have a Specific Site of Action

These are potent immunosuppressants and include CsA, FK-506, and rapamycin; their limiting side effect is nephrotoxicity. While mycophenolate mofetil decreases lymphocyte proliferation in general, its most desireable effect seems to be as an inhibitor of antibody production.[3,6,9,40,41]

Cyclosporin A: With the advent of CsA in the 1981, graft longevity improved dramatically; 1-year survival for kidney, liver, and heart transplant recipients improved from 50% to 80%. Prior to the cyclosporine era, immunosuppression for solid organ transplantation was dominated by the use of high-dose steroids and azathioprine. Long-term graft survival was uncommon and overwhelming systemic infection with opportunistic infections was a prominent source of morbidity. CsA is a cyclic decapeptide derived from the soil fungus *Tolypocladium inflatum.* Cyclosporine selectively inhibits T cell-dependent immune responses, mainly by preventing synthesis of IL-2 by blocking a late stage of the signaling pathway initiated by the T cell receptor. Inside the cell, cyclosporine binds to an immunophilin molecule called cyclophilin; the complex formed then binds to calcineurin, inhibiting its activity. Calcineurin is activated when intracellular calcium ion levels rise following T cell receptor binding to appropriate antigen: MHC complexes. Active calcineurin initiates a series of intracellular steps, resulting in transcription of the IL-2 gene. By blocking IL-2 synthesis, cyclosporine inhibits clonal expansion of T cells. The dominant effect appears to be on CD4 cells, with less effect on CD8 cells, and usually decreases the CD4/CD8 ratio. In vitro testing has shown that the addition of exogenous IL-2 will reverse cyclosporine-induced inhibition of T cell activation. For this reason, cyclosporine seems to provide excellent "prophylaxis" against rejection, but is inadequate therapy once the alloresponse (i.e., rejection) has begun. Because cyclosporine exerts a rather specific response on the immune system, it is usually used in conjunction with other drugs for chronic immunosuppression, and is not adequate for the treatment of acute rejection.

Cyclosporine is a highly lipophilic compound which may be administered orally or intravenously; serum or whole blood levels must be closely followed. Toxic overdosage can occur quickly, resulting in severe hypertension, headaches, visual disturbances (such as transient blindness or tunnel vision), and seizures. It is a potent vasoconstrictor, which may account for some of the manifestations of toxicity as well as the dose-related hypertension, which is commonly seen with cyclosporine administration. Nephrotoxicity, perhaps based on limitation of renal blood flow through vascular constriction, also occurs frequently, and may range from mild elevations in serum blood-urea-nitrogen (BUN) and creatinine levels to severe renal insufficiency. In these extreme cases, the coexistent administration of other nephrotoxic drugs or the occurrence of other renal-damaging phenomena must be explored. Unfortunately, the nephrotoxicity associated with chronic cyclosporine therapy is progressive and may eventually lead to renal failure; there are some reported cases of patients who have required renal transplantation. Concurrent with renal toxicity, cyclosporine also causes electrolyte disturbances such as hyperkalemia and magnesium wasting. Cyclosporine can also effect hepato-biliary function, causing elevations in serum transaminases, development of gallstones, and pancreatitis. Other side effects include hirsuitism, gingival hyperplasia, tremor, and breast fibroadenomas. The adverse psychologic effects of these "cosmetic" toxicities can be deleterious, especially to adolescent patients.

In common with other chronically administered immunosuppressive medications, cyclosporine is implicated in the development of post-transplant lymphoproliferative disease (PTLD). These types of lymphoproliferative disorders are usually of the B cell lineage, and have been epidemiologically linked to seroconversion for or documented infection with Ebstein-Barr virus. It is thought that cyclosporine inhibits T cell-mediated surveillance and cytotoxicity against transformed PTLD B cells. Most forms of PTLD can be effectively treated by diminution of current immunosuppression, however, they can be rapidly progressive and aggressive, necessitating the use of conventional chemotherapy.

Cyclosporine interacts with a multiplicity of drugs and it is, therefore, essential to be informed of any medication prescribed by a cotreating physician who may not be aware of cyclosporine's capricious nature. A partial list of medication interactions is found in Table 3. Serious drug interactions may be manifest by rapid increases in cyclosporine level, the result of diminished hepatic metabolism or renal clearance, and ultimate toxicity. Likewise, drugs which enhance cyclosporine metabolism may leave the transplant recipient with inadequate immunosuppression and the potential for rejection. Despite all this, cyclosporine is still the immunosuppressive mainstay of most solid-tissue organ transplantation regimens.

FK-506: While chemically unrelated to cyclosporine, FK-506 acts similarly to inhibit the immune response. In structure, FK-506 is similar to Rapamycin and both are produced by different species of the fungus, *Streptomyces*. FK-506 binds intracellularly to the immunophilin called FK-binding protein (FKBP); the chain of events resulting from this mimics that of the cyclosporine molecule binding to cyclophilin, and results in the inhibition of IL-2 production and the prevention of T cell expansion. FK-506 has also been shown to decrease the expression of IL-2 receptors by T lymphocytes in vitro, a function that has also been attributed to cyclosporin A. However, the suppression of CD8 cell activation by FK-506 is not reversed by addition of exogenous IL-2, indicating direct suppression of IL-2 receptor expression; addition of exogenous IL-2 will reverse cyclosporine-induced inhibition of T cell activation. It is perhaps this action of FK-506 which support its use as a *treatment* for moderate rejection; in a study published by Swenson et al,[40] episodes of grade II to IIIA rejection were reversed solely by increasing the oral dosage of FK-506. This study also points out that 80% of patients were successfully weaned from corticosteroids after switch to FK-506 from cyclosporine. Nephrotoxicity continues to be a problem in FK-506-treated patients. Modest elevations in BUN and creatinine do occur, to an extent similar to that found with cyclosporine therapy, however hypertension does not appear to be a problem. The nephrotoxicity may be a progressive phenomenon, and can result in overt renal failure. FK-506 has recently been FDA approved and released for general use. Its therapeutic use in children has been well documented.

Rapamycin: Like FK-506, rapamycin is produced by the fungus *Streptomyces,* and both compounds compete for binding to the same cellular receptor, the immunophilin FKBP. Rapamycin does not inhibit production of IL-2, because the FKBP-rapamycin complex does not bind calcineurin. Rapamycin acts to inhibit the signaling pathway initiated by IL-2 binding to the IL-2 receptor; rapamycin inactivates intracellular protein kinases, thereby blocking signal transduction and the propagation of T cell expansion. Because rapamycin binds to the FKBP, it exerts competitive inhibition on FK-506, and concomitant use of both drugs is not beneficial. Rapamycin and cyclosporin A

Table 3.

Cyclosporine A: Drug Interactions

Drug	Effect	Comment
ACE inhibitors	Hyperkalemia	Decreased aldosterone, potassium retention
Acyclovir	Increased CsA level	Increased nephrotoxicity
Aminoglycosides	Increased toxicity (Aminoglycosides and CsA)	Nephrotoxicity
Amphotericin	Increased toxicity (CsA)	Nephrotoxicity
Bactrim/TMP + Sulfa	Increased CsA level	Altered metabolism
Carbamazepine	Decreased CsA level	Increased metabolism
Cholestyramine	Decreased CsA level	GI binding
Cimetidine	Increased toxicity (CsA)	Nephrotoxicity
Ceftriaxone	Increased CsA level	Probable altered hepatic metabolism
Digoxin	Increased toxicity (Digoxin)	Hypomagnesemia
Diltiazem	Increased CsA level	Decreased metabolism
Erythromycin	Increased CsA level	Decreased metabolism
Food	Variable CsA levels	Effects absorption and bioavailability
Isoniazid	Decreased CsA level	Increased metabolism
Kaolinpectin	Decreased CsA level	GI binding
Ketaconazole	Increased CsA level	Decreased hepatic metabolism
Lovastatin	Rhabdomyolysis, acute renal failure	Unknown
Lisinopril	Extreme hyperkalemia	Probable renal toxicity
Metoclopramide	Decreased CsA level	Decreased GI absorption
Nifedipine	Possible effect on CsA level	Increased gingival hyperplasia
Nonsteroidal anti-inflammatory drugs (NSAIDs, e.g. ibuprofen)	Increased toxicity (CsA)	Diminished renal blood flow/ vasospasm
Oral contraceptives	Increased CsA level	Increased hepatotoxicity
Pancuronium	No effect on level	Potentiation of neuromuscular blockade
Pediazole/Erythro + TMP	Increased CsA level	Decreased metabolism
Phenobarbital	Decreased CsA level	Increased hepatic metabolism
Phenytoin	Decreased CsA level	Increased hepatic metabolism
Prednisone/ Methylprednisolone	Increased CsA level	Decreased clearance
Procarbazine	Increased CsA level	Unknown
Progesterone	Increased CsA level	Unknown; probable decreased hepatic metabolism of CsA
Rifampin	Decreased CsA level	Increased hepatic metabolism
Spironolactone	Hyperkalemia	Potassium retention
Sulfadimidine	Decreased CsA level	Unknown; probable increased metabolism
Theophylline	Increased CsA level	Decreased metabolism
Trimethoprim (TMP)-oral	Increased toxicity (CsA)	Unknown; probable decreased metabolism and increased nephrotoxicity
Trimethoprim (TMP)-intravenous	Decreased CsA level	Unknown; porbable increased metabolism
Vancomycin	Increased toxicity (CsA)	Increased nephrotoxicity

can be used together, however, as rapamycin does not bind to cyclophilin. Therefore, cyclosporine can inhibit IL-2 production and rapamycin will inhibit the response to any IL-2 that is already produced.

Mycophenolate Mofetil: Mycophenolate mofetil, or mycophenolic acid (MPA), is a lymphocyte-specific inhibitor of purine synthesis with antiproliferative effects on both T and B lymphocytes. Mycophenolate primarily affects the late events in lymphocyte activation, inhibiting glycoprotein synthesis in cells by depleting cellular guanosine triphosphate (GTP), thereby, altering membrane glycoprotein composition. Surface membrane glycoproteins are essential for lymphocyte adhesion and chemotaxis. Activation of T cells is dependent on GTP and is blocked by mycophenolate at high doses. Because of MPA's effect on B lymphocyte proliferation, antibody production is decreased. Various animal models have shown that MPA decreases the intimal hyperplasia characteristic of allograft CAD, suggesting that mycophenolate may be effective in preventing or attenuating antibody-mediated damage to the vascular endothelium.

Several recent human studies have substituted MPA for azathioprine in the conventional immunosuppression regimen postsolid organ transplant (i.e., cyclosporine and azathioprine, with or without prednisone). In theory and clinical practice, mycophenolate seems to be superior to azathioprine, which is not lymphocyte specific and inhibits purine synthesis in other replicating cells, thus causing more anemia, neutropenia, thrombocytopenia, stomatitis, and mucositis. In addition, azathioprine is a pro-drug and must undergo hepatic conversion to 6-MP, its active form; the by-products of this conversion are toxic metabolites which are potentially mutagenic. MPA seems to be effective in cardiac transplant recipients as chronic maintenance therapy, as well as a treatment for acute rejection. In a study by Taylor et al,[41] 17 patients were followed for a 3-year period. There were 28 episodes of mild rejection (grade IB or II), 9 of which were treated with oral pulse-steroid therapy, and 19 were treated with increasing MPA dose alone; 68%, or 13 of 19 episodes, resolved. This suggests that mycophenolate may be useful in treating acute cardiac rejection. Also for clinical consideration, is the fact that MPA is a potent inhibitor of EBV-stimulated lymphocyte proliferation, which may be of benefit in the treatment of post-transplant B cell lymphomas. However, malignancy continues to be a risk in chronic immunosuppression.

The majority of MPA's side effects seem to be gastrointestinal: nausea; vomiting; and diarrhea. Infectious complications do occur, however, the most prevalent are upper respiratory viruses, herpes zoster, and herpes simplex. Bone marrow suppression occurs with less frequency than with azathioprine treatment. Leukopenia, anemia, and thrombocytopenia occur rarely and then usually early in the course.

Broad Spectrum Immunosuppressive Agents

This class of drugs is used by many institutions as part of the daily immunosuppressive regimen. As expected, these nonspecific drugs have several undesirable side effects, and as with all broadly acting cytotoxic medications, inhibit both beneficial and harmful immune responses.[3,6,9,7,43,44]

Corticosteroids: Corticosteroids are potent inhibitors of the inflammatory response; the steroids used most frequently in transplant immunotherapy are prednisone and methylprednisolone. Systemic administration causes lysis of immature T lymphocytes, however, their major mechanism of action seems to be in preventing activation of the immune response by down-regulating transcription of cytokines. Postulated targets include IL-1, IL-2, IL-6, and TNF-α. It has also been suggested by recent studies that steroids may also affect allograft HLA expression. Steroids cause T cell sequestration and inhibit cytotoxic T cell function. They also inhibit chemotaxis and lysosomal enzyme release of macrophages and other phagocytic cells, further hampering the immune response. Steroids have a rather broad effect on cell-mediated immunity, but leave humoral immunity relatively intact.

There still exists a fair amount of controversy surrounding the chronic use of steroids in maintenance immunosuppressive therapy, and this discussion is carried out elsewhere in this text. It has been shown by several institutions that low-dose daily steroids are efficacious in reducing the incidence of graft CAD. However, prolonged use of steroids can cause the weakening of connective tissues and bone necrosis, and may cause atrophy of the adrenal glands and reduce the body's ability to respond to stress. Because of their general influence throughout the body, steroids exhibit numerous side effects which occur with even short-term use. This list includes sodium and water retention, enhanced appetite, weight gain, abnormal fat deposition in the face ("cushingoid appearance") and suprascapular areas ("buffalo hump"), growth retardation, steroid-induced diabetes, acne, cataracts, behavioral changes, and poor wound healing.

Steroids are often administered at an induction dose at the time of transplantation and then tapered to a minimal daily amount. Corticosteroids are also effective as a first line of defense in the treatment of acute rejection episodes. A frequently used and efficacious regimen strategy is daily triple immunosuppression with cyclosporine, steroids, and azathioprine.

Azathioprine: Azathioprine acts by inhibiting the growth and differentiation of immune cells. It is a pro-drug of 6-MP. After metabolism in the liver, azathioprine becomes incorporated into the recipient DNA, thereby inhibiting purine synthesis and metabolism, and RNA and DNA synthesis. The ultimate effect is to inhibit gene replication and cell division.

Azathioprine is useful for chronic therapy and effectively blocks primary immune responses, but is less effective in blocking secondary responses and acute rejection. Azathioprine inhibits cell-mediated hypersensitivity, suppresses most T cell functions, and blocks antibody-dependent cellular cytotoxicity. It also inhibits primary antibody synthesis, and decreases the numbers of granulocytes and monocytes in circulation. As azathioprine kills rapidly proliferating cell types, this includes bone marrow cells that produce cellular elements of blood, causing anemia, generalized leukopenia, and thrombocytopenia. Hence, its major side effect is myelosuppression, and the dosage of azathioprine must be adjusted to titrate blood components to acceptable numbers. Other side effects include macrocytic anemia, liver toxicity, pancreatitis, alopecia, nausea, vomiting, viral infection (especially with herpes viruses), and neoplasia. One notable drug interaction is the potentiation of the pharmacologic effect of azathioprine by concomitant use of allopurinol. Azathioprine dose should be decreased by 75% when administered with allopurinol.

Methotrexate: Methotrexate is a folic acid analog that competitively inhibits dihydrofolate reductase, interfering with purine formation and, therefore, DNA synthesis. Methotrexate has been used effectively, in addition to standard immunosuppression, as rescue therapy for severe or recalcitrant rejection, and has been shown to diminish the incidence of rejection episodes both during and after treatment. Methotrexate is administered orally or intravenously, and is usually given as weekly pulse therapy of several weeks to months duration. Leukopenia is the most common side effect, with the nadir occurring 3 weeks after initiation of the drug. Because of this, the dose of concomitantly administered azathioprine must be decreased in order to titrate the leukocyte count to acceptable levels. Despite methotrexate's efficacy in reversing rejection with short-term use, some data suggest that there is an increase in rejection during the subsequent year after termination of therapy. Therefore, methotrexate may be better used as a chronic immunosuppressive agent.

Antibody Preparations Directed Against T Cells

Immunosuppressive agents which specifically recognize T cell surface antigens include monoclonal (e.g., OKT3) or polyclonal (e.g., antithymocyte globulin, or antithymocyte serum) antibody preparations, generated in animals following immunization with T cells. These agents are highly specific for T cell antigens, are very potent, and are extremely effective in the treatment of acute or refractory rejection. Anti-T cell antibodies may also be used in induction therapy for rejection prophylaxis early after transplant, and may especially be considered in patients who have renal compromise and are unable to tolerate the nephrotoxic side effects of cyclosporine.[42-46]

There is also some discussion that OKT3 and antilymphocyte preparations may be linked to the subsequent development of post-transplant malignancies. Many authors have proposed that the increased incidence of PTLD is the result of relative overimmunosuppression from combination therapy. Costanzo-Nordin, et al[50] however, have published data indicating that induction therapy with OKT3, in and of itself, significantly increases the risk of later development of PTLD. In addition, the risk of lymphoma increases with increasing cumulative dose of OKT3. Immunologic monitoring, including T cell subtypes, and available drug levels, is an important part of immune therapy and should assist in individualizing care and preventing overtreatment.[39,40,46]

OKT3: OKT3 is also called Muromonab-CD3, or murine monoclonal antibody-CD3. This is a monoclonal antibody produced in the mouse and directed against the CD3 molecular complex on human T cells. The CD3 complex on the surface of the T cell consists of three invariant dimers which transduce signals from the antigen-specific T cell receptor into the cell. When OKT3 binds to the δ dimer, the antibody-CD3 complex is either internalized into the cell or shed from the cell surface. At this point, T cells are either removed from circulation by the reticuloendothelial system (T cell depletion), or are rendered incapable of recognizing antigenic targets (anergy). These responses occur within minutes after initiating OKT3 infusion. After several days of therapy, other T cell receptor subsets increase in circulating number while CD3 cells remain undetectable.

OKT3 is usually reserved for treatment of acute rejection that is refractory to pulse-steroid therapy. Some centers, however, use OKT3 as induction prophylaxis. OKT3 is administered intravenously and the typical course of treatment is 7 to 14 days. There are many side effects to OKT3 administration, and some can be quite severe. Aseptic meningitis, hyperpyrexia, headaches, vomiting, nausea, malaise, rash, arthralgias, and a serum-sickness-like illness can all occur. The most profound clinical symptoms are seen with the first two doses of the course, and are the result of lymphokines and other mediators of inflammation released with T cell cytolysis. Premedication with antipyretics (acetaminophen), antihistamines, and corticosteroids is strongly recommended in order to diminish the body's response to these preparations. An acute syndrome which is idiosyncratic to OKT3 use has been infrequently reported. This syndrome consists of respiratory distress, pulmonary edema, and hypertension; it is for this reason that the first few doses of the drug be administered in an intensive care or close-watch setting. After several days of treatment, antibodies develop against antigenic determinants of the murine monoclonal antibody. These antimouse antibodies may decrease the efficacy of the drug, and in 30% of patients, may result in "breakthrough rejection," requiring increased doses. It is also notable that children less than 10 years of age seem to have higher levels of antimurine antibodies than do older patients.[44,45]

Antithymocyte Globulin: Antithymocyte globulin (ATGam) is a polyclonal immune globulin prepared from horse sera after immunization with human thymocytes. This antithymocyte agent is highly efficacious in the treatment of acute rejection episodes and appears to have some benefit in rejection prophylaxis. Because it is a polyclonal preparation, many antibodies are present which react with cell surface antigens common to a variety of cell types. Consequently, in addition to depleting T cells, ATGam will also deplete B cells, granulocytes, and platelets. ATGam may also affect T cell activation or allorecognition by binding to molecules on the surface of T cells which mediate these functions. Other side effects of ATGam are similar to those manifested by OKT3. ATGam can cause a serum sickness-like illness and glomerulonephritis; pain at the site of infusion, and the generalized symptoms of fever, urticaria, and hypotension can be controlled by premedication with antipyretics, antihistamines, and corticosteroids.[3,43,46]

Antithymocyte Serum: Antithymocyte serum (ATS) is the serum fraction from the polyclonal T cell antibody preparation raised in rabbits immunized to human thymocytes. It has been used as rescue therapy for the treatment of steroid refractory rejection, and in some centers has been used as induction therapy. ATS depletes peripheral blood lymphocytes, specifically those of the CD2 and CD3 subsets. A recent study by Lebeck et al[46] investigated the use of ATS in pediatric patients. Decreasing percentage and absolute numbers of CD2 and CD3 cells corresponded to the duration of ATS therapy. ATS levels, which were measured by assay, were quite variable in their group of patients, emphasizing the need to follow levels in patients who did not show clinical improvement with standard dosing. The authors recommended a course of treatment for rejection of 7 to 10 days, and for induction of 5 days. ATS has similar side effects to ATGam and OKT3.[3,46]

Nonpharmacologic Immunosuppression

These modalities have been suggested for treatment of refractory cellular and humoral rejection, but are not currently used as part of the standard post-transplant regimen. T cell depleting modalities include total lymphoid irradiation (TLI) and photophoresis; antibody depleting modalities include plasmaphoresis.[38–44]

Total Lymphocyte Irradiation: TLI involves the administration of low-dose radiotherapy targeted at the major lymph node-bearing areas, including the cervical, axillary, mediastinal, periaortic, and iliofemoral nodes, as well as the spleen and thymus, with a shielding of nonlymphoid tissue. This modality has been used as an adjunct in the treatment of recurrent cardiac rejection in adults and children, and recent results are promising. Because all lymphoid tissue is treated with TLI, it is potentially efficacious as a treatment for humoral as well as cell-mediated rejection. In addition, the protective effect of this therapy has been demonstrated for as long as 24 months after termination. TLI can be administered during a 4- to 8-week period on an outpatient basis. The target dose of radiation is 800 cGy (1 cGy=1 rad), irrespective of body size, and is administered in weekly or biweekly fractions. It is a painless procedure; there is no need for intravenous access, and patients rarely require sedation. Patients continue to receive usual immunosuppression throughout the course of TLI, however, azathioprine dose may have to be reduced because of the potential for bone marrow suppression. Important side effects are thrombocytopenia and leukopenia; the nadir of leukopenia seems to be approximately 4 weeks after TLI is initiated. Thus far, there does not seem to be an increase in the incidence of malignancy after TLI treatment.[47,48]

Photophoresis: Photophoresis, or photochemotherapy, appears to specifically target activated T cells and removes them from the circulation. This modality requires central venous access and several hours of monitoring as blood is removed, circulated through an external rotor pump, and then returned to the patient. Photophoresis requires the use of the drug, 8-methoxysporalen, which forms a potent DNA cross-linking agent when exposed to ultraviolet light. Photo-treated T cells are returned to the patient and may circulate for up to 7 days prior to clearance from the body. The death of the irradiated cells in the recipient may initiate suppression of a previously unregulated alloresponse. Photophoresis has been used successfully in treatment of aggressive cutaneous T cell malignancies and autoimmune diseases such as psoriasis. It is used in transplantation for chronic rejection and significant immune reactivity.[49,50]

Plasmapheresis: Vascular damage to solid organ grafts can be mediated by humoral factors that can be removed from circulation by plasmapheresis or plasma exchange. Plasmapheresis has been shown to improve the outcome of vascular rejection episodes in cardiac allograft recipients, especially in the setting of a positive crossmatch (i.e., the presence in the recipient of preformed antibodies and autoantibodies). Usually, plasmapheresis is performed on a patient for 2 to 3 days each week, for several weeks or months, with monitoring of antibody levels and endomyocardial specimens for vascular rejection. The exchange of blood requires reliable venous access and a large-gauge catheter. Hypotension can be rate-limiting and may necessitate replacement with 5% albumin. The maintenance oral drug regimen is modified in the setting of plasmapheresis to include a medication that has more anti-B cell activity, such as cyclophosphamide, or cytoxan; the more general immunosuppressant, azathioprine, is usually eliminated.[51-53]

Conclusions and Considerations:
Whether Pigs Have Wings

Advancements in the understanding of the interplay between the various characters in the immunologic response may lead to improved forms of immunosuppression, and perhaps to true tolerance. Among the more promising approaches to manipulating the immune system are mixed chimerism, the possibility of modifying the recipient to become tolerant of the graft, or conferring properties on the donor which make it more like the recipient. In the near future, however, all these approaches will continue to require the use of continued immunosuppression.

Understanding the mechanisms of effective drugs such as cyclosporine and FK-506 is leading to the development of newer agents, which may exhibit less nephrotoxicity. The potential for further manipulation of the cytokine cascade, perhaps in the form of an IL-2 inhibitor, may provide additional immune support in the not-too-distant future. With enhanced understanding of the body's response to a transplanted organ, and improved methods of modulating that response, the goal seems clear: to improve the quality of life and absolute longevity of transplant recipients.

References

1. Medawar PB, Gibson T: The fate of skin homografts in man. *J Anatomy* 77:299–309, 1943.
2. Calne R: Has effective immunosuppresson eliminated the need for transplant immunology? *Transplant Proc* 24:2366–2368, 1992.
3. Janeway CA, Travers P: *Immunobiology: The Immune System in Health and Disease.* New York: Garland Publishing, Inc.; 11:30–32, 1994.
4. Janeway CA, Travers P: *Immunobiology: The Immune System in Health and Disease.* New York: Garland Publishing, Inc.; 1:24–25, 1994.
5. Nepom BS, Nepom GT: Immunogenetics and the Rheumatic Diseases. In: Kelley WN, Harris ED Jr, Ruddy S, Sledge CB (eds). *Textbook of Rheumatology.* 4th Ed. Philadelphia: WB Saunders, Co.; 90–97, 1993.
6. Krensky AM, Clayberger C: Transplantation immunology: clinical immunology. *Pediatr Clin North Am* 41:819–839, 1994.
7. Stepkowski SM: Transplantation immunobiology: horizons in organ transplantation. *Surg Clin North Am* 74:991–1013, 1994.
8. Costanzo MR: The role of histocompatability in cardiac allograft vasculopathy. *J Heart Lung Transplant* 14:S180–S184, 1995.
9. Jordan SC, Rosenthal P, Makowka L: Immunosuppression in organ transplantation. *Semi Pediatr Surg* 2:206–217, 1993.
10. Janeway CA, Travers P: *Immunobiology: The Immune System in Health and Disease.* New York: Garland Publishing, Inc.; 8:3,8:31, 1994.
11. Janeway CA, Travers P: *Immunobiology: The Immune System in Health and Disease.* New York: Garland Publishing, Inc.; 7:24–31, 1994.
12. Janeway CA, Travers P: *Immunobiology: The Immune System in Health and Disease.* New York: Garland Publishing, Inc.; 7:31–32, 1994.
13. Janeway CA, Travers P: *Immunobiology: The Immune System in Health and Disease.* New York: Garland Publishing. Inc.; 8:1–3, 1994.
14. Janeway CA, Travers P: *Immunobiology: The Immune System in Health and Disease.* New York: Garland Publishing, Inc.; 1:24–27, 1994.
15. Janeway CA, Travers P: *Immunobiology: The Immune System in Health and Disease.* New York: Garland Publishing, Inc.; 2:48–50, 1994.
16. Olerup O, Zetterquist H: HLA-DR typing by PCR amplification with sequence-specific primers (PCP-SSP) in 2 hours: an alternative to serological DR typing in clinical practice including donor-recipient matching in cadaveric transplantation. *Tissue Antigens* 39:225–235, 1992.
17. DiSesa VJ, Mull R, Daly ES, Edmounds LH, Mancini DM, Eisen HJ: Cardiac transplant donor heart allocation based on prospective tissue matching. *Ann Thorac Surg* 58:1050–1053, 1994.
18. Cocanougher B, Ballantyne CM, Pollack MS, et al: Degree of HLA mismatch as a predictor of death from allograft arteriopathy after heart transplant. *Transplant Proc* 25:233–236, 1993.
19. Addonizio LJ, Hsu DT, Douglas JF, et al: Decreasing incidence of coronary disease in pedi-

atric cardiac transplant recipients using increased immunosuppression. *Circulation* 88(Pt 2):224–229, 1993.

20. Zerbe T, Utretsky B, Kormos R, et al: Graft atherosclerosis: effects of cellular rejection and human lymphocyte antigen. *J Heart Lung Transplant* 11:S104–S110, 1992.

21. Wetzsteon P, Head MA, Fletcher MC, Norman DJ: Confidence levels assigned to serologic HLA-DR typing predict DNA HLA-DR typing discrepancies. *Transplant Proc* 24:2483–2484, 1994.

22. Costanzo-Nordin RM, Fisher SG, O'Sullivan EJ, et al: HLA-DR incompatibility predicts heart transplant rejection independent of immunosuppressive prophylaxis. *J Heart Lung Transplant* 12:779–789, 1993.

23. Costanzo-Nordin RM: Cardiac allograft vasculopathy: relationship with acute cellular rejection and histocompatibility. *J Heart Lung Transplant* 12:S90–S103, 1992.

24. Janeway CA, Travers P: *Immunobiology: The Immune System in Health and Disease.* New York: Garland Publishing, Inc. 11:30–48, 1994.

25. de Begona JA, Gundry SR, Nehlsen-Cannerella SL, et al: HLA matching and its effect on infant and pediatric cardiac graft survival. *Transplant Proc* 23:1139–1141, 1991.

26. Thomas LJ, Ryan US: Immunologic consequences of organ transplantation: implications for therapeutic development. *J Heart Lung Transplant* 14:938–944, 1995.

27. Hauptman PJ, Nakagawa T, Tanaka H, Libby P: Acute rejection: culprit of coincidence in the pathogenesis of cardiac graft vascular disease? *J Heart Lung Transplant* 14:S173–S180, 1995.

28. Billingham ME, Cary NRB, Hammond ME, et al: A working formulation for the standardization of nomenclature in the diagnosis of heart and lung rejection. *J Heart Lung Transplant* 9:587–593, 1990.

29. Rose EA, Pepino P, Barr ML, et al: Relation of HLA antibodies and graft atherosclerosis in human cardiac allograft recipients. *J Heart Lung Transplant* 11:S120–S123, 1992.

30. Hosenpud JD, Everett JP, Morris TE, Wagner CR, Shipley GD: Cellular and humoral immunity to vascular endothelium and the development of cardiac allograft vasculopathy. *J Heart Lung Transplant* 14:S185–S187, 1995.

31. Hammond EH, Yowell RL, Nunoda S: Vascular (humoral) rejection in heart transplantation: pathologic observations and clinical implications. *J Heart Lung Transplant* 8:430–443, 1989.

32. Zales VR, Crawford S, Backer CL, Patricia L, Benson DW, Mavroudis C: Spectrum of humoral rejection after pediatric heart transplantation. *J Heart Lung Transplant* 12:563–572, 1993.

33. Loy TS, Bulatao IS, Darkow VD, et al: Immunostaining of cardiac biopsy specimens in the diagnosis of acute vascular (humoral) rejection: a control study. *J Heart Lung Transplant* 12:736–740, 1993.

34. Nehlsen-Cannerella SL, Chang L: Immunology and organ transplantation in the neonate and young infant. *Crit Care Nurs Clin North Am* 4:179–191, 1992.

35. Charlton B, Auchincloss H Jr, Fathman CG: Mechanisms of transplantation tolerance. *Ann Rev Immunology* 12:707–734, 1994.

36. Sachs DH: Transplantation tolerance. *Ann Thorac Surg* 56:1221–1227, 1993.

37. Sharabi Y, Sachs DH: Mixed chimerism and permanent specific transplantation tolerance induced by a nonlethal preparative regimen. *J Exp Med* 169:493, 1989.

38. Ohajekwe OA, Chowdhury NC, Fiedor PS, Hardy MA, Oluwole SF: Transplantation tolerance to rat cardiac and islet allografts by posttransplant intrathymic inoculation of soluble alloantigens. *Transplantation* 60:1139–1143, 1995.

39. Purdy RE, Boucek MM, Boucek RJ, Jr: *Handbook of Cardiac Drugs.* 2nd Ed. Boston: Little, Brown and Co.; 322–335, 1995

40. Swenson JM, Fricker FJ, Armitage JM: Immunosuppression switch in pediatric heart tranpslant recipients: cyclosporine to FK-506. *J Am Coll Cardiol* 25:1183–1188, 1995.

41. Taylor DO, Ensley RD, Olsen SL, Dunne D, Renlund DG: Mycophenolate mofetil (RS-61443): preclinical, clinical and three-year experience in heart transplantation. *J Heart Lung Transplant* 13:571–582, 1994.

42. Bourge RC, Kirklin JK, White-Williams C, et al: Methotrexate pulse therapy in the treatment of recurrent acute heart rejection. *J Heart Lung Transplant* 11:1116–1124, 1992.

43. Cosimi AB: The clinical usefulness of antilymphocyte antibodies. *Transplant Proc* 15:583–589. 1983.
44. Schroeder TJ, Michael AT, First MR, et al: Variations in serum OKT3 concentration based upon age, sex, transplanted organ, treatment regimen, and anti-OKT3 antibody status. *Therapeutic Drug Monitoring* 16:361–367, 1994.
45. Swinnen LJ, Costanzo-Nordin MR, Fisher SG, et al: Increased incidence of lymphoproliferative disorder after immunosuppression with the monoclonal antibody OKT3 in cardiac transplant recipients. *N Engl J Med* 323:1723–1728, 1990.
46. Lebeck LK, Chang L, Lopez-McCormack C, et al: Polyclonal antithymocyte serum: immune prophylaxis and rejection therapy in pediatric heart transplantation recipients. *J Heart Lung Transplant* 12:S286–S292, 1993.
47. Kirklin JK, George JF, McGiffin DC, Naftel DC, Salter MM, Bourge RC: Total lymphoid irradiation: is there a role in pediatric heart transplantation? *J Heart Lung Transplant* 12:S290–S300, 1992.
48. Hunt SA, Strober S, Hoppe RT, Stinson EB: Total Lymphoid Irradiation for treatment of intractable cardiac allograft rejection. *J Heart Lung Transplant* 10:211–216, 1991.
49. Pepino P, Berger CL, Fuzesi L, et al: Primate cardiac allo and xenotransplantation: modulation of the immune response with photochemotherapy. *Eur Surg Res* 21:105–113, 1989.
50. Costanzo-Nordin MR, Hubbell EA, O'Sullivan EJ, et al: Reversal of heart transplant rejection with photopheresis (abstr). *J Heart Transplant* 10:177, 1991.
51. Partanen J, Nieminen MS, Krogerus L, Harjula ALJ, Mattila S: Heart transplant rejection treated with plasmapheresis. *J Heart Lung Transplant* 11:301–305, 1992.
52. Ratkovec MR, Hammond EH, O'Connell JB, et al: Outcome of cardiac transplant recipients with a positive donor-specific crossmatch-preliminary results with plasmapheresis. *Transplantation* 651–655, 1992.
53. Franco A, Anaya F, Niembro E, Ahijada F, Luno J, Valderrabano F: Plasma exchange in the treatment of vascular rejection: relationship between histological changes and therapeutic response. *Transplant Proc* 3661–3663, 1987.

Chapter 2

Infectious Complications of Heart and Lung Transplantation in Children

Marian G. Michaels, MD, MPH, Michael D. Green, MD, MPH

Introduction

Infections are a major cause of morbidity and mortality after heart, heart-lung, and lung transplantation. Although specific literature documenting the infectious profiles of pediatric heart and thoracic organ transplant recipients is limited, numerous reports summarizing the combined outcome of both adult and pediatric transplant recipients confirm the importance of infections. Infections account for approximately 20% of early and 40% of late deaths after cardiac transplant and 40% of all deaths in heart-lung transplant recipients.[1] The aim of this chapter is to provide the reader with a general approach to infectious complications arising after thoracic (heart, heart-lung, or lung) transplantation in children. While some complications are unique to patients receiving a given organ, the majority of infections will have similarities in the patterns and timing of their presentation.

Predisposing Factors

Factors which predispose to infection can be divided into those existing prior to transplant in the candidates or their donors and those secondary to intraoperative and post-transplant activities (Table 1).

Recipient Pretransplant Factors

The site of the organ transplant is one of the most important factors determining the location of postoperative infections, especially during the first 3 months after

From: Franco KL (ed). *Pediatric Cardiopulmonary Transplantation.* Armonk, NY: Futura Publishing Company, Inc.; © 1997.

Table 1.

**Predisposing Factors to Infection after
Thoracic Transplantation in Children**

I. Recipient pretransplant factors

Organ transplanted
Underlying disease
Severity of illness prior to transplant
   Malnutrition
   Requirement for intensive care
   Requirement for assist devices
Age
   Immunologic immaturity
   Primary exposure
   Immunization history

II. Donor factors

Latent infections
Colonization of respiratory tract*

III. Intraoperative factors

IV. Post-Transplant factors

Technical problems
Immunosuppression
Indwelling cannulas
Nosocomial exposure

*Heart-lung and lung transplant recipients

transplantation.[2] Patients undergoing a renal transplant are at increased risk for infections of the urinary tract, while those receiving a liver transplant are predisposed to intra-abdominal infections. Likewise, children who have undergone a heart or lung transplant are more likely to develop an infection within the thoracic cavity. Factors which predispose to a high frequency of infection at or near the site of transplantation are almost certainly the occurrence of local ischemic injury and bleeding, as well as potential soilage with contaminated material.[3]

The type and severity of the underlying illness leading to organ failure can influence the risk for infection. For example, bacterial or fungal colonization of the airways in patients with cystic fibrosis may predispose to infection after transplantation. Similarly, children with severe end-stage heart disease may require prolonged mechanical ventilation while awaiting transplantation, increasing the risk of colonization and subsequent disease with nosocomial respiratory pathogens. The presence of a pulmonary infarct pretransplant has been associated with an increased risk of developing pulmonary abscesses after heart transplantation.[4]

In addition to risks associated with specific conditions, patients with more severe disease in general at the time of transplantation are at increased risk for postoperative morbidity and mortality.[5] Adult heart transplant recipients who require the use of circulatory assist devices have been shown to have a significant increase in nonviral infections during the perioperative period.[5] Children who suffer long-standing malnutrition are predisposed to infections both before and after transplantation. These candidates may require central venous catheters to deliver parenteral hyperalimentation which may lead to frequent episodes of catheter-associated infection.

Age is another pretransplant factor to consider as it is an important determinant of susceptibility to certain pathogens, severity of expression of infection, and immune system maturity. Neonatal transplant recipients, similar to other young infants, may present with overwhelming infections in the absence of fever and be mistakenly treated for rejection. Likewise, neonates may experience severe systemic illness with coagulase negative staphylococci more readily than older children. Like all children less than 2 years of age, the young transplant recipient, particularly if unimmunized, is at an increased risk of developing infection with encapsulated respiratory organisms (*Haemophilus influenzae, Neisseria meningitides, Streptococcus pneumoniae*). On the other hand, pathogens such as *Cryptococcus neoformans* are uncommon causes of infection in young children.[6] Age is also an important factor governing clinical expression of infection with cytomegalovirus (CMV) and Epstein-Barr virus (EBV). In immunocompetent hosts, the younger the child, the milder the clinical manifestations of these infections. However, when transplants are performed in young children, there is a very high likelihood that they will be seronegative for CMV and EBV and, therefore, will be susceptible to primary infections which tend to be more severe than episodes of reactivation or reinfection in patients who are seropositive pretransplant.[7,8]

The number of protective immunizations that children will have received pretransplant is largely determined by their ages. Children who have not received their full complement of immunizations will require vaccination after transplantation, at a time when their ability to mount an immune response may be hampered, and the use of live vaccines is controversial.

Donor Infections

Transplant recipients are at risk for acquiring infections that may be active or latent within the donor at the time of organ harvesting. Perhaps the most dramatic example of this is CMV. This agent is the most frequent and important viral pathogen causing infection after solid-organ transplantation.[9–13] The link between positive CMV serologic status of the donor and development of disease in the seronegative recipient has been clearly established. Other pathogens noted as causing donor-associated infections include toxoplasmosis,[14,15] EBV,[16] and human immunodeficiency virus (HIV).[17]

The presence of bacteria or fungi colonizing the donor respiratory tract can cause infection in the lung or heart-lung transplant recipient. The recognition of the extremely high rate of pneumonia in these patients has led to the suggestion that positive tracheal aspirate cultures obtained from the donor (ordinarily considered to represent only tracheal colonization in the absence of inflammation) is considered subclinical pneumonia.[18] Quiescent infection in the donor such as tuberculosis, histoplasmosis, or coccidiomycosis can also potentially cause problems. Occult bacteremia or viremia in any donor prior to the time of organ harvesting, likewise, represents a risk to the recipient.

Intraoperative Factors

Operative factors may predispose to infectious complications in patients undergoing thoracic transplantation. For example, the anastomosis of the transected trachea in heart-lung transplant recipients provides a potential portal of entry for microorganisms either from the donor or the recipient.[18] Injury to the phrenic, vagal, or recurrent laryngeal nerves can affect pulmonary toilet and predispose to pneumonia.[18] Other technical factors affecting the risk of infection post-transplantation remain to be identified.

Post-Transplant Factors

Technical problems, immunosuppression, indwelling cannulae, and nosocomial exposures are the major postoperative risk factors for infectious complications. Mediastinal bleeding postoperatively may require subsequent reexploration, and lead to an increased risk of early and severe mediastinitis and sepsis in heart or heart-lung transplant recipients.[9]

The kind and amount of immunosuppression used to prevent or control allograft rejection is probably the most important postoperative factor predisposing to infection. Immunosuppressive regimens have evolved in an attempt to achieve more specific control of rejection with the least impairment of immunity. The introduction of cyclosporine, used in combination with low-dose corticosteroids, appears to have decreased the incidence of infections in cardiac transplant recipients, compared to those treated with a combination of azathioprine and prednisone,[2,19] or azathioprine, prednisone, and antilymphocyte preparations.[20,21] The introduction of tacrolimus (FK 506) may also affect infectious outcome in children undergoing thoracic transplantation. Treatment with this drug has allowed many patients to be managed without the chronic use of steroids.[22,23] Analysis at our center of pediatric heart and pediatric lung transplant recipients treated with FK 506 compared to children treated with conventional immunosuppression has not shown a change in infectious deaths.

Treatment of episodes of rejection with additional or higher doses of immunosuppressants leads to an increased risk of invasive and sometimes fatal infection. Of particular concern is the use of antilymphocyte preparations, especially OKT3, which is often indispensable in the treatment of steroid refractory rejection.[13,24]

The prolonged use of indwelling cannulae is an important cause of bacterial infection in all hospitalized patients. The presence of intravascular central venous catheters was associated with seven bacteremic episodes in 37 heart transplant recipients at our hospital (unpublished data). Similarly, the presence of urethral catheters increase the risk of urinary tract infections which occur in approximately 5% to 15% of nonrenal transplant recipients.[9,22] Bacterial pneumonia may be associated with prolonged nasotracheal or endotracheal intubation.

Nosocomial exposures constitute the final group of postoperative risk factors. Children who have undergone thoracic transplantation may be exposed to many common viral pathogens (e.g., rotavirus or respiratory syncytial virus [RSV]). They are also at risk of exposure to transfusion-associated pathogens (e.g., hepatitis B, C, CMV, or HIV). Finally, the presence in the hospital (especially during construction efforts) of contamination with Aspergillus, may increase the risk of invasive fungal disease in these patients.

Timing of Infections

The time of the onset of infection with various pathogens after transplantation tends to be predictable and is an important consideration in both devising prophylactic regimens and performing diagnostic evaluations when patients become ill. Much of the data on the timing of infectious complications is derived from adult reports; the smaller pediatric experience appears to bear out these temporal relationships.

The majority of clinically important infections occur within the first 180 days following thoracic transplantation.[9,24–26] The timing of infections can be divided into three intervals: early (0 to 30 days after transplantation); intermediate (30 to 180 days after transplantation); and late (greater than 180 days after transplantation). Additionally, some infections may occur throughout the postoperative course. This schema, while arbitrary, is generally useful in approaching a patient with fever after thoracic transplantation, and can be used as a guide to differential diagnosis.

Early Infections (0 to 30 Days)

Early infections tend to be associated with preexisting conditions and surgical manipulation. In general, these infections are caused by either bacteria or yeast. Examples of preexisting infections include tracheitis or pneumonia in a cystic fibrosis patient undergoing heart-lung or lung transplant. Herpes simplex infection, though more common in adult patients, can also reactivate and cause early symptomatic disease.[10,27]

Surgical manipulation predisposes to early bacterial infections. Green et al found that 8 of 10 episodes of bacterial infection in 27 children occurred within the first 30 days after heart or heart-lung transplantation.[9] Mediastinitis, associated with mediastinal bleeding and reexploration, was fatal in two cases. Similarly, bacterial infections in heart-lung transplant recipients occur during the early period of post-transplant, and are most likely to involve the lungs or thorax.[18,25]

Intermediate Period (31 to 180 Days)

The intermediate period is the typical time of onset of infections associated with donor transmission (either organ or blood product), reactivated viruses, and opportunistic infections. The onset of symptomatic CMV infection, the predominant virus causing disease in all types of organ recipients, peaks during this interval.[9–12] This period is also when many patients present with EBV infections, post-transplant lymphoproliferative disorders,[8,28] *Pneumocystis carinii* pneumonia (PCP),[29–32] and toxoplasmosis.[14,33,34]

Late Infections (>180 Days)

Late infectious complications after thoracic transplantation are less well characterized than other periods, because patients have usually been discharged from the transplant center to their respective homes, often quite far away. This makes the accurate accumulation of data on these late infections difficult. A high incidence of late onset chronic bronchiectasis, often due to *Pseudomonas sp.*, has been noted in adult heart-lung transplant recipients.[18] Experience with pediatric heart-lung transplant or lung transplant recipients shows that they too have problems with *Pseudomonas sp.* and fungal infections if bronchiolitis obliterans is present. EBV-associated lymphoproliferative disease (LPD) can occur in the late period, but at a decreased rate after the first year from the time of transplant [8,35]

Infections Occurring Throughout the Postoperative Course

Iatrogenic factors are an important cause of bacterial and fungal infections at all times, but predominate in the early transplant period. Central venous lines are maintained for a variable time; the risk of infection persists for the entire period that the catheter remains in place. Urethral catheters are used in the early postoperative periods. Resultant episodes of urinary tract infection tend to be temporally related to their use.

Nosocomial acquisition of community viruses, such as RSV, rotavirus, and influenza A, or B, can lead to infection if present in the community regardless of where the patient is in the postoperative course. These viruses spread easily in hospital environments from personnel or other hospitalized patients to transplant recipients. It is, therefore, important to modify diagnostic considerations according to local epidemiologic considerations.

Although incompletely documented,[36,37] most children who have received thoracic transplants experience the usual childhood respiratory and gastrointestinal illnesses without significant problems. This is especially true when they occur long after transplantation and are not associated with an episode of rejection. In contrast, early infection with community acquired viruses may result in profound illness. Review of our experience with RSV after pediatric liver transplantation, suggests that disease is more severe in children who acquire infection in the first 3 weeks after transplant surgery.[38] Our experience with other common viral infections (parainfluenza and influenza) suggests that pediatric solid-organ transplant recipients who develop infection during the early transplant period or at times of intense immunosuppression may be at risk for severe disease.[37] Likewise, adenovirus infection early after lung transplantation has a poor prognosis.[39]

Specific Infections

Bacterial Infections

Serious bacterial infections tend to occur early after transplantation. Similar to adult heart transplant recipients, children experience a high rate of mediastinitis and intrathoracic infections. Mediastinitis has been reported in 7% of adult cardiac recipients.[19,40] Enteric gram negative rods and staphylococcal species made up the majority of organisms. *Mycoplasma hominis* was also noted in several patients from one center.[41] Mediastinitis resulted in severe disease in 2 of 27 of our initial pediatric thoracic transplant recipients at our institution.[9]

The upper and lower respiratory tract was the most common site of infection in a 15-year review of pediatric heart transplantation undertaken at Stanford.[10] Thirty-eight bacterial infections involving this site occurred in 53 patients. Likewise, 5 of 10 proven bacterial infections in the Pittsburgh population included pneumonia or lung abscess.[9] In contrast, investigators from two other series identified only one child each with pneumonia in 18 and 43 pediatric heart transplant recipients, respectively.[36,12]

Infants undergoing heart transplantation may be at increased risk of developing serious bacterial infections compared to older children. Four serious bacterial infections occurred in 19 infant heart transplant recipients reported by Baker et al.[43] Ten of 14 infants less than 6 months of age transplanted at our center experienced serious infections, resulting in two deaths (unpublished data).

Pediatric heart-lung transplant recipients are also at a high risk for bacterial infections of the respiratory tract. In general, these children develop infections due to the same pathogens as heart transplant recipients.[44] Alternatively, patients who undergo lung or heart-lung transplant for cystic fibrosis are at increased risk of developing serious and sometimes fatal disease due to *Pseudomonas aeruginosa*.[45] The diagnosis of pneumonia may be difficult in a heart-lung (or lung) transplant recipient. Radiographic abnormalities, while nearly universal, present in children with proven pneumonia, were also observed in most patients with early rejection.[46] Similar observations have been made in adults.[47,48] A combination of transbronchial biopsy and bronchoalveolar lavage are often necessary for definitive diagnosis.

Fungal Infections

An overview of the common infectious syndromes due to bacterial and fungal infection after pediatric thoracic transplantation seen at the Children's Hospital of Pittsburgh is shown in Table 2.

Fungal infections appear to occur less frequently than bacterial disease after pediatric heart transplantation. However, infections due to fungal pathogens are remarkable for their severity. Ten fungal infections, half of which were due to *Aspergillus sp.,* developed in 53 pediatric heart transplant patients reported from Stanford.[10] Eight percent of pediatric heart transplant recipients at our center have experienced moderate to severe fungal infections. Pathogens included *Candida sp., Aspergillus fumigatus,* and *Cryptococcus neoformans.*

An increased rate of invasive candida infection has been observed among adult heart-lung transplant recipients compared to those who underwent heart transplantation.[48] Infection occurred most often in the first 6 weeks following transplantation in patients who were in the intensive care unit on multiple antibiotics. Similarly, 5 of 10 pediatric heart-lung transplant recipients from Stanford had fungal infections due to either *Candida* or *Aspergillus sp.*[44]

Aspergillus colonization in cystic fibrosis patients is quite common and represents a special concern for patients about to undergo immunosuppression. While the presence of a pulmonary aspergilloma has been considered an absolute contraindication for

Table 2.

Common Bacterial and Fungal Infections in Pediatric Thoracic Transplant Recipient at the Children's Hospital of Pittsburgh

Syndrome	Pathogen
Pneumonia Lung abscess	Enterobacteriaceae *Staphylococcus aureus* *Candida sp.* *Aspergillus fumigatus*
Mediastinitis	Enterobacteriaceae *Staphylococcus sp.*
Bacteremia	Enterobacteriaceae Coagulase negative Staphylococci *Haemophilus influenzae* type B *Streptococcus pneumoniae* *Candida sp.*
Urinary tract infection	Enterobacteriaceae *Candida sp.*

transplantation, the risk from colonization alone is less clear.[49] Recovery of aspergillus from a respiratory culture in a transplant patient should be aggressively treated with amphotericin B. Patients known to be colonized with aspergillus prior to transplantation should receive prophylaxis with antifungals early after transplantation. The use of prophylaxis prior to transplantation is more controversial because the waiting period duration is unpredictable.

Viral Infections

Cytomegalovirus

CMV is the most frequent and important viral infection occurring after solid-organ transplantation. An incidence of approximately 25% has been reported among pediatric heart and heart-lung transplant recipients.[9,10] Infection may be due to primary acquisition in a seronegative patient (either from the donor graft or blood products), reactivation of latent infection, or reinfection with a different strain in a previously seropositive patient. Primary infection is associated with an increased severity of disease.[7] CMV reactivation or reinfection occurs frequently in the seropositive patient after solid-organ transplantation, but is generally associated with more mild or even asymptomatic infection.[7] However, CMV pneumonia occurs frequently among heart-lung or lung transplant recipients who were seropositive pretransplant.[11] An increase in the severity of CMV (both in patients experiencing primary infection or reactivation or reinfection) has also been documented after the use of antilymphocyte agents in liver and kidney transplant recipients.[13,24,50] Similar increases in severity of infection may occur in patients who have been exposed to increased immunosuppression in general. The negative effect of these agents on CMV disease is likely to be seen in thoracic transplant recipients as well.

Symptomatic CMV disease will typically occur between 1 and 3 months after transplantation.[7,9–13] Patients may present with the "CMV syndrome" defined by the presence of one or more symptoms of varying severity including fever, rash, or hematologic abnormalities. Invasive CMV disease occurs involving the gastrointestinal tract, liver, or lungs. Recipients of thoracic transplantation are at an increased risk of developing pneumonia. Unlike patients with acquired immunde deficiency syndrome (AIDS), chorioretinitis due to CMV is uncommonly seen after solid-organ transplantation, although ophthalmologic evaluation at the time of CMV infection may be warranted.

In addition to the direct effects of CMV infection, secondary immunologic events leading to both increased rates of secondary infection and rejection have been attributed to infection with CMV. Symptomatic infection has been associated with increased susceptibility to bacterial and fungal superinfections among adult organ transplant recipients.[51] This has been explained by the observation that significant alterations of T lymphocyte subsets in patients with symptomatic CMV disease occur leading to depression of cellular immunity.[52] Alternatively, the increased rate of secondary infections may simply be an indication that these patients have been overly immunosuppressed. CMV infection has also been associated with an increased frequency of acute and chronic allograft rejection in heart and lung transplant recipients.[53,54] A possible explanation for this is provided by the hypothesis that infection with CMV alters the expression of class I major histocompatibility antigens predisposing to acute and chronic rejection.[53] However, a causal role for the increased rate of infection or rejection after CMV infection remains to be proven.

Experience over the first 10 years of pediatric thoracic organ transplants at the Children's Hospital of Pittsburgh with CMV is shown in Table 3.[55] Thirty-nine of 55 heart transplant recipients who survived for at least 2 weeks after transplantation were seronegative for CMV pretransplant, 11 were seropositive, and in 5 children, serologic status was unknown. Nine of 11 patients who developed symptomatic CMV disease experienced primary infection. Six of these nine infections were invasive; the lung was involved in five patients. Two episodes were associated with a fatal outcome. In contrast, only one of eight patients known to be seropositive pretransplant developed symptomatic infection. One additional child whose pretransplant status for CMV was unknown developed nonfatal CMV pneumonia. This experience is similar to that of Baum et al[10] who reported that 6 of 53 children developed severe, symptomatic CMV disease after heart transplantation, resulting in four deaths.

Twenty-four children surviving greater than 2 weeks after heart-lung or lung transplantation were evaluable.[55] Twenty-one of 24 were seronegative and three were seropositive for CMV pretransplant. CMV was recovered from BAL fluid of 7 of these 24 patients. Five of the 21 seronegative patients experienced primary symptomatic disease; one was fatal. All symptomatic infections developed within the first 6 months after transplantation. Seronegative recipients of an organ from a seropositive donor had an eightfold increased risk for CMV infection compared to those with a seronegative donor. CMV pneumonia developed, despite initial prophylaxis for 4 weeks with intravenous ganciclovir followed by high-dose oral acyclovir. A number of previously seropositive patients have CMV detected by early antigen presence from BAL fluid with no symptoms of disease. Only one patient who was previously seropositive developed CMV pneumonitis after steroid augmentation.

Reports describing the outcome of adult heart-lung transplant recipients also emphasize the significance of CMV pneumonia in these patients.[18,56] A high rate of

Table 3.

CMV Infection after Pediatric Heart and Heart-Lung/Lung Transplantation at the Children's Hospital of Pittsburgh (1982–1992)

	Heart	Heart-Lung Lung
Total Patients	55	24
Symptomatic infection	11	5
Primary infection	9	5
Invasive infection	7	3
Organ involvement		
GI tract	1	0
Liver	1	0
Lung	5	3
Heart	1	0
Fatal disease	2	1

CMV = cytomegalovirus; GI = gastrointestinal

pneumonitis has been observed in both high-risk patients (CMV-positive donor/CMV-negative recipients) experiencing primary infection, and those developing CMV disease due to either reactivation or reinfection. Fatal pneumonitis had been reported frequently in patients with primary CMV pneumonia prior to the introduction of ganciclovir.[18,56] In contrast, death was rare in patients who were seropositive pretransplant.[56]

Experience with ganciclovir documents an improved outcome of CMV infection in recipients of thoracic transplantation.[57–59] In a large published series, Smyth et al reported an 80% success rate in the treatment of CMV pneumonia in adult heart-lung transplant recipients.[57] It is important to note that both early and late recurrences have been observed after treatment with ganciclovir.[57,58] Our experience with ganciclovir has also been favorable.

The potential role of intravenous gamma globulin (either hyperimmune CMV immunoglobulin or standard preparations) in combination with ganciclovir has also been suggested for the treatment of CMV pneumonia by some investigators.[60] Retrospective data among bone-marrow transplant recipients experiencing CMV pneumonia suggests a benefit to this combined therapeutic approach.[61,62] The efficacy of this combination in the treatment of CMV disease of thoracic organ transplant recipients is questionable. Furthermore, the comparability of CMV pneumonia in bone marrow transplant recipients (where graft versus host disease is known to play a critical role in the development of pneumonitis) to thoracic transplant recipients is unclear. Given the overall excellent results obtained in the treatment of adult thoracic transplant recipients experiencing CMV pneumonia with ganciclovir alone,[57,58] we do not currently recommend this combined approach.

Epstein-Barr Virus

Infection due to EBV and EBV-associated LPD is an important problem after solid-organ transplantation.[9,63,64] The incidence of LPD in patients surviving more than 30 days has been reported as 3.4% after heart and 7.9% after heart-lung transplantation; a trend toward a significant difference was noted between the rates of LPD in these two patients groups (P = 0.08).[65] LPD is more common after primary EBV infection, placing children at higher risk than adults for developing this disease.[8] Ho et al reported a 63% overall frequency of EBV infection in 92 pediatric liver transplant recipients.[8] Primary infection occurred in 77% of seronegative children, while reactivation infection occurred in 33% of seropositive patients. These investigators found that 4% of children undergoing solid-organ (including thoracic) transplantation and 10% of children with primary EBV infection developed LPD between 1 month and 5 years after transplant. Armitage et al found that 9.7% of pediatric thoracic transplant recipients developed LPD.[65] More recently, Boyle et al reported a 6.7% and 17% incidence in cardiac and lung transplant recipients, respectively, at Children's Hospital of Pittsburgh.[35] Post-transplant LPD was associated with primary EBV infection in all of these cases. Although greater than 75% of cases of LPD may occur during the first post-operative year,[8] several investigators have identified that there is an on-going risk of developing this disease for each year of survival post-transplant.[28,65] Seven years after liver transplantation in children, the actuarial risk of developing LPD has been calculated as 20%.[28]

Several schemas describing the clinical syndromes of LPD have been proposed.[8,28,66] Ho et al identified three distinguishable presentations: a self-limited form of mononucleosis resembling illness in immunologically normal children; a similar often fatal syndrome progressing to widespread lymphoproliferation involving visceral organs; and isolated extranodal lymphoma.[8] In general, onset of the first and second syndromes is observed within the first year, while extranodal lymphoma occurs later. Heart-lung and lung transplant recipients appear to be at increased risk for early presentation and for development of disease involving the lung.[65] The initial histology of patients with a progressive infectious mononucleosis-like illness may not be predictive of outcome.

The management of patients with LPD is controversial and may need to vary depending on clinical presentation and histologic analysis. Reduction of immunosuppression is widely endorsed and recommended.[8,28,63] We currently reduce immunosuppression to the lowest tolerable level. Hanto et al reported benefit of intravenous acyclovir, however, this drug has not been evaluated in formal clinical trials.[67,68] Nonetheless, it is our usual practice to use 14 days of intravenous acyclovir or ganciclovir. Resection of tumor may also be of value in patients with lymphoma.[8] The potential role of chemotherapy in these tumors has not been established. Other therapeutic modalities include interferon, monoclonal antibodies, and cytotoxic lymphocytes. Formal clinical trials with this disease will be beneficial.

Herpes Simplex

Herpes simplex virus (HSV) has been a major problem following adult transplantation procedures, especially after augmentation of immunosuppression for treatment of rejection. Pneumonitis, which may be fatal, occurs more frequently in adult heart-lung patients compared to other solid-organ transplant recipients and develops despite the presence of serum antibodies against HSV.[27] An estimated 10% of pediatric patients will develop episodes of herpes stomatitis after solid-organ transplantation.[9,11–13] Disseminated disease due to HSV is uncommon. Oral acyclovir prophylaxis to prevent this problem is recommended, particularly in the first several months following transplantation.

Varicella

Many children who undergo solid-organ transplantation do so before they have had an exposure to varicella. Feldhoff et al found that 19 of 160 renal transplant patients developed varicella; eight of these children had severe disease including one death.[69] Similarly, McGregor et al found that varicella developed in 14 of 47 susceptible pediatric liver transplant recipients.[70] Thirteen of the 14 were treated with intravenous acyclovir. Two of these patients died, although the rest had only mild disease. Of note, almost half of the patients receiving varicella zoster immune globulin (VZIG) developed disease, including one of the fatal cases. Currently, we administer VZIG within 72 hours of a varicella exposure to our nonimmune patients. If varicella develops, we treat with intravenous acyclovir until no new lesions erupt and all lesions crust.

Opportunistic Infections

Pneumocystis Carinii

PCP is a well-documented cause of pneumonia in immunocompromised patients. Both reactivation of latent infection and person-to-person transmission have been proposed as mechanisms of disease development.[71,72] While this organism has been noted to cause pneumonia in recipients of each type of solid-organ transplantation,[28–32] it has a higher than anticipated attack rate in heart-lung patients.[31] Gryzan et al found evidence of PCP in 88% of consecutively followed adult heart-lung transplant recipients who were not on sulfamethoxazole/trimethoprim (SMZ/TMP).[31] Seventeen episodes occurred in 14 patients, of which 6 resulted in significant disease. Infections tend to occur within the first year after transplantation, but have on occasion been seen later. Symptoms range from fever alone to profound respiratory distress leading to death. PCP can be prevented with prophylaxis[73] and will be discussed in more detail later in the chapter.

Toxoplasma Gondii

Acquired toxoplasmosis, usually a benign disorder in a normal host, can lead to devastating consequences in immunocompromised patients.[14,74] It can on rare occasions cause disease in renal and liver transplant recipients,[24,75,76] but is more commonly found as a pathogen after cardiac transplantation.[33] In contrast to AIDS patients, in whom reactivation of dormant cysts occur, the transplant recipient experiences the most severe disease from primary infection associated with the transmission of toxoplasma via the donor organ.[77] The highest risk and most severe symptomatic disease occurs in seronegative heart transplant recipients of grafts from seropositive donors.[14,33,34,78,79] Review of the literature reveals 14 of 16 mismatched cardiac transplant patients had serious disease.[14] This compares with absent or mild symptoms and rising titers in 11 of 58 patients who were seropositive prior to transplantation and no symptoms in 93 seronegative recipients when the donor was also seronegative. Evidence of severe toxoplasmosis due to community acquisition post-transplantation has not been documented in the literature, but remains a concern in susceptible hosts.

Clinical presentation of toxoplasmosis most often occurs within 1 to 6 months after transplantation. Expression of infection can vary from asymptomatic seroconversion to severe disease with fever, chorioretinitis, myocarditis, neurologic abnormalities, or pulmonary compromise. We have cared for four children who developed primary seroconversion; two of these children had severe toxoplasmosis documented at autopsy.[14] Treatment is with pyrimethamine and sulfonamides. Folinic acid (leucovorin) should also be given to decrease the incidence of bone marrow depression. Prophylaxis of high risk adult patients with pyrimethamine is currently being studied with encouraging results.[78]

Management

Pretransplant Evaluation

Our infectious disease division is consulted on all potential transplant candidates for a pretransplant evaluation. In addition to helping to determine whether infectious contraindications to transplantation exist, this evaluation helps with planning special perioperative prophylaxis if needed and affords the family the opportunity to ask infectious disease-related questions. An outline of this evaluation is shown in Table 4. A complete history and physical examination is performed with particular attention to previous infections, immunizations, and drug allergies. An intermediate strength tuberculin skin test, along with an anergy panel, is applied during the pretransplant evaluation.

Pretransplant surveillance sputum cultures are obtained from children with cystic fibrosis or those with a prolonged intensive care stay just prior to transplantation in order to guide antimicrobial prophylaxis and treatment if needed. Colonization with *Burkholderia cepacia* or bacterial organisms resistant to all available antibiotics is currently a contraindication to lung transplantation at our institution.[80]

We recommend serologic testing for CMV, EBV, varicella, herpes simplex virus, RPR, toxoplasma, and HIV on all candidates at the time of pretransplant screening. If the actual date of transplantation is more than 1 month after this initial visit, we repeat any previously negative studies. Serologic tests on the donor should include HIV, hepatitis B and C, CMV, and toxoplasma. Although some European centers are currently accepting only CMV negative donors for patients who are CMV negative in an effort to prevent primary infections, the current shortage of donors in the United States precludes the routine use of this type of matching. However, knowledge of donor and recipient CMV serologic status allows the clinician to anticipate infection frequency and severity, and guides the diagnostic evaluation of fever. It may also identify high-risk patients for whom the development of prophylactic regimens would be of benefit.

Finally, those candidates in whom transplantation is not imminent should undergo an update of appropriate immunizations at the time of the pretransplant evaluation.

Table 4.

Management Guidelines for Children Undergoing Solid-Organ Transplantation at the Children's Hospital of Pittsburgh

Pretransplant evaluation

History
Physical exam
PPD with energy panel
Serologic screening for CMV, EBV, varicella, HSV, HIV, hepatitis A, B, C, measles, and toxoplasmosis
Update immunizations if transplant not imminent

Chronic prophylatic regimens

1. Nystatin
2. SMZ/TMP
3. Acyclovir[a]
4. Ganciclovir[b]
5. Immunizatons[c]
   Diptheria-pertusis-tetanus
   Inactivated poliomyelitis vaccine
   Haemophilus influenzae type B
   Influenza
   Measles-mumps-rubella[d]

[a]Given as HSV prophylaxis for first 3 months in seropositive patients.
[b]Initially given twice daily for 14 days, then once a day for 7 to 14 days in heart-lung or lung transplant recipients.
[c]Given 3 months post-transplant or 1 month post-treatment for rejection.
[d]Limited experience in patients living in areas with epidemic measles.
CMV = cytomegalovirus; EBV = Epstein-Barr virus; HIV = human immunodeficiency virus; HSV = herpes simplex virus; SMZ/TMP = sulfamethoxazole/trimethoprim.

This is especially true for the measles-mumps-rubella vaccine (MMR), since the use of this live viral vaccine after transplantation is currently discouraged. In the appropriate season, influenza vaccine should also be given prior to transplantation.

Prophylactic Regimens

Our prophylactic strategies are divided into perioperative and long-term prophylaxis (Table 4). They have evolved to reflect the infectious complications seen at our institution.

Perioperative prophylaxis is used in the hope of preventing intraoperative sepsis and wound infection. The choice of antimicrobial agents is based on the organ being transplanted, individual patient characteristics, expected normal flora, and a knowledge of the antimicrobial sensitivities of local pathogens. Because of the concern that prolonged intubation and subsequent airway colonization of the heart-lung transplant donor may lead to infection in the immunosuppressed recipient, we currently modify our perioperative prophylaxis based upon surveillance cultures of the donor graft.

Long-term prophylaxis against infections occurring beyond the perioperative period must take into consideration the risk and severity of infection, as well as the toxicity, cost, and efficacy of a given prophylactic strategy. Nystatin suspension is used in all pediatric transplant recipients in an effort to prevent oropharyngeal candidiasis for at least 3 months following transplantation.

SMZ/TMP is used to prevent PCP. It is given as a single daily dose or as a single dose on alternate days. The duration of prophylaxis for PCP is somewhat controversial. The majority of cases occur during the first year after transplant. However, because late exceptions do occur, we currently recommend using SMZ/TMP indefinitely.

The optimal antimicrobial choice for prophylaxis of PCP in children who cannot tolerate sulfa drugs is not known. Some institutions forego prophylaxis in these children and closely observe them for the development of pneumonia. Studies from adult patients with AIDS suggest that aerosolized pentamidine or dapsone (either alone or in combination with trimethoprim) may serve as alternative regimens.[81–84] Delivery of aerosolized drug in small children may be difficult and only a single small report on the use of aerosolized pentamidine in pediatric patients has been published.[85]

The frequency and severity of CMV infection in transplant recipients has prompted the consideration of several prophylactic strategies.[86–88] Studies in both bone marrow transplant[87] and adult renal transplant recipients[88] have suggested a role for high-dose acyclovir in the prevention or modification of CMV disease. In contrast, Dummer et al did not find a decrease in CMV disease in adult heart or heart-lung transplant recipients who received prophylaxis with acyclovir at 30 mg/kg per day.[11]

Several centers have evaluated intravenous immunoglobulin (both high-titer anti-CMV and commercially available products) in the prevention of CMV disease in adult solid-organ transplant recipients.[30,86,89,90] While their initial results are encouraging, reports of CMV disease in patients receiving IVIG prophylactic regimens have occurred. Further studies are required to determine the costs, benefits, dosage, duration, and efficacy of IVIG in modifying or preventing CMV disease in transplant recipients.

We currently use ganciclovir as CMV prophylaxis, in patients who are seropositive prior to transplantation or receive an organ from a seropositive donor. A multicenter trial describing ganciclovir prophylaxis in adult heart transplant recipients demonstrated decreased disease in seropositive recipients, but not in high-risk, previously seronegative patients.[91] Likewise, ganciclovir prophylaxis after lung transplantation of high-risk patients (seronegative recipient/seropositive donor) has not prevented CMV disease in our patient population.

Finally, the use of CMV negative blood products has been shown to decrease the transmission of CMV in patients whose organ donors are seronegative. We strongly recommend the use of CMV-negative blood products, or alternatively, leukocyte filtering devices, as an important method of decreasing the exposure of transplant recipients to CMV.

A discussion of prophylaxis would be incomplete without a comment on immunizations. Often, children undergo transplantation prior to completing a routine immunization series. In these cases, we recommend waiting 3 months after transplantation to resume the series. Diphtheria tetanus pertussis and conjugate vaccines against *Haemophilus influenzae* type b should be given as routinely prescribed. Inactivated polio vaccine should be substituted for oral polio vaccine in the patient and siblings. Influenza vaccine is also recommended for these children and their family members. The use of MMR, a trivalent live virus vaccine, is currently controversial. It has been used without adverse effects in children with AIDS.[92] We have given MMR without adverse effects to approximately 15 pediatric liver transplant recipients who were all at least 6-months post-transplant. Immunogenicity data on these children is incomplete at this time. Varicella vaccine, recently available, has the potential to be useful in susceptible children.

References

1. Kreitt JM, Kaye MP: The registry of the international society for heart transplantation: seventh official report—1990. _J Heart Transplant_ 9:323–330, 1990.
2. Dummer JS, Hardy A, Poorsattar A, Ho M: Early infections in kidney, heart and liver transplant recipients on cyclosporine. _Transplantation_ 36:259–267, 1983.
3. Ho M, Dummer JS: Infections in transplant recipients. In: Mandell GL, Douglas RG Jr, Bennett JE (eds). _Principles and Practice of Infectious Diseases._ 4th Ed. New York: Churchill Livingstone, Inc.; 2709–2717, 1995.
4. Young JN, Yazbeck J, Esposito G, Mankad P, Townsend E, Yacob M: The influence of acute preoperative pulmonary infarction on the results of heart transplantation. _J Heart Transpant_ 5:20–22, 1986.
5. Hsu J, Griffith BP, Dowling RD, et al: Infections in mortally ill cardiac transplant recipients. _J Thorac Surg_ 98:506–509, 1989.
6. Wittner M: Cryptococcosis. In: Feigin RD, Cherry JD (eds). _Textbook of Pediatric Infectious Diseases,_ 3rd Ed. Philadelphia: WB Saunders, Co.; 1934–1939, 1992.
7. Breinig MK, Zitelli B, Starzl TE, Ho M: Epstein-Barr virus, cytomegalovirus, and other viral infections in children after liver transplantation. _J Infect Dis_ 156:273–279, 1987.
8. Ho M, Jaffe R, Miller G, et al: The frequency of Epstein-Barr virus infection and associated lymphoproliferative syndrome after transplantation and its manifestations in children. _Transplantation_ 45:719–727, 1988.
9. Green M, Wald ER, Fricker FS, et al: Infections in pediatric orthotopic heart transplant recipients. _Pediatr Infect Dis J_ 8:87–93, 1989.
10. Baum D, Bernstein D, Starnes VA, et al: Pediatric heart transplantation at Stanford: results of a 15-year experience. _Pediatrics_ 88:203–214, 1991.
11. Dummer JS, White LT, Ho M, et al: Morbidity of cytomegalovirus infection in recipients of heart or heart-lung transplants who received cyclosporine. _J Infect Dis_ 152:1182–1191, 1985,
12. Trachman H, Weiss RA, Spigland I, Greifer I: Clinical manifestations herpesvirus infections in pediatric renal transplant recipients. _Pediatr Infect Dis J_ 4:480–486, 1985.
13. Bowman JS, Green M, Scantlebury VP, et al: OKT3 and viral disease in pediatric liver transplant recipients. _Clin Transplant_ 5:294–300, 1991.
14. Michaels MG, Wald ER, Fricker FJ, Del Nido PJ, Armitage J: Toxoplasmosis in pediatric heart transplant recipients. _Clin Infect Dis_ 14:847–857, 1992.
15. Ryning FW, Mcleod R, Maddox JC, Hunt S, Remington JS: Probable transmission of Toxoplasma gondii by organ transplantation. _Ann Intern Med_ 90:47–49, 1979.
16. Cen H, Breinig MC, Atchinson RW, et al: Epstein-Barr virus transmission via the donor-organ in solid-organ transplantation: polymerase chain reaction and restriction fragment length polymorphism analogue of IR2, IR3, IR4. _J Virol_ 65:976–980, 1991.
17. Dummer JS, Siegfried E, Breinig MK, et al: Infection with human immunodeficiency virus in the Pittsburgh transplant population. _Transplantation_ 47:134–139, 1989.
18. Dummer JS: Infectious complications. In: Cooper DKC, Novitzky D (eds). _The Transplantation and Replacement of Thoracic Organs._ Kluwer Academic Publishers; 325–332, 1990.
19. Hofflin JM, Potasman I, Baldwin JC, et al: Infectious complication in heart transplant recipients receiving cyclosporine and corticosteroids. _Ann Intern Med_ 106:209–216, 1987.
20. Andreone PA, Olivari MT, Elick B, et al: Reduction of infectious complications following heart transplantation with triple-drug immunotherapy. _J Heart Transplant_ 5:13–19, 1986.
21. Najarian JS, Fryd DS, Strand M, et al: A single institution, randomized, prospective trial of cyclosporine versus azathioprine-antilymphocyte globulin for immunosuppression in renal allograft recipients. _Ann Surg_ 201:142–157, 1985.

22. Green M, Tzakis A, Reyes J, Nour B, Todos, Starzl TE: Infectious complications of pediatric liver transplantation under FK 506. *Transplant Proc* 3:3038–3039, 1991.
23. Todo S, Fung JJ, Starzl TE, et al: Liver, kidney, and thoracic organ transplantation under FK 506. *Ann Surg* 212:295–307, 1990.
24. Kusne S, Dummer JS, Singh N, et al: Infection after liver transplantation: an analysis of 101 consecutive cases. *Medicine* 67:132–143, 1988.
25. Griffith BP, Hardesty RL, Trento A, et al: Heart-lung transplantation: lessons learned and future hopes. *Ann Thorac Surg* 43:6–16, 1987.
26. Morduchowicz G, Pitlik SD, Shapira Z, et al: Infections in renal transplant recipients in Israel. *Isr J Med Sci* 21:791–797, 1985.
27. Smyth RL, Higenbottam TW, Scott JP, et al: Herpes simplex virus infection in heart-lung transplant recipients. *Transplantation* 49:735–739, 1990.
28. Malatack JJ, Gartner JC, Urbach AH, Zitelli BJ: Orthotopic liver transplantation, Epstein-Barr virus, cyclosporine and lymphoproliferative syndrome ∫ a growing concern. *J Pediatr* 118:667–675, 1991.
30. Schafers HJ, Cremer J, Wahlers T, et al: *Pneumocystis carinii* pneumonia following heart transplantation. *Eur J Cardiothorac Surg* 1:49–52, 1987.
31. Gryzan S, Paradis IL, Zeevi A, et al: Unexpectedly high incidence of *Pneumocystis carinii* after lung-heart transplantation. *Am Rev Respir Dis* 137:1268–1274, 1988.
32. Hardy AM, Wajszczuk CP, Suffredini F, et al: *Pneumocystis carinii* pneumonia in renal transplant recipients treated with cyclosporine and steroids. *J Infect Dis* 149:143–147, 1984.
33. Luft BJ, Naot Y, Araujo FG, et al: Primary and reactivated toxoplasma infection in patients with cardiac transplants. *Ann Intern Med* 99:27–31, 1983.
34. Nagington J, Martin AL: Toxoplasmosis and heart transplantation. *Lancet* 2:679, 1983.
35. Boyle GJ, Michaels MG, Webber S, et al: Post-transplant disorders in pediatric thoracic organ recipients. *J Pediatr* 1996. (In press.)
36. Bailey LL, Wood M, Razzouk A, et al: Heart transplantation during the first 12 years of life. *Arch Surg* 124:1221–1226, 1989.
37. Apalsch AM, Green M, Ledesma-Medina J, Nour B, Wald ER: Parainfluenza and influenza virus infections in pediatric organ transplant recipients. *Clin Infect Dis* 20:394–399, 1995.
38. Pohl C, Green M, Wald ER: RSV infection after pediatric liver transplantation. *J Infect Dis* 165:166–169, 1992.
39. Ohori NP, Michaels MG, Jaffe R, Williams P, Yousem SA: Adenovirus pneumonia in lung transplant recipients. *Human Pathol* 26:1073–1079, 1995.
40. Trento A, Dummer JS, Hardesty RL, et al: Mediastinitis following heart transplantation: incidence, treatment, and results. *Heart Transplant* 3:336–340, 1984.
41. Steffenson DO, Dummer JS, Granick MS, et al: Sternotomy infections with Mycoplasma hominis. *Ann Intern Med* 106:204–208, 1987.
42. Braunlin EA, Canter CE, Olivari MT, et al: Rejection and infection after pediatric cardiac transplantation. *Ann Thorac Surg* 49:385–390, 1990.
43. Baker CC, Zales VR, Harrison HL, Idriss FS, Benson DW, Mavroudis C: Intermediate term results of infant orthotopic cardiac transplant from two centers. *J Thorac Cardiovasc Surg* 101:826–832, 1991.
44. Starnes VA, Marshall SE, Lewiston NJ, Theodore J, Shumway NE: Heart-lung transplantation in infants, children and adolescents. *J Pediatr Surg* 26:434–438, 1991.
45. Whitehead B, Helms P, Goodwin M, et al: Heart-lung transplantation for cystic fibrosis. II. Outcome. *Arch Dis Child* 66:1018–1021, 1991.
46. Scott JP, Higenbottam TW, Smyth RL, et al: Transbronchial biopsies in children after heart-lung transplantation. *Pediatrics* 86:698–702, 1990.
47. Millet B, Higenbottam TW, Flower CDR, et al: The radiographic appearances of infection and acute rejection of the lung after heart-lung transplantation. *Am Rev Respir Dis* 140:62–67, 1989.
48. Starnes V, Theodore J, Oyer PE, et al: Pulmonary infiltrates after heart-lung transplantation: evaluation by serial transbronchial biopsies. *Cardiovasc Surg* 98:945–950, 1989.
49. Dummer JS, Montero CD, Griffith BP, Hardesty RL, Paridis IL, Ho M: Infections in heart-lung transplant recipients. *Transplantation* 41:725–729, 1986.

50. Bunchman TE, Nevins TE, Mauer SM, Chavers BM: Viral complications of OKT3 monoclonal antibody in children undergoing renal transplantation. *Transplant Proc* 21: 1761–1762, 1989.

51. Gorensek MJ, Stewart RW, Keys TF, McHenry MC, Babiak T, Goormastic M: Symptomatic cytomegalovirus infection as a significant risk factor for major infections after cardiac transplantation. *J Infect Dis* 158:884–887, 1988.

52. Schooley RT, Hirsch MS, Colvin RB, et al: Association of herpes virus infections with T-lymphocyte subset alterations, glomerulopathy, and opportunistic infections after renal transplantation. *N Engl J Med* 308:307–313, 1983.

53. Grattan MT, Moreno-Cabral CE, Starnes VA, Oyer PE, Stinson EB, Shumway NE: Cytomegalovirus infection is associated with cardiac allograft rejection and atherosclerosis. *JAMA* 261:3561–3566, 1989.

54. Keenan RJ, Lega ME, Dummer JS, et al: Cytomegalovirus serologic status and postoperative infection correlated with risk of developing chronic rejection after pulmonary transplantation. *Transplantation* 51:433–438, 1991.

55. Michaels MG, Green M, Wlad E, et al: Cytomegalovirus in pediatric heart and heart-lung or lung transplant recipients (abstr). *32nd ICAAC,* Anaheim, CA: 1428:329, 1992.

56. Smyth RL, Scott JP, Higenbottam TW, et al: Experience of Cytomegalovirus infection in heart-lung transplant recipients. *Transplant Proc* 22:1822–1823. 1990.

57. Smyth RL, Scott JP, Borysiewicz, et al: Cytomegalovirus infection in heart-lung transplant recipients: risk factors, clinical associations and response to treatment. *J Infect Dis* 164:1045–1050, 1991.

58. Cerrina J, Bavoux E, Le Roy Ladurie F, et al: Ganciclovir treatment of cytomegalovirus infection in heart-lung and double-lung transplant recipients. *Transplant Proc* 23:1174–1175, 1991.

59. Behrend M, Steinhoff G, Wagner TOF, Haverich A: Reactivation of CMV in human lung transplants. *Transplant Proc* 22:1824–1825, 1990.

60. Duncan SR, Cook DJ: Survival of ganciclovir-treated heart transplant recipients with cytomegalovirus pneumonitis. *Transplantation* 52:910–913, 1991.

61. Reed EC, Bowden RA, Dandliker PS, Lilleby KE, Meyers JD: Treatment of cytomegalovirus pneumonia with ganciclovir and intravenous cytomegalovirus immunoglobulin in patients with bone marrow transplants. *Ann Intern Med* 109:783–788, 1988.

62. Schmidt GH, Kovacs A, Zaia JA, et al: Ganciclovir/immunoglobulin combination therapy for the treatment of human cytomegalovirus-associated interstitial pneumonia in bone marrow allograft recipients. *Transplantation* 46:905–907, 1988.

63. Starzl TE, Porter KA, Iwatsuki S, et al: Reversibility of lymphomas and lymphoproliferative lesions developing under cyclosporin-steroid therapy. *Lancet* 1:583–587, 1984.

64. Touraine JL, Bosi E, El Yafi MS, et al: The infectious lymphoproliferative syndrome in transplant recipients under immunosuppressive treatment. *Transplant Proc* 17:96–98, 1985.

65. Armitage JM, Kormos RL, Stuart RS, et al: Post-transplant lymphoproliferative disease in thoracic organ transplant patients: ten years of cyclosporine-based immunosuppression. *J Heart Transplant* 10:877–886, 1991.

66. Hanto D, Frizzer G, Gajl-Peczalska K, Simmons R: Epstein-Barr virus, immunodeficiency, and B cell lymphoproliferation. *Transplantation* 39:461–470, 1985.

67. Hanto DW, Frizzera GF, Gajl-Peczalska KJ, et al: Epstein-Barr virus-induced B-cell lymphoma after renal transplantation. *N Engl J Med* 306:913–918, 1982.

68. Hanto DW, Frizzera G, Gajl-Peczalska KJ, et al: Acyclovir therapy of Epstein-Barr virus-induced post-transplant lymphoproliferative disorders. *Transpl Proc* 17:89–91, 1985.

69. Feldhoff CM, Balfour HH, Simmons RL, et al: Varicella in children with renal transplants. *J Pediatr* 98:25–31, 1981.

70. McGregor RS, Zitelli BJ, Urbach AH, et al: Varicella in pediatric orthotopic liver transplant recipients. *Pediatrics* 83:256–261, 1989.

71. Bensousan T, Garo B, Islam S, et al: Possible transfer of *Pneumocystis carinii* between kidney transplant recipients. *Lancet* 1:1066–1067, 1990.

72. Pifer LL, Hughes WT, Stagno S, Woods D: *Pneumocystis carinii* infection: evidence for high prevalence in normal and immunosuppressed children. *Pediatrics* 61:35–41, 1978.

73. Hughes WT, Rivera GK, Schell MJ, et al: Successful intermittent chemoprophylaxis for *Pneumocystis carinii* pneumonitis. *N Engl J Med* 316:1627–1632, 1987.
74. Ruskin J, Remington JS: Toxoplasmosis in the compromised host. *Ann Intern Med* 84:193–199, 1976.
75. Jacobs F, Depierreux M, Goldman M, et al: Role of bronchoalveolar lavage in diagnosis of disseminated toxoplasmosis. *Rev Infect Dis* 13:637–641, 1991.
76. Mason JC, Ordelheide KS, Grames GM, et al: Toxoplasmosis in two renal transplant recipients from a single donor. *Transplantation* 44:588–591, 1987.
77. Wreghitt TG, Cory-Pearce R, English TAH, Wallwork J: The impact of donor-transmitted CMV and *Toxoplasma gondii* disease in cardiac transplantation. *Transplant Proc* 18:1375–1376, 1986.
78. Hakim M, Esmore D, Wallwork J, et al: Toxoplasmosis in cardiac transplantation. *Br Med J* 292:1108–1109, 1986.
79. Rose AG, Uys CJ, Novitsky D, et al: Toxoplasmosis of donor and recipient hearts after heterotopic cardiac transplantation. *Arch Pathol Lab Med* 107:368–373, 1983.
80. Michaels MG, Kurland G, Fricker FJ, et al: Infectious complications of lung transplantation in children with cystic fibrosis (abstr). *Infectious Disease Society of America*. San Francisco, CA: (A27):23, 1995.
81. Leoung GS, Feigal DW, Montgomery B, et al: Aerosolized pentamidine for prophylaxis against *Pneumocystis carinii* pneumonia. *N Engl J Med* 323:769–775, 1990.
82. Hughes WT, Kennedy W, Dugdale M et al: Prevention of *Pneumocystis carinii* pneumonitis in AIDS patients with weekly dapsone. *Lancet* ii:1066, 1990.
83. Medina I, Mills J, Leoung G, et al: Oral therapy for *Pneumocystis carinii* pneumonia in the acquired immunodeficiency syndrome. *N Engl J Med* 323:776–782, 1990.
84. Mills J, Leoung G, Medina I, et al: Dapsone treatment of *Pneumocystis carinii* pneumonia in acquired immunodeficiency syndrome. *Antimicrob Agents Chemother* 32:1057–1060, 1988.
85. Katz BZ, Rosen C: Aerosolized pentamidine in young children. *Pediatr Infect Dis J* 10:958, 1991.
86. Snydman DR, Werner BG, Heinze-Lacey B, et al: Use of cytomegalovirus immune globulin to prevent cytomegalovirus disease in renal-transplant recipients. *N Engl J Med* 317:1049–1054, 1987.
87. Meyers JD, Reed EC, Shepp DH et al: Acyclovir for prevention of cytomegalovirus infection and disease after allogeneic marrow transplantation. *N Engl J Med* 318:70–75, 1988.
88. Balfour HH, Chace BA, Stapleton JT, et al: A randomized, placebo controlled trial of oral acyclovir for the prevention of cytomegalovirus disease in recipients of renal allografts. *N Engl J Med* 320:1381–1387, 1989.
89. Saliba F, Arulnaden JL, Gugenheim J, et al: CMV hyperimmune globulin prophylaxis after liver transplantation: a prospective randomized controlled study. *Transplant Proc* 21:2260–2262, 1989.
90. Fehir KM, Decker T, Samo T, et al: Immune globulin (GAMMAGARD) prophylaxis of CMV infections in patients undergoing organ transplantation and allogeneic bone marrow transplantation. *Transpantl Proc* 21:3107–3109, 1989.
91. Merrigan T, Renlund D, Keay S, et al: A controlled trial of ganciclovir to prevent cytomegalovirus disease after heart transplantation. *N Engl J Med* 326:1182–1186, 1992.
92. McLaughlin M, Thomas P, Onoratto I, et al: Live virus vaccines in human immunodeficiency virus-infected children: a retrospective survey. *Pediatrics* 82:229–233, 1988.

Chapter 3

Pathology of Heart and Lung Transplantation

Richard N. Eisen, MD

Introduction

Much of what has been learned regarding the pathology of heart and lung transplantation has come from the experience in adults gained over the last two decades. The early but expanding data accumulated from pediatric recipients indicates that the pathology of rejection, infection, and other processes is similar or identical to that in older patients. The purpose of this chapter is to acquaint the reader with the major pathologic changes observed in cardiac and lung transplant recipients, and the techniques and criteria used to determine these processes. Where known, differences between pediatric and adult patients will be highlighted.

Cardiac Transplantation

Perioperative Evaluation

The pathologic evaluation may begin with pretransplant endomyocardial biopsies to establish a clinical diagnosis of cardiomyopathy (including endocardial fibroelastosis) or myocarditis. Subsequently, the native heart is examined to confirm the nature of the patient's underlying disease, usually cardiomyopathy or congenital heart disease of varying types. The predominant specimen sent to the pathologist, of course, is the endomyocardial biopsy beginning at 1 week postoperatively. Increasingly, the biopsy technique is being used in young children and infants with similar low risk as seen in adults.[1,2] A minimum of four to five biopsies should be obtained and placed in room temperature 10% buffered formalin. Twelve-step sections are cut and intermediate levels are stained with hematoxylin and eosin, PAS, and Masson-trichrome.

From: Franco KL (ed). *Pediatric Cardiopulmonary Transplantation.* Armonk, NY: Futura Publishing Company, Inc.; © 1997.

When indicated, additional biopsy fragments may be snap-frozen in liquid nitrogen or isopentane cooled in liquid nitrogen and submitted for immunoperoxidase or immuno-fluorescence studies.[3]

Nonrejection-related changes often seen in biopsies in the first few weeks include ischemic/reperfusion changes, catecholamine effect, and prior biopsy site reaction. The latter occurs in up to 70% of all biopsies.[4] Ischemic injury manifests as focal, small areas of myocyte necrosis that are eventually replaced by small scars. Early changes include shrinkage of myocytes with nuclear pyknosis followed sequentially by cell drop out, sparse mixed inflammatory infiltrate, and fibrosis (Figure 1). Severe or widespread changes often correlate with postoperative cardiac dysfunction, which may be more prominent on the right side in patients with underestimated pulmonary hypertension.[5]

Catecholamine myocardial injury due to inotropic support results in very small zones of damage to a few myocytes with a mixed infiltrate. Biopsy site reaction is perhaps the most easily confused with acute rejection.[3] Cellular granulation tissue underlying fibrin, with disarray of myocytes at the base, is typical of the reaction 1 to 2 weeks after the biopsy, and distinguishes it from rejection (Figure 2). Later, biopsy sites exhibit scarring and persistent myocyte disarray.

Acute Rejection

Although acute rejection most commonly presents in the third or fourth week post-transplant and the majority of episodes occur in the first 3 months,[1] it may be detected in biopsies as early as the first week and years later. The rate of rejection appears equivalent to that in adults[1,4] although this may not be the case in the infant population.[6] Hyperacute rejection is fortunately quite rare and is usually mediated by preformed cir-

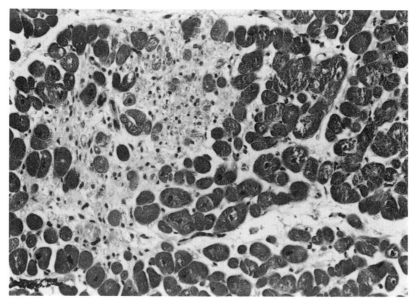

Figure 1. Ischemic reperfusion injury. Microscopic focus of myofiber dropout with healing changes (H & E, × 200).

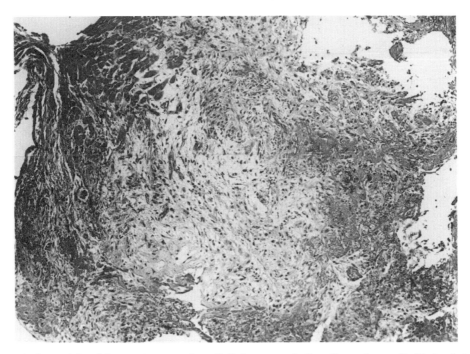

Figure 2. Organizing biopsy site reaction. Cellular granulation tissue beneath fibrin clot (H & E, × 100).

culating antibodies in the recipient serum.[7] Early or immediate graft failure correlates with diffuse hemorrhage, vascular thrombosis, neutrophilic infiltrate, and abundant myocyte necrosis. Immunofluorescence studies often detect immunoglobulin and complement deposition in small vessels. Acute rejection, on the other hand, is a progressive, largely cellular immune-mediated destruction of the graft that begins as a perivenular process. Although various grading schemes have been proposed and utilized by different centers, the ones most widely used are those of Billingham[8] or its minor modifications. In 1990, the International Society for Heart Transplantation (ISHT) proposed a uniform grading scheme, not designed to replace existing ones, but to ensure more uniform data for comparison[9] (Table 1). Grading of rejection is vital to management and treatment, as endomyocardial biopsy has not yet been replaced by other noninvasive techniques such as cytoimmunologic monitoring of peripheral or coronary sinus blood,[10,11] echocardiography,[12] or antimyosin scintigraphy.[13] Generally, moderate or severe (grades IIIA, IIIB, and IV) rejection is treated by augmented immunosuppression.

Mild acute rejection manifests as a patchy perivenular (IA) or sparse diffuse (IB) mononuclear cell infiltrate composed of activated lymphoid cells and macrophages. Myocyte injury or necrosis should be absent (Figure 3). Progression to grade III moderate rejection (in 30% to 50% of cases) is depicted by the appearance of interstitial and increased perivascular infiltrate with myocyte destruction. Helpful clues are lining up of lymphocytes against the myocyte membrane and "aggressive" displacement of myocytes (Figure 4). Grade II or focal moderate rejection has been defined as circumscribed dense mononuclear cell infiltrate associated with myocyte injury. Recent debate has arisen as to the validity of grade II acute rejection (see below). Prominent

Table 1.

Grading of Acute Cardiac Rejection

Billingham			*ISHT[a]*	
I	Mild		IA	(mild, perivascular)
			IB	(mild, diffuse)
II	Moderate		II	(focal moderate)
			IIIA	(diffuse moderate)
			IIIB	(borderline severe)
III	Severe		IV	(severe)
	Resolving		Resolving	

[a]International Society for Heart Transplantation (ISHT), 1990.
(Modified with permission from Reference 9.)

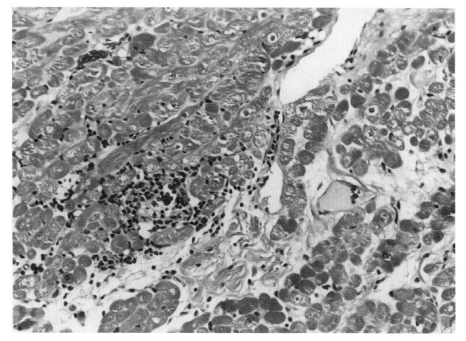

Figure 3. Grade IA (mild) acute rejection. Perivascular lymphoid infiltrate without myocyte injury or necrosis (H & E, × 200).

myocyte necrosis, interstitial hemorrhage, neutrophils and/or eosinophils in the infiltrate and/or vasculitis characterize severe acute rejection (Figure 5). Eosinophils, however, may be seen in varying numbers in otherwise typical lower grades of rejection and may be more prevalent in rejection in very young recipients (Dr. Arthur Hauk, Loma Linda University, personal communication). Although not currently in the ISHT grading scheme, a category of acute vascular rejection has been proposed by Hammond and colleagues at the University of Utah. They have demonstrated vascular rejection by detecting imunoglobulin and/or complement deposition in vessels using immuno-

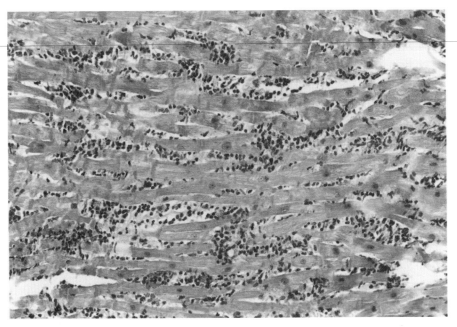

Figure 4. Grade IIIA (moderate) acute rejection. Interstitial infiltrate with multiple foci of myocyte destruction (H & E × 200).

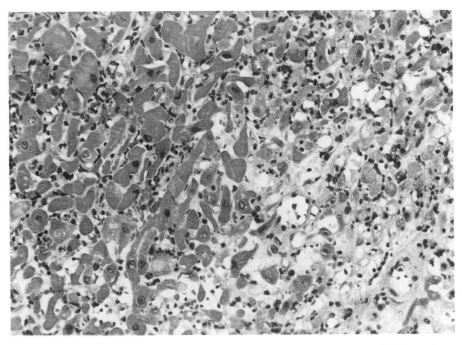

Figure 5. Grade IV (severe) acute rejection. Mixed interstitial infiltrate with large focus of myocyte necrosis (H & E, × 200).

fluorescence staining in up to one fourth of their adult recipients.[14] The process often presents with cardiac dysfunction, despite minimal or subtle perivascular or interstitial cellular infiltrate on biopsy. This phenomenon may be associated with an increased rate of graft loss and poor outcome; however, these preliminary findings need to be confirmed by other centers as well, as in the pediatric recipient.

Post-treatment diminution of cellular infiltrate with early fibrosis comprises the picture of resolving rejection, which may persist in biopsies for a few weeks in cyclosporine-treated patients (Figure 6). Histologically, biopsy site reaction (see *Perioperative Evaluation*) and quilty effect may be misinterpreted as acute rejection. The latter, named after the first patient in whom the process was described, is an endocardial-based, usually dense and focal infiltrate of lymphoid cells. The infiltrate is most often limited to the endocardial surface. When occasionally extending down around or displacing myocytes, or tangentially cut, it may be confused with acute rejection (Figure 7). Quilty effect occurs in approximately 9% of cyclosporine-treated adults and its etiology is still unclear.[3] Some studies have shown that the lesion is composed of T-cells, focal collections of B cells, and macrophages at its base.[15] It may be more exuberant in pediatric patients (Dr. Arthur Hauk, Loma Linda University, personal communication). Recent studies including the behavior of grade II acute rejection on subsequent biopsies[16] and serial sections of such biopsies,[17] indicate that grade II rejection likely represents a form of quilty lesion.

Recent advances in the immunology of rejection, both experimental and clinical, have laid the groundwork for potential aids to its diagnosis and treatment. These include expression of adhesion molecules,[18] cytotoxic T cell proteins,[19,20] and cytokine gene transcripts.[21]

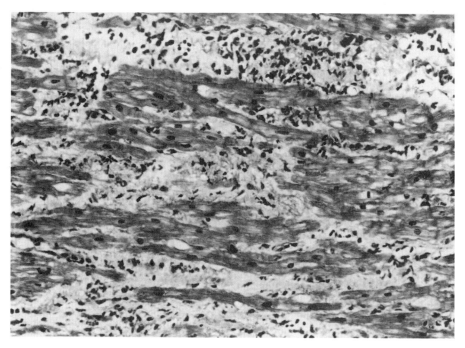

Figure 6. Resolving rejection. Diminished lymphoid infiltrate with early fibrosis. (Trichrome, × 200).

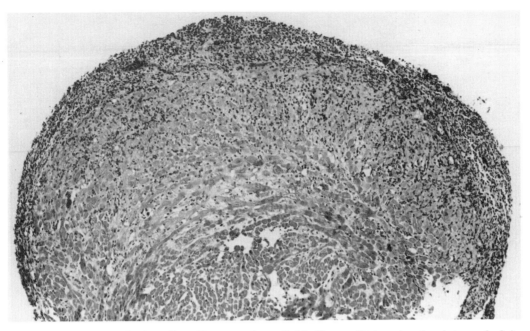

Figure 7. Prominent Quilty effect. Dense endocardial infiltrate. Note extension into underlying myocytes. Remaining myocardium away from surface was free of infiltrate (18-month-old female) (H & E, × 100).

Accelerated Graft Arteriosclerosis (Chronic Rejection)

The major cause of late graft loss and patient death appears to be accelerated graft arteriosclerosis. The vast majority of the data and experience regarding this complication has been gleaned from the adult population, in which approximately 50% have angiographic disease at 5 years. When examined pathologically, the incidence in adults is virtually 100% by 2 years.[22] Its occurrence has now been well documented in the pediatric cardiac recipient,[1,12,23,24] although its incidence appears to be lower than in adults.[1,6,24] The omission of steroids from maintenance regimens may also be beneficial in reducing the incidence.[5,6]

Patients usually present with silent ischemia manifesting as progressive congestive heart failure, arrhythmias, sudden death, or asymptomatic decrease in ejection fraction. Endomyocardial biopsy is exceedingly insensitive in this disease which affects the middle third and distal epicardial, as well as large intramyocardial, coronary arteries. Concentric, obliterative, fibromuscular intimal hyperplasia is observed, not infrequently with an intact internal elastic lamina (Figure 8). Lymphocytic infiltrate is variable, but commonly prominent beneath the endothelial lining, and macrophages are abundant in the deeper portions of the lesion. Frank vasculitis, although unusual, can occur with concomitant moderate to severe cellular rejection in the myocardium.[25]

The pathogenesis of accelerated coronary artery disease (CAD) is still unknown and its risk factors are still being identified.[26-28] However, mounting evidence, including the ability to culture lymphocytes from coronary arteries and endomyocardial biopsies in these patients,[28,29] supports an immunologic etiology. In situ studies of the cellular infiltrate, including T cells and activated endothelial cells, in these lesions further point to a form of chronic cell-mediated rejection.[30,31]

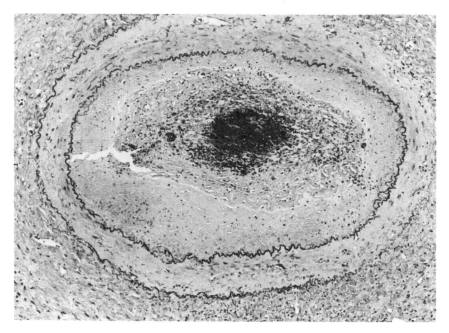

Figure 8. Chronic rejection/accelerated coronary arteriosclerosis. Distal epicardial artery with concentric intimal proliferation and superimposed thrombosis. Note intact internal elastica. (EVG, × 100).

Infection

As with acute rejection, the rate of infection is roughly equivalent to that in adults, approximately 75%.[12,32] However, in some series, the incidence of infection appears to be lower in the pediatric population.[33] Most of these are intrathoracic, and particularly pulmonary in location, and are due to a variety of bacteria. Viral, protozoan, and fungal infections are the most likely to result in pathologic specimens for evaluation which include bronchiolo-alveolar lavage, transbronchial or endoscopic gastric and intestinal biopsies, and others as dictated by the clinical setting. A high degree of suspicion should be born in mind when evaluating biopsies or tissue from these recipients and correlation with serologic data, and culture results are paramount. The time-course post-transplant should also be kept in mind, as most bacterial and fungal infections appear in the first few months and the incidence of viral infection rises thereafter. It would also appear that the pulmonary infection rate is higher in lung allografts than in cardiac-only recipients.[34] Among the viral infections, cytomegalovirus (CMV) is the most common, affecting up to 25% of patients[12] and accounting for 63% of viral infections.[32] Little inflammatory response may be present, so that careful search for typical viral inclusions should be performed (Figure 9). Ancillary techniques to identify CMV include immunoperoxidase staining using antibodies to early antigens,[35] in situ hybridization,[36] and more recently, the polymerase chain reaction.[37] These, and in particular the latter, are highly sensitive and specific techniques, and must be interpreted in light of clinical findings, careful histologic/cytologic evaluation and/or rapid culture technique.[38] Other viral infections include herpes simplex virus (HSV), Epstein-Barr virus (EBV), and respiratory

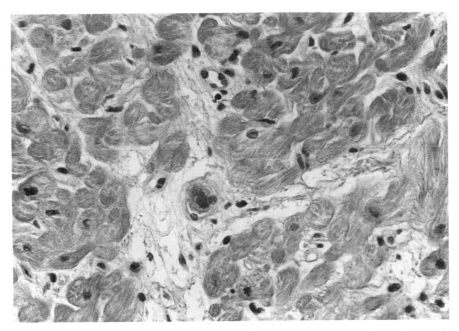

Figure 9. Cytomegalovirus (CMV) infection. Cardiac biopsy: cytomegalic inclusion in an endothelial cell. Note paucity of inflammatory reaction (H & E, × 400).

syncytial virus (RSV). Fortunately, the rate of viral infection in the cardiac allograft itself is relatively low, but may be seen in endomyocardial biopsies.[3,5]

Less common infections include nocardia, fungal (14% of registry patients), protozoan (6%), and others. Most protozoan infections are caused by pneumocystis carinii and Toxoplasma gondii, the latter occasionally causing myocarditis with a focal infiltrate of neutrophils and eosinophils. Cysts may be difficult to find and are often located away from areas of infiltrate.[3] Pneumocystis carinii is easily diagnosed with bronchiolo-alveolar lavage by looking for the characteristic granular eosinophilic exudate containing cysts that stain strongly with silver methenamine (Figure 10). Aspergillus and candida comprise the majority of fungal infections and unfortunately may be diagnosed late with disseminated and/or fatal disease[32,34] (Figure 11).

Other Complications

It has been known since the early days of organ transplantation that adult patients have an increased incidence of neoplasia. The majority appear to be lymphoproliferative disorders followed in incidence by cutaneous and genital tract squamous cell and basal cell carcinomas.[39] Post-transplant lymphoproliferative disorders (PTLD) have a higher incidence in cyclosporine-treated patients versus conventional immunosuppression (28% of all cancers versus 11%).[40] It is not yet known what the incidence of neoplasia will be in the pediatric population. However, PTLDs have been reported in children and may be slightly higher in frequency than in adults.[41] The disease spectrum ranges from severe EBV-like illnesses (particularly weeks post-transplant) to solitary

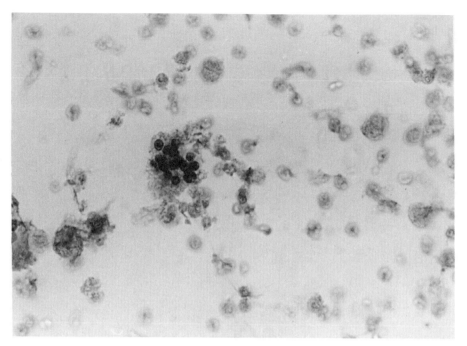

Figure 10. Pneumocystis carinii infection. Bronchiolo-alveolar lavage stained with methenamine silver. Group of silver stained cysts in proteinaceous exudate (× 800).

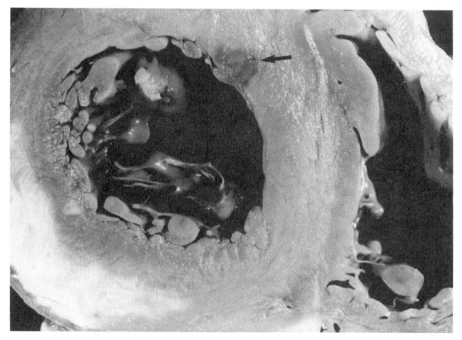

Figure 11. Myocardial aspergillosis: Large intramyocardial fungal abscess secondary to aspergillus endocarditis. Note smaller embolic lesion (**arrow**).

or multiple tumors often extranodal and localized to the lungs or gastrointestinal tract.[42] The tumors may be composed of a polymorphous proliferation of B cells, frequently with immunoblastic and plasmacytoid features (Figure 12), or monomorphous large cell immunoblastic or less commonly small noncleaved cell types.[42] These tumor masses may also exhibit prominent zones of necrosis. Both polyclonal and occasionally monoclonal tumors respond to reduction in immunosuppression with or without conservative surgery. Failure to recognize the disease early may lead to a rapid fatal course due to disseminated disease or secondary infection. The etiology of PTLD, in the vast majority of cases, is primary or reactivation infection with EBV.[41,42] It has been suggested that the repeated use of monoclonal antibodies such as OKT3 may play a role in its development.[44] Fortunately, cardiac allograft involvement is exceedingly rare.[3]

Renal biopsies may be performed in long-term survivors to evaluate declining renal function, and often exhibit tubulointerstitial nephritis and fibrosis.[12] These changes reflect chronic cyclosporine injury to the kidney, although complete loss of function is unusual from cyclosporine alone.

Lung Transplantation

Perioperative Changes

As compared to cardiac replacement, an even greater percentage of what is known about the pathology of lung transplantation comes from the adult experience

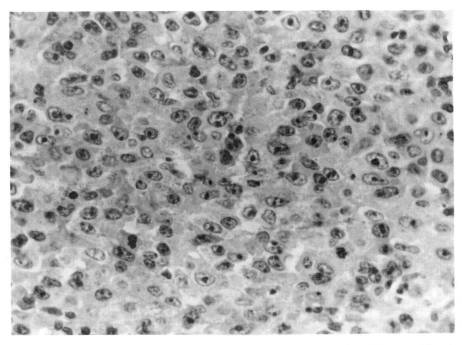

Figure 12. Post-transplant lymphoproliferative disorder. Polymorphous immunoblastic proliferation with plasmacytoid differentiation (H & E, × 200).

in both heart-lung and single lung recipients. Pathologic evaluation begins with examination of native lungs, usually confirming changes related to primary or secondary pulmonary hypertension or cystic fibrosis, the most common pediatric indications for allografting. Early post-transplant, the lungs may exhibit alveolar edema and dilated lymphatics. This correlates with radiographic interstitial infiltrate and edema, and has been termed the implantation response.[45] Severe preservation/reperfusion injury may lead to diffuse alveolar damage and loss of the graft (Figure 13). Other complications include severe perioperative hemorrhage due to adhesions from prior surgery and tracheal or bronchial anastomotic dehiscence or stenosis. These problems have been much reduced by careful patient selection, improved operative techniques, including sequential bilateral lung allografting and judicious use of steroids.

Acute Rejection

In heart-lung allografts, acute cardiac rejection is a relatively minor problem,[45] and very rarely occurs in the absence of pulmonary rejection. Early management of acute rejection was largely based on radiographic and clinical lung function evaluation, but has more recently been aided by the relatively safe use of either protocol or directed transbronchial biopsies.[46] The sensitivity of detection of acute rejection appears to increase with larger biopsies and great sampling, although the exact number of biopsies needed is debated.[47,48] Characteristic histologic changes occur both experimentally and in humans, and form the basis for the current ISHT lung rejection grading scheme (Table 2).[49]

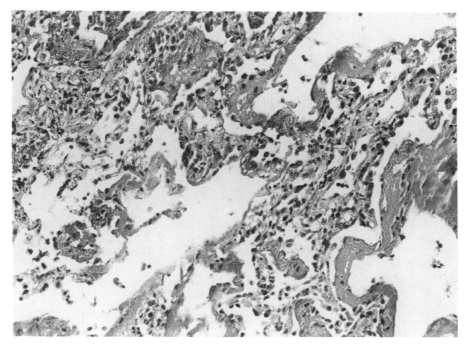

Figure 13. Transbronchial lung allograft biopsy. Diffuse alveolar damage. Edema and mild interstitial infiltrate with hyaline membranes.

Table 2.

Grading of Pulmonary Rejection[a]

	Acute	Chronic
Grade	Description[b]	
I	Minimal, perivascular	Obliterative bronchiolitis, active, subtotal or total
II	Mild, perivascular endothelialitis early interstitial	Obliterative bronchiolitis, inactive, subtotal or total
III	Moderate, II + alveolar septae	
IV	Severe, III + alveolitis neutrophils necrosis vasculitis	

[a]International Society for Heart Transplantation (ISHT), 1991. (Modified with permission from Reference 49.)
[b]Acute rejection may or may not be associated with bronchiolar inflammation.

Acute rejection is at least as, and probably more, frequent in lung recipients than cardiac transplant patients.[50,51]

Rejection begins as in other organs as a perivascular mononuclear infiltrate (minimal, grade I). This pattern has been reported in pulmonary infection, particularly with CMV,[52] although a recent study comparing CMV detection by PCR with perivascular infiltrates has cast further debate on this issue.[53] Acute rejection can be diagnosed with relative certainty when perivascular infiltrate occurs with endothelialitis and interstitial infiltrate (mild, grade II) or grade II changes, plus alveolar septal involvement (moderate, grade III)(Figure 14). Severe or grade IV rejection is present with the addition of alveolitis, neutrophilic infiltrate, vasculitis, necrosis, and/or hemorrhage. Lymphocytic bronchiolitis may or may not be seen, but is more often present with increasing grade of rejection. Eosinophils are often present (more frequently than in the cardiac rejection) and also increase in number with increasing grade.

Diminution in the density of infiltrate and ultimate resolution of normal lung architecture signals resolving and resolved rejection, respectively. Careful search for infection, including routine use of silver stains, should be performed in all transbronchial or open-lung biopsies, particularly in the case of mild rejection. Elastic-von-Gieson stains are quite useful in highlighting perivascular and peribronchiolar infiltrates, and corroborating a diagnosis of acute rejection. Though lavage specimens are useful in diagnosing infection, differential cell counts do not distinguish rejection from infection with needed sensitivity.[54] As with cardiac rejection, immune monitoring has not replaced other diagnostic modalities, though serial cytokine measurements such as serum interleukin-6 (IL-6) levels hold some promise.[55]

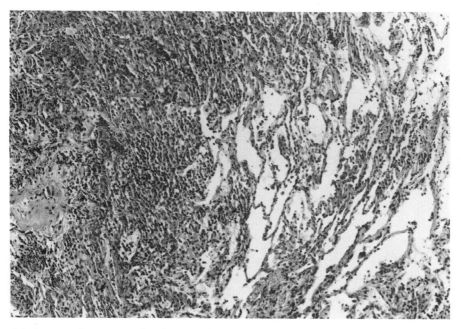

Figure 14. Acute pulmonary rejection, grade II. Dense perivascular infiltrate (**left**) with early interstitial extension (H & E, × 200).

Chronic Rejection/Obliterative Bronchiolitis

The most significant problem in the long-term lung allograft survivor is obliterative bronchiolitis (OB), occurring in 30% to 50% of adult patients.[56] Uniform occurrence had not been reported between centers thus far in pediatric patients,[50,51] although a more recent study in a larger number of recipients suggests near equal incidence to adults.[57] Clinically detected decrease in flow rates and shortness of breath, with or without cough, usually correlate well with histologic changes, although the latter may be seen in asymptomatic patients. Transbronchial biopsy is insensitive in providing a pathologic diagnosis of this condition.[58] Growing evidence indicates that OB is a form of chronic rejection[59,60,61] (immunologically mediated), although other risk factors/mechanisms (CMV, etc.) may play a role.[69]

The disease affects the distal airway, beginning as an active lymphocytic bronchiolitis, followed by epithelial injury/ulceration, lumenal granulation tissue and scarring, with or without obliteration of the lumen (Figure 15). Distal to the obstructed airway, foamy macrophages may accumulate in the alveoli. End-stage disease may result in complete fibrous replacement of the bronchioles and proximal airway dilatation, or bonchiectasis is described.[62,63] Intimal lesions of pulmonary arteries and veins, as seen in accelerated CAD in heart allografts may also be present. Despite the infrequent association with acute cardiac rejection, OB may be correlated with accelerated CAD in heart-lung grafts.[64]

Although not strictly correlated with OB, proximal airway changes include chronic bronchitis with intraepithelial leukocytes and apoptosis, atrophy or replacement of the submucosal glands, and bronchial cartilage changes.[56,65]

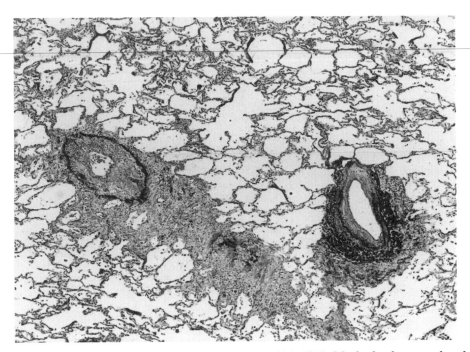

Figure 15. Chronic lung rejection: obliterative bronchiolitis (OB). Marked submucosal and peribronchiolar fibrosis with narrowing of the lumen. Note intimal thickening of pulmonary artery on the **right** (EVG, × 40).

Infection

The spectrum of agents to which pulmonary allograft recipients are prone is similar to that of cardiac patients, although the number of intrapulmonary infections may be higher.[66] Pneumocystis carinii infection is particularly prevalent in the absence of prophylaxis.[50] Diffuse alveolitis in the absence of prominent perivascular infiltrate should be highly suspect for infection, particularly viral.[68] All bronchiolo-alveolar lavage and biopsy specimens should be routinely stained for bacteria, and fungi and viral inclusions should be diligently searched for. Immunohistochemical stains for viral antigens are a useful adjunct for detection and results should be correlated with the clinical and other lab findings, including culture results.

Other Complications

As discussed in the section on cardiac transplantation, specimens containing PTLD and renal biopsies may come to the attention of the pathologist. Data from adult recipients has suggested that the rate of PTLD may be higher in heart-lung recipients than others.[70] As experience grows in the pediatric age group, one may postulate that PTLD may be more of a problem due to the higher rate of primary EBV infection.[41,43]

References

1. Baum D, Bernstein D, Starnes VA, et al: Pediatric heart transplantation at Stanford: results of a 15-year experience. *Pediatrics* 88:203–214, 1991.
2. Backer CL, Zales IF, Harrison HL, et al: Intermediate term results of infant orthotopic cardiac transplantation from two centers. *J Thorac Cardiovasc Surg* 101:826–832, 1991.
3. Billingham ME: Endomyocardial biopsy diagnosis of acute rejection in cardiac allografts. *Prog Cardiovasc Dis* 33:11–18, 1990.
4. Sibley RK, Olivari M-T, Bolman RM, Ring WS: Endomyocardial biopsy in the cardiac allograft recipient: a review of 570 biopsies. *Ann Surg* 203:177–187, 1986.
5. Trento A, Griffith BP, Fricker FJ, Kormos Rl, Armitage J, Hardesty RL: Lessons learned in pediatric heart transplantation. *Ann Thorac Surg* 48:617–623, 1989.
6. Boucek MM, Kanakriyeh MS, Mathis CM, Franklin Trimm R III, Bailey LL, Loma Linda University Pediatric Heart Transplant Group: Cardiac transplantation in infancy: donors and recipients. *J Pediatr* 116:171–176, 1990.
7. Hait DN: The effects of antibodies on organ allograft survival. *Heart Transplant* 2:143, 1983.
8. Billingham ME: Endomyocardiocardial biopsy detection of acute rejection in cardiac allograft recipients. *Heart Vessels* 1:86–90, 1985.
9. Billingham ME, Cary NRB, Hammond ME, et al: A workingformulation for the standardization of nomenclature in the diagnosis of heart and lung rejection: heart rejection study group. *J Heart Lung Transplant* 9:587–592, 1990.
10. Garner RJ, Springgate C, Hoyt T: Immune monitoring of blood in heart transplant recipients: application of flow cytometry. *Sem Diagn Pathol* 6:83–90, 1989.
11. Holzinger C, Zuckermann A, Laczkovics A, et al: Monitoring of mononuclear cell subsets isolated from the coronary sinus and the right atrium in patients after heart allograft transplantation. *J Thorac Cardiovasc Surg* 102:215–223, 1991.
12. Berstein D, Starnes VA, Banm D: Pediatric heart transplantation. *Adv Pediatr* 37:413–439, 1990.
13. Schutz A, Fritsch S, Kugler C, et al: Indium-lll monoclonal antimyosin for diagnosis of cardiac rejection. *Transplant Proc* 22:1464–1465, 1990.
14. Hammond EH, Ensley RD, Yowell RL, et al: Vascular rejection of human cardiac allografts and the role of humoral immunity in chronic allograft rejection. *Transplant Proc* 23:26–30, 1991.
15. Kottke-Marchant K, Ratliff NB: Endomyocardial lymphocytic infiltrates in cardiac transplant recipients. *Arch Pathol Lab Med* 113:690–698, 1989.
16. Milano A, Livi U, Caforio ALP, et al: Behavior of Internal Society for Heart and Lung Transplantation grade 2 cardiac rejection. *Transplant Proc* 26:2724, 1994.
17. Bell G, Lones M, Czer LSC, et al: Grade 2 cellular rejection: does it exist (abstr)? *Mod Pathol* 7:26A, 1994.
18. Griscoe DM, Schoen FS, Rice GE, Bevilaqua MP, Ganz P, Pober JS: Induced expression of endothelial-leukocyte adhesion molecules in human cardiac allografts. *Transplantation* 51:537–539, 1991.
19. Hameed A, Truong LD, Price V, Kruhenbuhl O, Tschopp J: Immunohistochemical localization of granzyme B antigen in cytotoxic cells in human tissues. *Am J Pathol* 138:1069–1075, 1991.
20. Kataska K, Naomoto Y, Snidzaki S, Matsuno T, Sakagami K: Infiltration of perforin-positive mononuclear cells into the rejected kidney allograft. *Transplantation* 53:240–241, 1992.
21. Dallman MJ, Larsen CP, Morris PJ: Cytokine gene transcription in vascularised organ grafts: analysis using semiquantitative polymerase chain reaction. *J Exp Med* 174:493–496, 1991.
22. Johnson DE, Alderman EL, Schroeder JS, et al: Transplant coronary artery disease: histopathologic correlations with angiographic morphology. *J Am Coll Cardiol* 17:449–457, 1991.
23. Pahl E, Fricker FJ, Armitage J, et al: Coronary arteriosclerosis in pediatric heart transplant survivors: limitation of long-term survival. *J Pediatr* 116:177–183, 1990.

24. Berry GJ, Rizeq MN, Weiss LM, Billingham ME: Graft coronary disease in pediatric heart and combined heart-lung transplant recipients: a study of fifteen cases. *J Heart Lung Transplant* 12:S309–319, 1993.

25. Johnson DE, Gao SZ, Schroeder JS, DeCampli WM, Billingham ME: The spectrum of coronary artery pathologic findings in human cardiac allografts. *J Heart Lung Transplant* 8:349–359, 1989.

26. Suciu-foca N, Reed E, Marboe C, et al: The role of anti-HLA antibodies in heart trnasplantation. *Transplantation* 51:716–724, 1991.

27. Grattan MT, Moreno-Cabral CE, Starnes VA, et al: Cytomegalovirus infection is associated with cardiac allograft rejection and atherosclerosis. *JAMA* 261:3561–3566, 1989.

28. Young JB, Lloyd KS, Windsor NT, et al: Elevated soluble interleukin-2 receptor levels early after heart transplantation and long-term survival and development of coronary arteriopathy. *J Heart Lung Transplant* 10:243–250, 1991.

29. Kaufman C, Zeevi A, Zerbe T, et al: In vitro culture of infiltrating lymphocytes from coronary arteries and endomyocardial biopsies: association with graft coronary disease. *Transplant Proc* 23:1142–1143, 1991.

30. Hruban R, Beschorner WE, Baumgartner WA, et al: Accelerated atherosclerosis in heart transplant recipients is associated with a T-lymphocyte mediated enothelialitis. *Am J Pathol* 137:871–882, 1990.

31. Salomon RN, Hughes CCW, Schoen FJ, et al: Human coronary transplant-associated arteriosclerosis; evidence for a chronic immune reaction to activated graft endothelial cells. *Am J Pathol* 138:791–798, 1991.

32. Green M, Wald ER, Fricker FJ, Griffith BP, Trento A: Infections in pediatric orthotopic heart transplant recipients. *Pediatr Infect Dis J* 8:87–93, 1989.

33. Braunlin EA, Canter CE, Olivari MT, Ring WS, Spray TL, Bolman RM III: Rejection and infection after pediatric cardiac transplantation. *Ann Thorac Surg* 49:385–390, 1990.

34. Kurland G, Orenstein DM: Complications of pediatric lung and heart-lung transplantation. *Curr Opin Pediatr* 6:262–271, 1994.

35. Jiwa SM, Raap AK, Van de Rijke FM, et al: Detection of cytomegalovirus antigens and DNA in tissues fixed in formaldehyde. *J Clin Pathol* 42:749–754, 1989.

36. Weiss LMN, Movhed LA, Berry GJ, Billingham ME: In situ hybridization studies for viral nucleic acids in heart and lung allograft biopsies. *Am J Clin Pathol* 93:675–679, 1990.

37. Gerna G, Zipeto D, Parea M, et al: Monitoring of human cytomegalovirus infections and ganciclovir treatment in heart transplant recipients by determination of viremia, antigenemia, and DNAemia. *Infect Dis* 164:488–498, 1991.

38. Kemnitz J, Haverich A, Gubernatis G, Cohnert TR: Rapid identification of viral infections in liver, heart, and kidney allograft biopsies by in situ hybridization. *Am J Surg Pathol* 13:80–82, 1989.

39. Penn I: Cancers following cyclosporine therapy. *Transplant Proc* 19:2211–2213, 1987.

40. Stephanian E, Gruber SA, Dunn DL, Matas AJ: Post-transplant lymphoproliferative disorders. *Transplant Reviews* 5:120–129, 1991.

41. Ho M, Jaffe R, Miller G, et al: The frequency of Epstein-Barr virus infection and associated lymphoproliferative syndrome after transplantation and its manifestations in children. *Transplantation* 45:719–727, 1988.

42. Nalesnik MA, Jaffe R, Starzl TE, et al: The pathology of posttransplant lymphoproliferative disorders occurring in the setting of Cyclosporine A-prednisone immunosuppression. *Am J Pathol* 133:173–192, 1988.

43. Preiksaitis JK, Diaz-Mitoma F, Mirzayans F, Roberts S, Tyrrell DLJ: Quantitative oropharyngeal Epstein-Barr virus shedding in renal and cardiac transplant recipients: relationship to immunosuppressive therapy, serologic responses and the risk of posttransplant lymphoproliferative disorder. *J Infect Dis* 166:986–994, 1992.

44. Swinnen LJ, Costanzo-Nordin MR, Fisher SG, et al: Increased incidence of lymphoproliferative disorder after immunosuppression with the monoclonal antibody OKT3 in cardiac-transplant recipients. *N Engl J Med* 323:1723–1728, 1990.

45. Tazelaar HD, Yousem SA: The pathology of combined heart-lung transplantation: an autopsy study. *Hum Pathol* 19:1403–1416, 1988.

46. Scott JP, Fradet G, Smyth R, et al: Prospective study of transbronchial biopsies in the management of heart-lung and single lung transplant patients. *J Heart Lung Transplant* 10: 626–637, 1991.

47. Scott JP, Higenbottam TW, Smyth RS, et al: Experience with transbronchial biopsies in children after heart-lung transplantation. *Pediatrics* 86:698–702, 1990.

48. Kurland G, Noyes BE, Jaffe R, Atlas AB, Armitage J, Orenstein DO: Bronchoalveolar lavage and transbronchial biopsy in children following heart-lung and lung transplantation. *Chest* 104:1043–1048, 1993.

49. Yousem SA, Berry GJ, Brunt EM, et al: A working formulation for the standardization of nomenclature in the diagnosis of heart and lung rejection: lung rejection study group. *J Heart Lung Transplant* 9:593–601, 1990.

50. Starnes VA, Marshall SE, Lewiston NJ, Theodore J, Stinson EB, Shumway NE: Heart-lung transplantation in infants, children, and adolescents. *J Pediatr Surg* 26:434–438, 1991.

51. Smyth RL, Scott JP, Whitehead B, et al: Heart-lung transplantation in children. *Transplant Proc* 22:1470–1471, 1990.

52. Tazelaar HD: Perivascular inflammation in pulmonary infections: implications for the diagnosis of pulmonary rejection. *J Heart Lung Transplant* 10:437–441, 1991.

53. Flint A, Frank TS: Cytomegalovirus detection in lung transplant biopsy samples by PCR. *J Heart Lung Transplant* 13:38–42, 1994.

54. Clelland C, Higenbottam T, Stewart S, et al: Bronchoalveolar lavage and transbronchial lung biopsy during acute rejection and infection in heart-lung transplant patients. *Am Rev Respir Dis* 147:1386–1392, 1993.

55. Yoshida Y, Iwaki Y, Pham S, et al: Benefits of posttransplantation monitoring of interleukin 6 in lung transplantation. *Ann Thorac Surg* 55:89–93, 1993.

56. Yousem SA, Paradis IL, Pauber JA, et al: Large airway inflammation in heart-lung transplant recipients—its significance and prognostic implications. *Transplantation* 43:654–656, 1990.

57. Whitehead B, Rees P, Sorensen K, et al: Incidence of obliterative bronchiolitis after heart-lung transplantation in children. *J Heart Lung Transplant* 13:903–908, 1994.

58. Kramer MR, Stoehr C, Whang JL, et al: The diagnosis of obliterative bronchiolitis after heart-lung and lung transplantation: low yield of transbronchial biopsy. *J Heart Lung Transplant* 12:675–681, 1993.

59. Taylor PM, Rose ML, Yacoub MH: Expression of MHC antigens in normal human lungs and transplanted lungs with obliterative bronchiolitis. *Transplantation* 48:506–510, 1989.

60. Holland VA, Cagle PT, Windsor NT, Noon GP, Greenberg SD, Lawrence EC: Lymphocyte subset populations in bronchiolitis obliterans after heart-lung transplantation. *Transplantation* 50:955–959, 1990.

61. Hertz MI, Henke CA, Nakhleh RE, et al: Obliterative bronchiolitis after lung transplanation: a fibroproliferative disorder associated with platelet derived growth factor. *Proc Natl Acad Sci USA* 89:10385-10389, 1992.

62. Yousem SA: Heart-lung transplantation. In: Abramowsky CR, Colvin RB (eds). *Organ Transplant in Children. Perspect Pediatr Pathol* Easel, Karger; 13:82–104, 1989.

63. Novick RJ, Ahmad D, Menkis AH, et al: The importance of aquired diffuse bronchomalacia in heart-lung transplant recipients with obliterative bronchiolitis. *J Thorac Cardiovasc Surg* 101:643–648, 1991.

64. Kawai A, Paradis IL, Keenan RJ, et al: Chronic rejection in heart-lung transplant recipients: the relationship between obliterative bronchiolitis and coronary artery disease. *Transplant Proc* 27:1288–1289, 1995.

65. Yousem SA, Dauber JH, Griffith BP: Bronchial cartilage alterations in lung transplantation. *Chest* 98:1121–1124, 1990.

66. Brooks RG, Hofflin JM, Jamieson SW, Stinson EB, Remington JS: Infectious complications in heart-lung transplant recipients. *Am J Med* 79:412–422, 1985.

67. Gryzan S, Paradis IL, Zeevi A, et al: Unexpectedly high incidence of pneumocytis carinii infection after lung-heart transplantation. *Am Rev Respir Dis* 137:1268–1274, 1988.

68. Stewart S, Higenbottam TW, Hutter JA, Penketh ARL, Zebro TJ, Wallwork J: Histopathology of transbronchial biopsies in heart-lung transplantation. *Transplant Proc* 20:764–766, 1988.

69. Abernathy EC, Hruban RH, Baumgartner WA, Reitz B, Hutchins GM: The two forms of bronchiolitis obliterans in heart-lung transplant recipients. *Hum Pathol* 22:1102–1110, 1991.

70. Randhawa PS, Yousem SA, Paradis IL, Dauber JA, Griffith BP, Locker J: The clinical spectrum, pathology, and clonal analysis of Epstein-Barr virus-associated lymphoproliferative disorders in heart-lung transplant recipients. *Am J Clin Pathol* 92:177–185, 1989.

Chapter 4

Mechanical Assistance for Cardiopulmonary Failure

D. Glenn Pennington, MD
Marc T. Swartz

Introduction

For decades, clinicians have sought a reliable mechanical device to partially or totally support cardiac and/or pulmonary function. During the decade of the 1980s, dramatic improvements in patient selection and postoperative management of adults and children undergoing advanced mechanical circulatory support led to wider clinical application.[1-12] Unfortunately, technological advances have been targeted largely at the adult population. Intra-aortic balloon pumps are available for children and infants, but their efficacy in this patient population is questionable, therefore limiting their use.[7,13-16] Concurrent with these improvements in mechanical circulatory support, cardiopulmonary transplantation in children also gained clinical acceptance.[17-23] The merger of these two technologies has led to a small experience of supporting infants and children as a bridge to cardiopulmonary transplantation, for graft failure in the immediate postoperative period, or for late severe rejection. Devices are currently available to support the cardiac and/or pulmonary function of infants and children for periods of several weeks. More advanced cardiac assist devices have been used in some adolescents for longer intervals. Since the current pediatric devices can provide support for only a few weeks, their most appropriate application may be for situations in which myocardial recovery is expected. Due to the long periods of time necessary to locate donor organs, present technology makes bridging to transplantation in children less feasible than in adults.

The ability to mechanically support the circulation was first demonstrated clinically in the early 1950s with the development of cardiopulmonary bypass.[24] Several of the early attempts at prolonged cardiopulmonary support involved children. In 1963, Spencer et al supported a 6-year-old girl in whom severe cardiac failure developed secondary to pulmonary hypertension after repair of a ventricular septal defect.[25] She was

From: Franco KL (ed). *Pediatric Cardiopulmonary Transplantation*. Armonk, NY: Futura Publishing Company, Inc.; © 1997.

successfully supported with venoarterial bypass for approximately 24 hours, but unfortunately died of arrhythmias. In 1967, DeBakey supported a 16-year-old girl with a left atrial-axillary ventricular assist device (VAD) for severe cardiac failure following mitral valve replacement.[26] The device performed well and she was a long-term survivor. The use of portable cardiopulmonary bypass or extracorporeal membrane oxygenation (ECMO) in children with severe cardiopulmonary failure was introduced in the 1970s.[27] Although early results of cardiac support were disappointing, these techniques were attempted again in the early 1980s with modest success. This activity rapidly expanded and is presently considered conventional therapy for children with refractory cardiorespiratory failure.[2-7,9-12] VADs have been occasionally employed in children over the last decade, but there has been renewed interest in their use. Although the sophisticated pulsatile devices are not available for infants and small children, centrifugal pumps have been used effectively.[8]

This chapter reviews the mechanical cardiac and cardiopulmonary support systems currently available for children, and summarizes the clinical results in patients younger than 18 years of age who have undergone mechanical support in conjunction with either heart, heart-lung, or lung transplantation. Some of the data contained in this chapter were obtained from the Registry for Mechanical Assist Devices and Total Artificial Hearts sponsored by the American Society for Artificial Internal Organs (ASAIO), and the International Society of Heart and Lung Transplantation (ISHLT), reports from the Extracorporeal Life Support Organization (ELSO), as well as a literature review.

Devices and Methods

Extracorporeal Membrane Oxygenation

Portable cardiopulmonary bypass or ECMO has been used for cardiorespiratory support in infants and children since it was first described by Bartlett et al (Figure 1).[27] ECMO is currently the most widely used technique of advanced mechanical circulatory support in children. This is due mainly to its availability, but there are other advantages, including its effectiveness for combined cardiac and pulmonary problems, and the fact that many children's hospitals have well-trained personnel to carry it out. Ultrafiltration or dialysis can be performed via the ECMO circuit for patients who are volume overloaded or have renal complications. However, the disadvantages of ECMO include the need for systemic heparinization, limited mobility of the patient who in most cases would be sedated and bed-bound, and the necessity to closely monitor the system with specially trained nursing and perfusion personnel.

Venoarterial ECMO is the most popular technique, because it provides the greatest degree of cardiac as well as respiratory support. There are multiple options for cannulation with venoarterial ECMO that include jugular vein to carotid artery, right atrium to aorta, and femoral vein to femoral artery. All three cannulation techniques provide adequate support, and the type of cannulation utilized often depends upon the patient's clinical situation. For example, patients who are being bridged to heart or lung transplantation may be best served by either jugular vein to carotid, or femoral vein to femoral artery cannulation, leaving the chest unopened until the transplant is performed. Patients who undergo surgical correction of congenital lesions and are unable

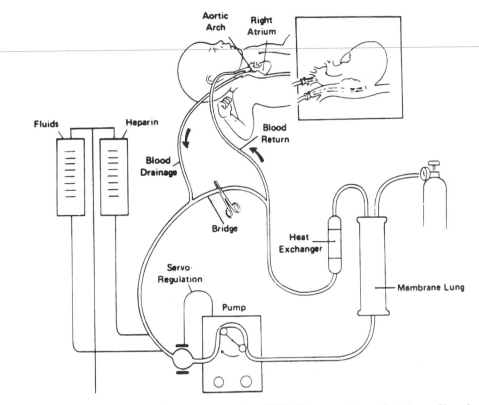

Figure 1. Extracorporeal membrane oxygenation (ECMO) set-up for pediatric cardiopulmonary failure. (Reproduced with permission from Bartlett RA, et al: ECMO for neonatal respiratory failure. *Surgery* 92:425–433, 1982.)

to be weaned from cardiopulmonary bypass may be candidates for cardiac transplantation. If these patients are to be supported with ECMO, right atrial to aortic cannulation may be preferred since the chest has already been opened.

The effects of ECMO on an ischemic, failing myocardium are not yet fully understood. However, it is clear that ECMO significantly decreases right heart preload, resulting in a dramatic decrease in pulmonary blood flow and pulmonary artery pressure. Left heart preload is also reduced, however, some patients continue to maintain high left atrial and left ventricular end-diastolic pressures due to the left ventricle's inability to eject against the ECMO-induced increased afterload.[7] This increased afterload is a result of oxygenated blood being returned from the ECMO circuit into the aorta.[28,29] Despite the apparent adverse effects of ECMO on the left ventricle, many postcardiotomy patients with stunned hearts have recovered normal ventricular function while being supported with ECMO. In the bridge to transplant patient population, myocardial recovery is not a major concern. Therefore, the level of perfusion and oxygenation provided by ECMO is usually adequate to support a patient until transplantation can be accomplished. Unfortunately, some patients are rejected for transplantation on the basis of ECMO-related complications, including bleeding, infection, or thromboemboli. More often, major organ dysfunction that developed prior to the initiation of ECMO, such as renal, hepatic, or neurologic failure is the primary reason for exclusion.

Venovenous ECMO can be accomplished by cannulating the jugular and femoral veins, or placing a double lumen catheter through the jugular vein and positioning it in the right atrium. Venovenous ECMO provides oxygenation to the venous blood, often resulting in a decrease in pulmonary vascular resistance. For venovenous ECMO to be effective, cardiac function must be normal. Since venovenous ECMO does not provide any cardiac support, it is often considered to be less effective than venoarterial. In addition, some patients with respiratory failure who are treated with venovenous ECMO need to be switched to venoarterial ECMO due to hemodynamic deterioration or continued hypoxemia.

Ventricular Assist Devices and Total Artificial Hearts

The use of these devices has been limited in the pediatric population due to the lack of sophisticated systems designed especially for children. VADs have been available in a limited way for children since the late 1970s. The development of the smaller Biomedicus Medtronic centrifugal pumps in the mid-1980s provided a method of temporary VAD support for infants and children (Figure 2). The major limitation of centrifugal devices is their lack of ability to support patients for the long durations necessary to locate a donor organ. A few older children have been supported with some of the more sophisticated devices such as the Thoratec (Thoratec Laboratories, Inc., Berkeley, CA), Novacor (Novacor Division-Baxter Healthcare Corporation, Oakland,

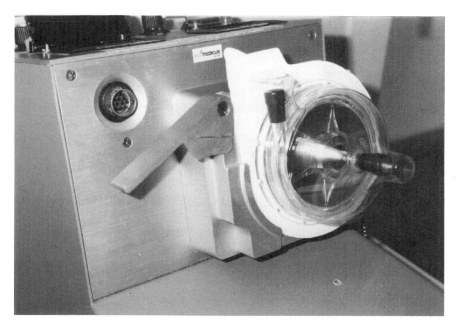

Figure 2. Medtronic Biomedicus centrifugal pump with pediatric head used in children for temporary ventricular assistance.

CA), Thermo Cardiosystems (Thermo Cardiosystems, Inc., Woburn, MA), and Abiomed (Abiomed, Inc., Danvers, MA) VADs (Figure 3), or the Symbion-Jarvik (Symbion, Inc., Tempe, AZ) total artificial heart (TAH). However, for the most part, these have been children older than 12 years.[30-34] For infants and children less than one square meter of body surface area, there are presently no sophisticated cardiac support devices available in the United States.

Centrifugal and pulsatile devices require a sternotomy for insertion. Devices which can utilize atrial cannulation (centrifugal, roller, Thoratec, and Abiomed) can be inserted without cardiopulmonary bypass in stable patients, while systems requiring left ventricular cannulation (Novacor, Thermocardiosystems) and TAHs must be placed during cardiopulmonary bypass.

External centrifugal and roller pumps are commercially available and do not require special approval by the United States Government. These devices are readily available, relatively inexpensive, and have been used extensively in adults. Roller pumps and centrifugal pumps have both been used extensively in ECMO circuits. These devices are positioned extracorporeally and attached to cannulae that may be

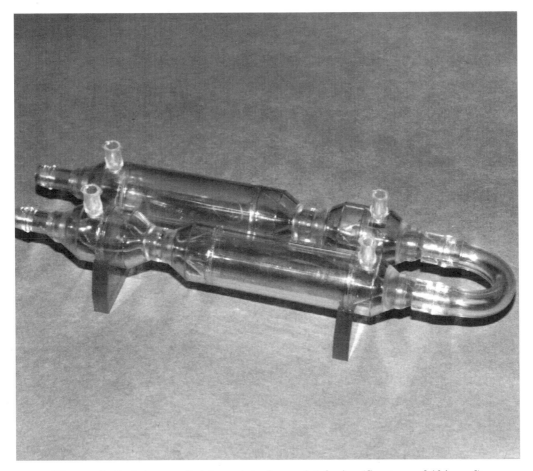

Figure 3. Prototype pediatric ventricular assist device (Courtesy of Abiomed).

placed in any of the cardiac chambers to provide the desired type of support. Furthermore, insertion of these devices does not require complicated techniques, and in many cases does not require cardiopulmonary bypass. Due to the size, weight, and extracorporeal nature of these devices, the patient's mobility is limited. The patients are usually confined to bed or to getting up in a chair. Because of the limitation of mobility and the requirement for continuous intravenous heparin, the results with these devices are best if the duration of support is less than 2 weeks.

External pulsatile assist devices are now being used worldwide. The Pierce-Donachy VAD developed at Pennsylvania State University and manufactured by Thoratec Medical Corporation has been used in more than 378 patients. However, only a small percentage of these patients have been younger than 18 years of age. The Thoratec cannulae are generally too large to place in an individual with a body surface area of less than one square meter. This device is positioned paracorporeally on the upper portion of the abdominal wall and, therefore, allows for considerable patient mobility. It can be used to support the right, left, or both sides of the heart, and atrial or left ventricular cannulation is available. This device uses compressed air to eject blood from an ultrasmooth polyurethane sac and contains Bjork-Shiley Monostrut valves. While it has good blood-contacting characteristics, anticoagulation is advised if support is continued for more than a few days.

The Abiomed (BVS 5000) is different in configuration to the Thoratec VAD. It is located extracorporeally and, like centrifugal and roller pumps, it impairs patient mobility. It utilizes atrial cannulae and can provide right, left, or biventricular support. The Abiomed BVS 5000 fills by gravity and provides pulsatile flow by utilizing polyurethane valves.

Implantable left ventricular assist systems are currently being used as bridges to transplantation. Several manufacturers are also developing permanent implantable systems. The two devices currently used clinically, the Novacor left VAD and the Thermocardiosystems left VAD are both implanted in the abdomen. Due to the size and nature of these devices, it is unlikely that many patients younger than 18 years of age would have sufficient body mass to house this device. These devices provide only left ventricular support. The energy source for the Novacor left ventricular assist system is electricity, while the Thermocardiosystems device has two models, one which is powered by electricity and one which uses compressed air. Both the Novacor and the Thermocardiosystems devices utilize bioprosthetic valves. The Novacor device has an ultrasmooth polyurethane blood sac, while the Thermocardiosystem's device has a textured blood sac which promotes development of a pseudointimal layer within the pump to reduce the risk of thromboembolism.

Between 1985 and 1990, several pneumatic TAHs (biventricular replacement devices) were available throughout the world. The most publicized and the most commonly used of these devices was the Symbion Jarvik 7, which was used in more than 180 cases of bridging to transplantation worldwide. This system is not currently available as the Symbion device, but is being reintroduced as the Cardiowest (Cardiowest Corporation, Tucson, AZ) TAH. With these devices, two compressed air drivelines exit the upper abdomen so the patient is relatively mobile. One of the primary concerns with TAHs is size. Earlier designs were severely compromised by nonanatomic fit. The Jarvik 7 solved some of these problems, and by introducing a 70-cc version of this device, even smaller patients could be supported. It is unlikely that a patient with a body surface area of less than 1.2 m² would be able to have·a 70 cc TAH implanted, and allow for proper closure of the sternum. Therefore, infants, small children, and even some adolescents would not be candidates for this device.

Clinical Results

Bridge to Cardiac Transplantation

The results in 11 patients who were bridged to cardiac transplantation with ECMO are outlined in Table 1. The mean age of these 11 patients was 8.7 years, with only three patients being less than 1 year of age. Duration of ECMO ranged from 0.7 to 15.4 days, with a mean of 4.6 days. Seven patients (64%) were transplanted and three (27%) patients survived.

In Table 2, the results of 30 patients bridged to cardiac transplantation with VADs or TAHs are presented. Of the 30 patients, 21 (70%) were transplanted and 13 (43%) survived. The best results were in patients who received pneumatic biventricular assist devices (100% survival).

In Table 3, the complications encountered in these 30 VAD and TAH patients are listed. Major complications were common in both survivors and nonsurvivors. However, there was no statistically significant difference in the incidence of bleeding, renal failure, infection, or respiratory failure in survivors when compared to nonsurvivors.

ECMO for Post-Transplant Support

The results in 28 patients who were supported with ECMO after cardiac transplantation for acute rejection or ischemic graft failure are presented in Table 4. The ages

Table 1.

Results of Bridging to Cardiac Transplantation with ECMO

Pt#	Age	Duration of ECMO (Days)	Transplanted	Survived
1	5 years	2.4	Yes	No
2	8 months	5.6	Yes	Yes
3	6 months	0.7	Yes	No
4	13 years	1.3	Yes	Yes
5	14 years	3.0	Yes	No
6	15 years	2.9	No	No
7	18 years	1.5	No	No
8	6 years	8.2	No	No
9	18 years	15.4	No	No
10	5.1 years	7.6	Yes	Yes
11	6 months	1.5	Yes	No
		0.7 − 15.4 (mean 4.6)	7(64%)	3(27%)

ECMO = extracorporeal membrane oxygenation

Table 2.

Results of Bridging to Transplantation with Ventricular Assist Devices and Total Artificial Hearts*

Device	# of Patients	# Transplanted	# Survived
1) RVAD			
Centrifugal	5	3	1
Pneumatic	0	0	0
2) LVAD			
Centrifugal	2	1	0
Pneumatic	6	3	0
3) LVAS	2	1	1
4) BVAD			
Centrifugal	4	4	2
Pneumatic	5	5	5
5) TAH	6	4	4
Total	30	21	13

*American Society for Artificial Internal Organ=International Society for Heart and Lung Transplantation Registry. RVAD=right ventricular assist device; LVAD=left ventricular assist device; LVAS=left ventricular assist system; BVAD=biventricular assist device; TAH = Total artificial heart.

Table 3.

Complications of Bridging to Transplantation with Ventricular Assist Devices and Total Artificial Hearts*

Complication	% Survivors (n=13)	% Nonsurvivors (n=17)	p value**
Bleeding	46	62	NS
Renal failure	31	54	NS
Infection	15	31	NS
Respiratory failure	23	38	NS

*American Society for Artificial Internal Organs -International Society for Heart and Lung Transplantations Registry
** chi square analysis
NS=not significant

of these 28 patients ranged from 7 days to 17 years, with at least 10 patients being less than 1 year of age. At least 14 patients were switched from routine cardiopulmonary bypass to an ECMO circuit in the operating room at the time of transplantation. All of the remaining patients were placed on ECMO within 30 hours of cardiac transplantation. The duration of ECMO ranged from 0.25 to 10.5 days (mean 3.8 days). One patient was retransplanted and died, and 14 (50%) survived.

ECMO for Late Cardiac Rejection

In Table 5, the results are presented of 10 patients who were supported with ECMO for cardiac rejection after their initial transplant hospitalization. The ages

Table 4

ECMO for Immediate Post-Transplant Support

Pt#	Age	Transplant to ECMO (Hours)	Duration of ECMO (Days)	Retransplanted	Survived
1	3.5 years	12	5	No	No
2	10 years	24	1	No	Yes
3	7 years	OR	2	No	No
4	2 years	OR	1.1	No	No
5	7 days	OR	8	No	No
6	1.2 years	12	3.8	No	Yes
7	1.5 years	20	0.25	No	No
8	26 days	12	2.3	No	No
9	3 months	16	3.25	No	Yes
10	7 months	8	2.6	No	Yes
11	6 months	NA	2.7	No	No
12	17 years	NA	4.7	No	No
13	7 months	30	2.7	No	Yes
14	6 months	NA	1.5	No	No
15	7 days	OR	6.9	No	No
16	16 months	OR	9	Yes	No
17	16 months	12	2	No	Yes
18	37 months	OR	10.5	No	No
19	19 days	OR	0.5	No	No
20	34 months	OR	10.1	No	Yes
21	2 months	OR	1.5	No	Yes
22	NA	NA	NA	No	Yes
23	NA	OR	NA	No	Yes
24	NA	OR	NA	No	No
25	NA	OR	NA	No	Yes
26	NA	OR	NA	No	Yes
27	NA	OR	NA	No	Yes
28	NA	NA	NA	No	Yes
			0.25 − 10.5 (mean 3.8)	1 (3.6%)	14 (50%)

OR = operating room; NA = not available; ECMO = extracorporeal membrane oxygenation.

Table 5.

ECMO for Late Cardiac Rejection

Pt#	Age	Duration of ECMO (Days)	Re-Transplanted	Survived
1	12 years	3.3	No	Yes
2	10 months	5	Yes	Yes
3	3 years	3	No	Yes
4	7 months	2	No	No
5	1.5 months	0.9	No	No
6	17 months	4.7	No	No
7	3 months	2.9	No	Yes
8	3 years	3	No	Yes
9	17 years	4.9	No	No
10	2 months	4.1	No	Yes
		0.9 − 5 (mean 3.0)	1 (10%)	6 (60%)

ECMO = extracorporeal membrane oxygenation

ranged from 2 months to 17 years. Duration of ECMO ranged from 0.9 to 5 days (mean 3.0 days). One patient was retransplanted and survived, and five additional patients were weaned and survived.

Discussion

From the preceding data, it is apparent that ECMO is the most commonly used method of circulatory support in the pediatric cardiac transplant population. The popularity of ECMO is due in part to its availability and the familiarity in most pediatric transplant centers with this technique. It is effective in the neonatal period, as well as in older children and adolescents. However, in bridging to cardiac transplantation, ECMO has not been as effective in children as VADs and TAHs have been in adults. From the sparse data available in this review, the success rate of bridging with ECMO in children has been poor. Although 64% were transplanted, only 43% of those transplanted survived. In the adult population, several large series of patients bridged with VADs have reported survival rates among those transplanted in the 80% to 90% range.[30-32] The poor results in children are in large part related to the long periods necessary for donor hearts to become available, and the inadequacy of ECMO to provide long-term support. While ECMO may be effective for a period of days, or 1 to 2 weeks, bridging to transplant often requires effective support for several weeks or months. Furthermore, the waiting period should be used as a period of rehabilitation during which patients with chronic cardiac failure can gain strength, improve their nutrition, and undergo reversal of organ dysfunction, so that by the time they are transplanted they are much better candidates. Such rehabilitation is unlikely to occur with ECMO, because the system does not allow for the mobility and strenuous exercise which can be achieved with VADs or TAHs. More sophisticated devices are needed to support children for extended periods prior to transplantation. The Berlin heart has been used successfully in children and the Japanese experience with pneumatic VADs includes several children who were successfully supported with assist devices.[7] Some preliminary work is under way to design an artificial heart for children.[35] However, clinical trials are not anticipated within the next few years.

From these data, the use of ECMO for immediate post-transplant cardiac failure produced a 50% survival rate. The precise etiology of the post-transplant cardiac failure was not known in most instances. However, it was known that many of the patients required ECMO in the operating room at the time of transplantation, and that some of them were transferred directly from cardiopulmonary bypass to ECMO. That suggests that primary graft failure was the most common problem. The salvage rate of 50% is quite remarkable, considering that these were immunosuppressed patients having just undergone an extensive cardiac operation with cardiopulmonary bypass. The survival rate of 50% is somewhat better than that of postcardiotomy ECMO for the other congenital heart defects.[2-6] While infection undoubtedly occurred in a significant number of patients, it did not preclude survival in most of them. It is also important to note that of the 28 patients supported during the acute period, only one was retransplanted and that patient did not survive. These data emphasize the importance of myocardial recovery in these patients and the unlikelihood of repeat transplantation. In fact, it is not clear that retransplantation should be considered an option in these patients, since their outcome would be anticipated to be poor, even if a donor heart could be obtained.

The best results with advanced mechanical circulatory support associated with cardiac transplantation were in children with late cardiac rejection who were supported with ECMO. Of the 10 patients supported, 6 were long-term survivors, one of whom was successfully retransplanted. These results are also unusual in that there are no published comparable series in adults. While the results of retransplantation in adults have been better in patients with chronic rejection, the need for mechanical circulatory support was a significant mortality risk factor.

As with adults, it is clear that cardiac transplantation cannot provide enough donor hearts to satisfy the need for cardiac support and/or replacement in the younger population. Therefore, work must progress toward the development of more sophisticated temporary and permanent devices for infants and children.

The experience with bridging to lung transplantation in children is very limited with only one case reported in the literature,[9] although there have been several cases reported of adults bridged to lung transplantation with ECMO systems.[36] However, many lung transplant centers consider transplantation in acutely ill patients to be unwise. It seems clear that patients who suffer severe, acute pulmonary deterioration requiring ECMO support, prior to lung transplantation, are at a significantly higher mortality risk than more stable patients.[37] ECMO has been used in several centers for post-transplant lung failure. The early experience with lung transplantation in Toronto included a patient with paraquat poisoning who was treated with ECMO.[38]

At present, there is not a suitable intraoperative method to determine the degree or potential reversibility of myocardial or pulmonary dysfunction. Therefore, we believe that virtually every patient should be offered some method of mechanical cardiopulmonary support after transplantation. Currently, ECMO seems to be the best device available. Intra-aortic balloon pumps may be helpful in some cardiac transplant patients with predominant left heart failure, however, this would be an extremely small population. Scaled down versions of pulsatile pneumatic ventricular assist devices and intravascular oxygenators seem to hold the most promise. Until such devices are available, ECMO will remain the primary method of cardiopulmonary support in children. As techniques are perfected and better devices become available, survival rates for children requiring temporary support should improve. At the same time, we must work toward the development of more sophisticated permanent devices for infants and children since transplantation cannot provide enough donor organs to satisfy the current needs.

References

1. Pennington DG, Swartz MT: Assisted circulation and the mechanical heart. In: Braunwald E (ed). *Heart Disease. A Textbook of Cardiovascular Medicine.* 4th Ed. Philadelphia: WB Saunders, Co.; 535–550, 1992.
2. Raithel SC, Pennington DG, Boegner E, Fiore A, Weber TR: Extracorporeal membrane oxygenation in children after cardiac surgery. *Circulation* 86(suppl II):II-305-II-310, 1992.
3. Andersen HL, Attorri RJ, Custer JR, Chapman RA, Bartlett RH: Extracorporeal membrane oxygenation for pediatric cardiopulmonary failure. *J Thorac Cardiovasc Surg* 99:1011–1021, 1990.
4. Klein MD, Shaheen KW, Whittlesey GC, Pinsky WW, Arcinegas E: Extracorporeal membrane oxygenation for the circulatory support of children after repair of congenital heart disease. *J Thorac Cardiovasc Surg* 100:498–505, 1990.
5. Rogers AJ, Trento A, Siewers RD, et al: Extracorporeal membrane oxygenation for postcardiotomy shock in children. *Ann Thorac Surg* 47:903–906, 1989.
6. Weinhaus L, Carter C, Noetzel M, McAlister W, Spray TL: Extracorporeal membrane oxygenation for circulatory support after repair of congenital heart defects. *Ann Thorac Surg* 48:206–212, 1989.
7. Pennington DG, Swartz MT: Circulatory support in children. In: Mavroudis C (ed). *Innovations in Congenital Heart Surgery. State of the Art Reviews; Cardiac Surgery.* Philadelphia: Hanley and Belfus; 381–391, 1989.
8. Karl TR, Sano S, Horton S, Mee RBB: Centrifugal pump left heart assist in pediatric cardiac operations, indications, technique and results. *J Thorac Cardiovasc Surg* 102:624–630, 1991.
9. Hunkeler MN, Canter CE, Donle A, Spray TL: Extracorporeal life support in cyanotic congenital heart disease before cardiovascular operation. *Am J Cardiol* 69:790–793, 1992.
10. Galantowicz ME, Stolar CJH: Extracorporeal membrane oxygenation for perioperative support in pediatric heart transplantation. *J Thorac Cardiovasc Surg* 102:148–152, 1991.
11. Custer JR, Bartlett RH: Recent research in extracorporeal life support for respiratory failure. *ASAIO J* 38:754–771, 1991.
12. Zwischenberger JB, Cox CS: ECMO in the management of cardiac failure. *ASAIO J* 38:751–753, 1992.
13. Veasy LG, Webster HW, Boncek MM, et al: Pediatric use of intra-aortic balloon pumping. In: Doyle EF, Engle MA, Gersony WM, et al (eds). *Pediatric Cardiology.* New York: Springer-Verlag; 600–602, 1986.
14. Pollack JC, Charlton MC, Williams WG, Edmonds JF, Trusler GA: Intra-aortic balloon pumping in children. *Ann Thorac Surg* 29:522–528, 1980.
15. Del Nido PJ, Swan PR, Benson LN, et al: Successful use of intra-aortic balloon pumping in a 2-kilogram infant. *Ann Thorac Surg* 46:574–576, 1988.
16. Christensen DW, Veasy LG, McGough EC, Dean JM: Intra-aortic balloon counterpulsation in children: a review of 29 patients. *Crit Care Med* 19(suppl 4):S75, 1991.
17. Pennington DG, Sarafian JE, Swartz MT: Heart transplantation in children. *J Heart Transplant* 4:441–445, 1985.
18. Starnes VA, Bernstein D, Oyer PE, et al: Heart transplantation in children. *J Heart Transplant* 8:20–26, 1989.

19. Bailey LL, Gundry SR, Razzouk AJ, et al: Bless the babies: one hundred fifteen late survivors of heart transplantation during the first year of life. *J Thorac Cardiovasc Surg* 105:805–815, 1993.
20. Pennington DG, Noedel N, McBride LR, Naunheim KS, Ring WS: Heart transplantation in children: an international survey. *Ann Thorac Surg* 52:710–715, 1991.
21. Tweddell JS, Canter CE, Bridges ND, et al: Predictors of operative morality and morbidity after infant heart transplant: early results of infant heart transplantation. *Ann Thorac Surg* 58(4):972–977, 1994.
22. Starnes VA, Marshall SE, Lewiston NJ, et al: Heart-lung transplantation in infants, children and adolescents. *J Pediatric Surg* 26:434–438, 1991.
23. Spray TL, Mallory GB, Canter CE, et al: Pediatric lung transplantation for pulmonary hypertension and congenital heart disease. *Ann Thorac Surg* 54:216–225, 1992.
24. Gibbon JH: Application of a mechanical heart and lung apparatus to cardiac surgery. *Minn Med* 37:171, 1954.
25. Spencer FC, Eiseman B, Trinkle JK, Rossi NP: Assisted circulation for cardiac failure following intracardiac surgery with cardiopulmonary bypass. *J Thorac Cardiovasc Surg* 49:56–73, 1965.
26. DeBakey ME: Left ventricular bypass pump for cardiac assistance: clinical experience. *Am J Cardiol* 27:3–11, 1971.
27. Bartlett RH, Gazzaniga AB, Fong SW, Roohk HB, Haidue N: Extracorporeal membrane oxygenator (ECMO) for cardiorespiratory failure: experience with 28 cases. *J Thorac Cardiovasc Surg* 73:375–386, 1977.
28. Martin GR, Short BL: Doppler echocardiographic evaluation of cardiac performance in infants on prolonged extracorporeal membrane oxygenation. *Am J Cardiol* 62:929–934, 1988.
29. Bavaria JE, Ratcliffe MB, Gupta KB, et al: Changes in left ventricular wall stress during biventricular circulatory assistance. *Ann Thorac Surg* 45:526–532, 1988.
30. Farrar DJ, Hill JD: Univentricular and biventricular Thoratec VAD support as a bridge to transplantation. *Ann Thorac Surg* 55:276–282, 1993.
31. Ramasamy N, Portner PM, Novacor LVAS: Results with bridge to transplant and chronic support. In: OHRA, Gutfinger DE, Gazzaniga AB (eds). *Cardiac Surgery: State of the Art Reviews*. Philadelphia: Hanley and Belfus, Inc.; 363–376, 1993.
32. Frazier OH, Rose EA, Macmanus Q, et al: Multicenter clinical evaluation of the Heartmate 1000 IP left ventricular assist device. *Ann Thorac Surg* 53:1080–1090, 1992.
33. Champsaur G, Ninet J, Vigneron M, et al: Use of the Abiomed BVS system 5000 as a bridge to cardiac transplantation. *J Thorac Cardiovasc Surg* 100:122–128, 1990.
34. Johnson KE, Prieto M, Joyce LD, Pritzker M, Emery RW: Summary of the clinical use of the Symbion total artifical heart: a registry report. *J Heart Lung Transplant* 11:103–116, 1992.
35. Koppert E, Holfert GW, Dew PA, et al: Preliminary in vitro evaluation of the first neonatal total artificial heart. *Trans Am Soc Artif Intern Organs* 36:M122–128, 1991.
36. Jurmann MJ, Haverich A, Demertzis S, et al: Extracorporeal membrane oxygenation as a bridge to lung transplantation. *Eur J Cardio-Thorac Surg* 5:94–98, 1991.
37. Spray TL, Huddleston CB: Pediatric lung transplantation. In: Patterson GA, Croper JD (eds). *Chest Surgery Clinics of North America*. Philadelphia: WB Saunders, Co.; 123–144, 1993.
38. The Toronto Lung Transplant Group: Sequential bilateral lung transplantation for paraquat poisoning. *J Thorac Cardiovasc Surg* 89:734–742, 1984.

Chapter 5

Myocardial Preservation for Pediatric Cardiac Transplantation

Valluvan Jeevanandam, MD

Introduction

Since the early 1980s, heart transplantation has evolved into an effective and rational therapy for infants and children with terminal cardiomyopathy or uncorrectable congenital disease. Despite excellent long-term survival with the introduction of cyclosporin A, and improved management of infections and rejections, the perioperative mortality rate in children remains at 10%.[1] Apart from technical factors with reoperations and the pretransplant condition of recipients, primary donor, heart dysfunction is the chief cause of mortality.[1-3] Graft failure (right ventricular, left ventricular, or biventricular) is usually secondary to either myocardial injury in the donor, poor myocardial preservation, graft reperfusion injury, or all of these. Therefore, it is quite reasonable to expect that improved myocardial preservation will improve immediate donor heart function, decrease the need for inotropic support and temporary mechanical assistance, hasten the recovery period, and, perhaps, decrease other noncardiac complications. Improved myocardial preservation may also be expected to shorten intensive care unit and hospital stays, and to decrease perioperative mortality. In addition, improved myocardial preservation could extend hypothermic ischemic times.[4]

Since the proliferation of cardiac transplantation centers has reduced the number of donors offered from outside regional programs, improved methods of myocardial preservation may not increase the donor pool; however, improved methods would allow a greater safety margin in cases of delayed preparation of the recipient for surgery or in cases of difficult reoperations. As in adult cardiac transplantation, there is now a shortage of pediatric donor organs. Improved preservation and pretreatment of donors would allow for the use of marginally acceptable hearts and, thus, effectively expand the donor pool.

Currently, myocardial preservation in most centers is accomplished by hypothermic cardioplegic arrest and static storage.[2] This technique yields acceptable ischemic periods of about 4 hours, with some reports of up to 8 hours of safe storage.[5,6] If the ischemic

From: Franco KL (ed). *Pediatric Cardiopulmonary Transplantation.* Armonk, NY: Futura Publishing Company, Inc.; © 1997.

time could be expanded to 24 to 48 hours, as achieved in renal and liver transplantation, then other benefits would be possible, including scheduled elective surgery and possibly even human leukocyte antigen (HLA) matching.[7]

HLA matching, especially in the DR locus, has resulted in longer graft survival following kidney transplantation. Data for heart transplantation is controversial especially since HLA matching, with the limitations imposed by the nature of current heart transplantation procedure (i.e., shorter ischemic times and no living-related donors), is not possible. However, on theoretical grounds, better HLA matching should decrease the severity and number of rejection episodes, decrease the intensity of immunosuppression, and perhaps even retard the accelerated atherosclerotic process.

In summary, improved methods of myocardial preservation would be valuable clinical tools, and significant research has been devoted to their realization. The ultimate aim is long-term storage with complete preservation of graft function. This goal could be accomplished by optimizing heart function in the donor, maintaining the myocardium during storage, and decreasing injury during reperfusion. Most advances in this area have been made in adult "conventional" surgery and transplantation; however, the physiologies of adult and pediatric myocardia differ significantly, and important therapeutic principles do not invariably apply to both. In this chapter, differences in mature and immature myocardia are reviewed, as well as current practices in both adult and pediatric cardiac transplantation, with a glimpse into future developments.

Characteristics of the Immature Myocardium

Unlike the mature organ, many characteristics of the immature myocardium affect preservation. The most striking morphologic differences in immature hearts are the smallness of the myocytes and the paucity of T tubules.[8-10] Cell size increases exponentially following birth and by fivefold upon maturity. Similarly, T tubules, which allow interstitial fluid to be in contact with a larger portion of the myocytes, develop with increasing myocyte size, thus maintaining the surface-to-volume relationship. This has significant implications, as the surface-to-volume relationship is critical in cardioplegia distribution and cooling, and hence in myocardial protection.

Intracellular structures also undergo maturation. Myofibrils, which initially have incomplete sarcomeres and are oriented randomly, coalesce and make up a larger volume density in the mature myocyte.[11] Mitochondria increase in number, develop cristae, and organize within myofibrils.[12] The sarcoplasmic reticulum grows at the same rate as the myocytes.[13] Maturation of these organelles coincides with the metabolic and functional maturity of the heart, and probably corresponds to the heart's decreased tolerance of ischemic insult.[14]

During early embryonic life, energy production is dependent upon glycolysis as the enzymes for oxidative phosphorylation are not yet developed.[15] The transition from glucose-dependent energy production to fatty acid-dependent energy production begins in utero as gas exchange is initiated. This process eventually decreases the need for glucose as an energy source in the adult myocardium.[12,16] The maturation from glycolysis parallels the development of the mitochondria as seen ultrastructurally.

Since the immature myocyte cannot use fatty acid precursors, glucose in the form of glycogen is stored in large quantities, significantly larger than those contained in the adult heart. Glycogen stores serve as a readily available energy source for the ischemic heart and are, therefore, an advantage for the immature heart. A direct correlation between myocardial glycogen stores and ability to survive a period of anoxia has been reported. Glycogen permits a higher rate of anaerobic glycolysis, which leads to better preservation of adenosine triphosphate (ATP) levels. Therefore, investigators have been able to show improved recovery of contractility and greater compliance of the immature ventricle compared to the adult ventricle after an ischemic event.[17,18]

Preservation of the total adenine nucleotide pool, not necessarily the postischemic concentration of ATP, has also been correlated with myocardial preservation following ischemia. ATP hydrolyzes during ischemia to produce adenosine diphosphate (ADP) and adenosine monophosphate (AMP). These products, which cannot diffuse out of cells, accumulate during ischemia. As substrate level phosphorylation of AMP and ADP comprises the major pathway for ATP synthesis in the postischemic period, loss of these precursors inhibits postischemic recovery.[19,20] Mature myocardia demonstrate a rapid rise in AMP during the initial periods of ischemia. AMP can be lost during ischemia by the conversion of the enzyme 5'nucleotidase to adenosine. Adenosine can freely diffuse across the cellular membrane, resulting in a net loss of the total nucleotide pool, a decrease in substrate available for postischemic ATP synthesis, and, ultimately, hindered recovery of ventricular contractility. 5'Nucleotidase is less active in the immature myocardium and, therefore, during ischemia, immature myocardial tissue can maintain higher levels of total adenine nucleotides.[21,22]

The approximate age at which humans attain mature 5'nucleotidase levels has not been determined. Myocardial tissue obtained from children ranging in age from 2 to 18 months demonstrated an increased level of AMP, indicating that 5'nucleotidase levels had not reached mature levels. During experiments with adult myocardium, administration of adenosine or inhibition of 5'nucleotidase, or both, increased protection from ischemia.[23,24] Whether these findings are directly applicable to the immature myocardium is still not clear.

The mechanisms of storage and use of glycogen and the preservation of the nucleotide pool have direct relevance to heart transplantation, and have formed the basis for the expectation that immature hearts should be better able to survive the ischemic/hypoxic events associated with donor procurement. This is demonstrated in immature hearts by consistently longer periods of successful hypothermic storage and the ability to resuscitate immature donor hearts even after prolonged periods of cardiopulmonary resuscitation, as reported by the Loma Linda group.[6,25]

In addition to 5'nucleotidase levels, calcium metabolism also differs in the immature heart. Due to poorly developed sarcoplasmic reticulum and a relative inability to adequately store calcium, the immature heart is very dependent on external calcium for excitation coupling and tension development. The integrity of the glycocalyx, the outermost layer of the cell membrane, is dependent upon calcium bridging. At low calcium levels, integrity of the membrane is lost, causing massive injury to the cell. Furthermore, calcium serves as a coenzyme for many cellular reactions and regulates cross-bridging of myosin to actin. Therefore, maintaining optimum calcium levels during arrest and reperfusion contributes to acceptable preservation of the immature heart. This is especially true in periods of normothermia as minor variations in calcium concentrations, deviating from a range of 1 mM to 2.4 mM, result in significant depression of ventricular function.

In periods of hypothermia, however, the role of calcium is undetermined.[26-28] Caspi et al,[29] in a report using newborn pigs, demonstrated decreased ventricular recovery after hypothermic ischemia, with increasing calcium concentrations in cardioplegic solution. Increase in calcium has been postulated as one of the mechanisms for "rapid cooling contracture" of the myocardium. The high calcium concentration during periods of hypothermia leads to increased cytosol calcium, which promotes myofilament cross-linkage, which in turn leads to ventricular stiffness and decreased postrecovery performance. Therefore, at least during periods of hypothermia, it would seem prudent to minimize cytosolic calcium by decreasing the concentration in the cardioplegia or by adding calcium channel blockers to the storage solution, or both. Reperfusion, after the period of hypothermia, should be initiated with normocalcemic solution; high calcium may cause "calcium paradox" and a hypercontractile state.

Characteristics of myocardial function also differ in the immature heart. Since there is reduced fetal myocyte size and myofibril volume density, isolated heart muscle preparations have less ability to generate active tension in immature heart muscle. This results in diminished myocardial shortening velocity and increased myocardial resting tension.

There are similar differences in the intact ventricles. The immature right ventricle is significantly less compliant than the adult right ventricle, although it is more compliant than the left ventricle at all stages of development. The reduced compliance causes a decrease in ventricular performance with volume loading. The stroke volume is subsequently fixed, and the only method of increasing cardiac output is by increasing heart rate. In addition, the immature heart may be limited by operating under maximal adrenergic stimulation with limited inotropic reserve.[8,30]

When considered in terms of transplantation and preservation, adult and immature myocardia differ in many ways. Immature hearts should be better able to tolerate ischemia, especially if they have normal levels of myocardial glycogen before the stress period. However, immature hearts are very sensitive to calcium fluxes, both during storage and reperfusion, and due to functional limitations are less compliant and have less inotropic reserve after procurement. This point emphasizes the necessity for optimal myocardial preservation of immature hearts to ensure adequate function after hypothermic storage.

Myocardial Preservation

As presented by Buckberg,[31] preservation during transplantation can be divided into four distinct phases: preharvest, cardioplegic arrest, storage, and reperfusion. Each period offers specific opportunities to improve preservation. It will be impractical and probably unnecessary to implement all of the potentially beneficial techniques, since with reasonably good heart function, simple cardioplegic arrest and a short, cold ischemic period is sufficient to obtain an adequately functioning organ. However, with the increasing shortage of donor hearts and the resultant increasing use of marginally acceptable organs, optimal preservation is critical, and the clinician should at least be acquainted with the many facets of maintaining good organ function.

Donor Preharvest Management

This period offers the opportunity to resuscitate and optimize the heart for transplantation. Brain death causes the loss of the anterior and posterior pituitary function. Hence, after brain death, there is a loss of cranioneural innervation, and decreases in the level of cortisol, antidiuretic hormone (ADH), and active thyroid stimulating hormone occur. The donors subsequently become hypovolemic, acidotic, and hemodynamically unstable, and their myocardial function inexorably declines. The longer it takes to pronounce the patient brain dead, determine distribution of organs, and obtain consent, the greater the chance of not being able to harvest donor organs.

Circulation can generally be supported with volume replacement, correction of acidosis, and steroids. Intracellular energy can be supplied by infusing glucose and insulin, but this is controversial. Two hormones, ADH and thyroid, also play a critical role. Diabetes insipidus, due to a decrease in ADH production, is a constant feature of brain death. The resultant polyuria results in dehydration, hypernatremia, hyperosmolarity, and hypokalemia—a general defect of extracellular homeostasis. Yoshioka and associates[32-33] have shown a dramatic effect of synthetic arginine vasopressin in brain-dead donors. Antidiuretic hormone, administered by constant infusion at one to two units per hour, potentiated the effect of epinephrine and ensured prolonged hemodynamic maintenance. Total peripheral resistance and mean blood pressure were increased, and the mean time to asystole after brain death was increased from 2 days to over 3 weeks. Antidiuretic hormone is routinely used at the present time for donor management.[32-35]

In the normal setting, thyroxine (T4) is converted by peripheral tissue to triiodothyronine (T3), the active form of the hormone. However, after brain death, T4 follows the alternative pathway and is converted to reverse T3, which is metabolically inactive. T3 possesses no intrinsic inotropic activity in normal hearts; however, T3 infusion improves ventricular function after ischemia. The rapidity of this activity suggests extranuclear effects and direct inotropy. T3 binding to myocyte plasma membrane or sarcoplasmic reticulum receptors increases calcium-ATPase activity, cyclic adenosine monophosphate (cAMP), and sodium channel activity. These events increase intramyocardial calcium and increase myocardial contractility. T3 has also been shown to increase myocardial adenine nucleotide translocase activity on the inner mitochondrial membrane. This process increases cytosol ATP (enhancing myocardial activity) and mitochondrial ADP, which stimulates oxidative phosphorylation and, hence, aerobic metabolism. Additionally, T3 may act at the peripheral level to decrease the breakdown of catecholamines and activate conversion of alpha to beta receptors. If so this would increase the activity of endogenous and exogenous inotropes.[36,37]

Studies have shown that more than 85% of donors are T3 deficient. In this setting, T3 replacement can rapidly reverse myocardial dysfunction.[38] In our experience, and in that of Novitsky, marginal hearts with large pressor requirements and significant dysfunction can be salvaged and transplanted successfully.[39,40] We use a 0.2 to 0.4, µg/kg bolus of synthetic triiodothyronine, liothyronine sodium (Triostat™, SmithKline Beecham Pharmaceuticals, Pittsburgh, PA, USA) repeated hourly for a maximum of three doses, and have shown dramatic donor response with excellent short- and long-term allograft function. As an extension of the study, we, in conjunction with our procurement agency, initiated a study of routine infusion of T3 to all donors. Preliminary data reveals a significant improvement in post-transplant myocardial function, manifested by decreases in the amount and duration of pressor requirements.

In summary, brain death leads to a significant deterioration in myocardial function. Correction of metabolic and hormonal imbalances can improve function and optimize the milieu to allow long-term preservation with good graft function.

Cardioplegic Arrest

After metabolic and hemodynamic optimization, the heart is arrested and explanted. The period in which cardioplegia is introduced is the best time to uniformly distribute a solution throughout the heart, either to cool the heart or to distribute agents that can improve or, at least, maintain subsequent heart function.

Cardioplegia Delivery

The donor cardiectomy starts with a median sternotomy and creation of a pericardial well. The heart is examined for contusions, abnormalities of venous drainage, coronary arteries, and ventricular wall motion. If a decision is made to proceed, the inferior and superior venae cavae and aorta are encircled and heparin is administered. Depending on the size of the donor, either the ascending aorta or innominate artery are cannulated for administration of cardioplegia. Excessive delivery pressure may cause endothelial bed damage, which can later be manifested as myocardial edema, decreased coronary artery flow, and primary graft dysfunction. Drinkwater et al found that infusion pressures of more than 120 mm Hg have caused marked dysfunction in a neonatal piglet model.[41] Therefore, cardioplegia should be administered at less than 80 mm Hg for a total volume of 10 to 15 mL/kg. After cross-clamping and arrest, topical cold saline is used to cool the heart externally. The heart is then explanted and stored until transplantation.

Cardioplegia Solutions

Cardioplegic solutions can be categorized as colloid or crystalloid, and of intracellular or extracellular electrolyte composition. Many formulations are available (i.e., St. Thomas, Plegisol, Bretschneider, etc.) and they all provide reasonable preservation over a short ischemic period. Three specific formulations will be discussed in detail: Stanford solution; University of Wisconsin solution (UWS); and Roe's solution (Table).

The most commonly used crystalloid/extracellular solution is Stanford solution[2] the composition of which is presented in Table. It is a simple solution mixed by institutional pharmacies and consists of an aqueous solution with moderate dosages of potassium as the cardiac arresting agent, sodium bicarbonate as buffer, mannitol for osmotic effects, and glucose as substrate for glycolysis. With the use of this solution, the safe period for clinical heart preservation is approximately 4 hours. After this period of time, Billingham et al have documented a correlation between ischemic time

Table

Composition of Cardioplegic Preservation Solutions

A. Composition of Stanford Solution.[46]

	Stanford Solution
Hydroxyethyl starch (Pentafraction)	—
Lactobionic acid	—
Potassium phosphate	—
Magnesium sulfate	—
Raffinose	—
Adenosine	—
Allopurinol	—
Glutathione	—
Dexamethasone	—
Glucose	50 gm/L
Mannitol	12.5 gm/L
Potassium	30 mEq/L
Sodium	30 mEq/L
Bicarbonate	30 mEq/L
Total osmolarity	431 mOsm
pH	7.8

B. Composition of University of Wisconsin Solution (UWS).[46]

	UWS
Hydroxyethyl starch (Pentafraction)	50 gm/L
Lactobionic acid	100 mmol/L
Potassium phosphate	25 mmol/L
Magnesium sulfate	5 mmol/L
Raffinose	30 mmol/L
Adenosine	5 mmol/L
Allopurinol	1 mmol/L
Glutathione	3 mmol/L
Dexamethasone	16 mg/L
Insulin	100/L
Glucose	0.06 mmol/L
Mannitol	—
Potassium	113 mEq/L
Sodium	30 mEq/L
Bicarbonate	—
Total osmolarity	323
pH	7.4

C. Composition of Roe's Solution.[6]

	Roe's Solution
NaCl	27 mEq
KCL	20 mEq
$MgSO_4$	3 mEq
Methylprednisolone (Solu-Medrol)	250 mg
5% dextrose in water	1000 mL
Adjusted to pH 7.4 with $NaHCO_3$	
Important: Store at 4°C	

and ultrastructural injury seen by electron microscopy, even after 3 hours of storage.[42] This is manifested clinically as donor graft dysfunction and a greater likelihood of operative mortality. These data are in agreement with the International Society for Heart Transplantation Registry and the Cardiac Transplant Research Database, both of which show an increase in 30-day mortality, with increasing organ ischemic time reaching more than 18% for ischemic hearts for 4 to 5 hours.[3]

UWS (ViaSpan DuPont critical care, Wilmington, DE, USA), developed by Southard and Belzer, provides extended preservation periods for kidney, liver, and pancreas in clinical and experimental transplantation. It is basically an intracellular/colloid solution that contains many agents that have potential, but unproven benefit in cardiac transplantation. It is a "shot gun" approach to preservation, based upon the principle that if elements are beneficial individually, then a combination may be even better.

UWS is a high potassium, low sodium solution that approximates the electrolyte concentration of the intracellular milieu. Hence, the gradient for sodium and potassium across the cellular membrane is decreased. This is beneficial on two fronts. During hypothermia, Na-K ATPase decreases in activity, allowing a flux of potassium out of the cell and sodium into the cell. Water is transported along with sodium, resulting in cellular edema. Subsequently, the cell attempts to compensate by using ATP to drive the Na-K ATPase pump and correct the gradient. Hence, decreasing the gradient by using intracellular electrolytes decreases myocardial swelling and preserves the ATP that would otherwise have been used to correct the electrolyte imbalance.[43-45] The concept of an "intracellular" solution was first introduced by Collins et al and Reitz in the early 1970s for kidney preservation[46,47] and by Greipp for heart preservation.[48] Most investigators have found improved preservation with "intracellular" versus "extracellular" solutions. However, there is still some controversy concerning the superiority of intracellular solutions, as cardiac function is preserved when the electrolyte composition of UWS has been reversed. Furthermore, reports of damage to endothelium and cardiac cells by high potassium containing cardioplegia agents, such as the Melrose solution, are present in the literature.[49,50] The potassium concentrations of these solutions were greater than 200 mEq/L and were hyperosmolar. Initial and late cardiac function were depressed and these solutions were not used for cardioplegia. Gharagozloo and colleagues[51] have shown that solutions with potassium concentrations between 20 and 30 mEq/L were associated with the least cardiac damage, but the investigators used a normothermic ischemia model. Kohno et al[52] reported better myocardial function after initial arrest with a solution having a lower potassium content and then storage in an intracellular (Collins) solution. However, hearts arrested and stored in UWS (both experimentally and clinically) have neither demonstrated depression in initial myocardial function nor potassium-induced myocardial cellular injury.[44,45] Perhaps this can be attributed to the rapid arrest of the hearts with adenosine, and the fact that UWS is isosmolar and contains impermanents that prevent cellular injury and edema.

Other components of UWS also contribute to organ preservation. Lactobionate, raffinose, and hydroxyethyl starch decrease transcapillary and osmotic fluid transport, and decrease the edema associated with hypothermic storage. Experimentally, hearts treated with UWS did not change in weight during preservation, and histological study revealed minimal increase in the intracellular space and mitochondrial swelling.

Allopurinol suppresses the generation of oxygen-derived free radicals by inhibition of xanthine oxidase. This, along with glutathione, which acts by reducing the level of cytotoxic oxidants, decreases the level of injury induced during reperfusion. Adenosine acts as a rapid arrest agent, and facilitates the regeneration of ATP during reperfusion. Magnesium is also present and perhaps improves preservation by stabilizing the membranes, reducing transmembrane magnesium efflux, and reducing the influx of calcium.[53,54]

Two studies have compared UWS and Stanford solution in a randomized blinded fashion for adult heart preservation with normal ischemic periods of under 4 hours. The results were similar.[45,55] Hearts preserved in UWS solution regained function faster with less cardiac enzyme leakage, but with similar hemodynamic and ultrastructural profiles. The improvements with UW solution were subclinical, especially within this short ischemic period. This result could have been predicted, since conventional crystalloid cardioplegia has been routinely used for thousands of transplants with excellent results. Recently, at Temple Universtiy, we have studied 15 patients who had ischemic times of greater than 4 hours. When compared to patients with shorter ischemic times, myocardial function, patient survival, and inotrope use were similar. This outcome is more favorable than those reported in national data, in which prolonged ischemic times were a predictor of poor outcome. Therefore, the value of UWS will probably only be manifested in marginally functional donor hearts or in cases of extended periods of preservation.

With regard to clinical pediatric heart preservation, the bulk of the literature is from the pioneering Loma Linda group. This group uses a very simple solution, Roe's solution with excellent results. Roe's solution is a crystalloid, slightly hypertonic glucose-based solution containing steroids, potassium, and magnesium. The Loma Linda group's incidence of primary donor heart function is low, and they have used some marginal donors, some even after prolonged cardiopulmonary resuscitation. When they compare results between donor ischemic times of 2 hours to 6 hours, there is a slight effect on immediate function with the longer ischemic group, but the difference disappears after 1 week. Given the compelling data, it is clear that Roe's solution with donor glucose pretreatment certainly preserves pediatric hearts even with prolonged ischemic times.[6,25]

It is important to note that all of the cardioplegic agents we have discussed can only preserve the heart; they cannot make a marginally acceptable heart better. The cardioplegic agents minimize ischemic injury and, at best, return myocardial function to the preprocurement level. Buckberg[31] has proposed a method to "resuscitate" these organs with warm-blood cardioplegic solution and make the hearts more capable of sustaining the subsequent period of ischemia. Substrate-enhanced (aspartate, glutamate) warm cardioplegia is initially infused, and is followed after arrest with hypothermic cardioplegia. This method has been shown clinically to be useful for energy-depleted hearts and experimentally for transplantation.[56,57] The proposed mechanism of action is tolerance of myocardium to ischemia, especially in young hearts, due to glycogen stores and anaerobic metabolism. Mitochondrial ATP synthesis may proceed during periods of hypoxia or ischemia, augmenting the energy derived from glycolysis. This mitochondrial ATP synthesis involves the transamination of aspartate and glutamate, producing oxaloacetate and alpha glutamate, which enter the mitochondria and generate ATP through substrate level phosphorylation. Therefore, supplying the substrate for ATP synthesis helps replete the energy profile of these ischemic hearts. Although this fact is theoretically appealing and clinically useful in surgery involving ischemic myocardium, its application to transplantation has yet to be tested. The biggest obstacle appears to be the instrumentation required to administer blood cardioplegia in a donor setting.

Organ Storage

The phase of organ storage is critical, especially if extended ischemic periods are required, because further ischemic injury cannot be permitted. Hypothermia is an essential component of the storage process. The principle of hypothermia-induced decrease in metabolic rate was first used in the 1950s by Bigelow et al,[58] who demonstrated that a 10°C drop in temperature decreases the metabolic rate by 50%. Lower et al achieved extended ischemic times using simple hypothermia in initial canine heart transplant experiments.[59] Later studies revealed that cardioplegic arrest combined with hypothermia improved the ability to protect subcellular organelles, sarcoplasmic reticulum, and myofibrils. Hence, the concepts of potassium-induced cardioplegia and hypothermia were applied in heart transplantation.

Single flush with cold cardioplegia followed by storage in either saline, dextrose-enhanced saline, Ringer's lactate, or the cardioplegia solution is the most commonly used preservation technique.[2] The technique, referred to as static storage, is simple, safe, and reproducible with an ischemic period of up to 6 hours. The optimal temperature is between 4° to 6°C. Cooler temperatures may cause crystallization injury to the myocardium, and have been associated with sinus node dysfunction. Warmer temperatures may increase metabolic requirements and increase ischemic damage. A report by Takahashi's group[60] suggests that temperature should be lowered gradually as the heart is prepared for cold storage. Mechanisms such as impaired calcium flux and edema, caused by sudden cold paralysis of the Na-K ATPase pump, may cause increased coronary resistance from vessel spasm or rheologic effects on red blood cells. However, the practical aspects with regard to human transplantation still remain doubtful.

Continuous perfusion techniques, initially used for kidney transplantation with ischemic periods of up to 72 hours, have also been attempted for cardiac preservation. In a primate autotransplantation model, Wicomb et al[61] have demonstrated preservation of up to 48 hours with acceptable ultrastructural preservation and good hemodynamic function. A hyperosmotic extracellular-type perfusate was used with continuous oxygenation and low-pressure perfusion at 4° to 6°C. Although there would appear to be no contraindication of its trial in clinical transplantation, the complexity of the apparatus and the lack of utility for long-term preservation limit its use. With the increase in the number of transplant centers, ischemic times are shortening, not increasing; and, unless hearts are nationally allocated by HLA matching, as in kidney transplantation, preservation up to 48 hours would pose an unnecessary risk. Currently, perfusion could only be justified if preservation within an ischemic period of 6 hours could be shown to be superior to static storage, and that has yet to be demonstrated.

Other perfusion techniques have been reported. Prieto and associates[62] have kept organs viable with continuous normothermic perfusion using oxygenated blood. Although primate survival experiments were not performed, recovery of immediate myocardial function in a canine model was reported. Subsequently, a compact perfusion apparatus was developed, but the complexity of the circuit, requiring constant electrolyte and blood monitoring, and blood volume replacement in order to achieve significant improvement in preservation, made it impractical. Other investigators have tried compromise solutions: either intermittent reperfusion while in static storage or very slow microperfusion.[63] Theoretically, these techniques allow wash-out of metabolic by-products while allowing for repletion of substrates for energy stores. Although initial reports were encouraging, they have not been applied clinically.

Reperfusion

The final phase of myocardial preservation is the period of reperfusion. Most studies show that ischemia makes the heart vulnerable to damage with myocardial and endothelial membrane destabilization, and that the damage becomes evident on revascularization. The irreversible damage that may occur relates to the introduction of calcium, oxygen, and cellular elements such as neutrophils into the ischemic myocardium. Therefore, low calcium levels should be maintained during the reperfusion phase (0.3 to 0.5 mM/L). Oxygen damage results from the migration of highly toxic oxygen-free radicals (OFR) into the myocardial and endothelial cells, which are depleted of protective enzymes after ischemia. When added to the reperfusate, OFR scavengers, such as superoxide dismutase and catalase, can help in obtaining improved recovery of ischemic myocardium.[64-66]

Cellular elements are also important, as activated neutrophils can cause a significant amount of myocardial injury. Drinkwater and associates[43,67] have demonstrated significant improvement in both ultrastructural and functional parameters by depleting the reperfusate of leukocytes. In randomized studies on adult transplant recipients, they found significant ultrastructural, biochemical (CPK-MB, thromboxane B2), and functional improvement using the technique of leukocyte filtration during reperfusion. They have extended this technique in pediatric and neonatal hearts after prolonged periods of ischemia with good results.

Low-pressure reperfusion probably leads to less edema and better myocardial function. Retrograde cardioplegia techniques allow the reperfusion process to begin with low pressure, to help in flushing debris and air out of the coronary circulation, and to ensure uniform distribution of cardioplegia. The coronary sinus can be easily cannulated after completion of the right atrial anastomosis, and reperfusion can be initiated while the pulmonary and aortic anastomoses are being completed. This method allows limited ischemia and evenly distributed reperfusate.

In summary, warm retrograde reperfusion initiated 5 minutes before cross-clamp release with aspartate- and glutamate-enriched, leukocyte-depleted cardioplegia is currently the best method for minimizing reperfusion injury. The method of adding OFR scavengers and antioxidants to further decrease injury is presently undergoing trials.

Another important task during reperfusion is to supply the heart with appropriate hormonal support. Studies have shown that recipients in heart failure develop a "sick euthyroid state," in which there is a decrease in free T3. This sick euthyroid state, combined with the effects of cardiopulmonary bypass that decrease T3 levels, sets up an environment of significant T3 deficiency during the immediate postimplantation period.

At Temple University, we have studied the effects of exogenous T3 treatment after heart transplantation in a randomized, blinded study of 19 recipients. The T3 reperfused group demonstrated a decrease in post-transplant inotrope requirements and less myocardial lactate production from coronary sinus specimens. Interestingly, four placebo patients, who failed weaning from cardiopulmonary bypass and would have required intra-aortic balloon insertions, were successfully managed with T3 crossover. Hence, to optimize preservation, reperfusion must be controlled and the appropriate hormonal environment must be prepared for optimal function of the donor heart.

Conclusion

The phases of donor heart preservation, in addition to proper donor and recipient management, are essential for an adequately functioning graft. Currently available techniques include donor treatment with steroids, correction of acidosis and electrolytes, infusion of ADH, and repletion of T3. Until equipment is available for warm substrate-enhanced blood cardioplegia, arrest is induced by either UWS or Roe's solution as outlined by the Loma Linda group. The donor heart is then immersed in either UWS or in a glucose-enhanced saline solution. This immersion will help to avoid contracture injury and maximize cardiac function. Reperfusion of the donor heart is initiated with warm aspartate/glutamate-enhanced, leukocyte-depleted retrograde cardioplegia about 3 to 5 minutes before cross-clamp release. Calcium levels are maintained in the 0.3 to 0.5 mM/L range during the operation and reperfusion. Calcium is then administered at the end of bypass to a level of 1 to 1.2 mM/L; this method is designed to reduce ischemic contracture injury. T3 can also be administered (0.4 µg/kg bolus followed by 0.8 µg/kg infusion over 6 hours), especially in recipients with free T3 deficiency, those with high pulmonary vascular resistance, or those with long cardiopulmonary bypass runs. It is understood that not all of these techniques need be used for every patient. Thousands of heart transplants have been performed with simple crystalloid cardioplegia without any reperfusion additives. However, in order to decrease mortality associated with primary donor heart failure, to increase the use of marginally acceptable donor organs, and to allow a reasonable safety net for extended preservation periods, these and other developing procedures, such as cryopreservation and perfusion techniques, must be employed. Such measures will be necessary if we are to successfully advance pediatric heart transplantation to the next frontier.

References

1. Bailey L, Gondrey S, Razzouk A, Wang N: Pediatric heart transplantation: issues related to outcome and results. *J Heart Lung Transplant* 11:S267–S271, 1992.
2. Wheeldon D, Sharples L, Wallwork J, English T: Donor heart preservation survey. *J Heart Lung Transplant* 11:986–993, 1992.
3. Kriett JM, Kaye MP: The registry of the International Society for Heart and Lung Transplantation—8th official report, 1991. *J Heart Lung Transplant* 10:491–498, 1991.
4. Swanson DK, Pasaoglui, Berkoff HA, et al: Improved heart preservation with UW preservation solution. *J Heart Lung Transplant* 7:456–467, 1988.

5. Thomas FT, Szentepetery SS, Mammana RE, et al: Long distance transportation of human hearts for transplantation. *Ann Thorac Surg* 26:344–350, 1978.

6. Kawauchi M, Gundry S, Alonzo DeBegona J, et al: Prolonged preservation of human pediatric heart for transplantation: correlation of ischemic time and subsequent function. *J Heart Lung Transplant* 12:55–58, 1993.

7. Ploeg RJ, Goossens D, Vreugdenhil P, McAnulty JF, Southard JH, Belzer FO: Successful 72-hour cold storage kidney preservation of UW solution. *Transplant Proc* 20:935–938, 1988.

8. Stein DG, Laks H, Drinkwater DC: Myocardial protection in children. *Adv Surg* 3:113–133, 1992.

9. Anversa P, Olivetti G, Loud A: Morphometric study of early postnatal development in the left and right ventricular myocardium of the rat. *Circ Res* 46:495–502, 1980.

10. Hirakow R, Kraus W: Postnatal differentiation of ventricular myocardial cells of the opossum and T-tubular formation. *Cell Tissue Res* 210:95–100, 1980.

11. Legato M: Cellular mechanisms of normal growth in the mammalian heart. *Circ Res* 44:250–262, 1979.

12. Smith H, Paige E: Ultrastructural changes in rabbit heart mitochondria during the perinatal period: neonatal transition to aerobic metabolism. *Dev Biol* 57:109–117, 1977.

13. Forbes M, Sperelakis N: The presence of transverse and axial tubules in the ventricular myocardium of embryonic and neonatal guinea pigs. *Cell Tissue Res* 166:83–90, 1976.

14. Hopkins S, McCutcheon E, Wekstein D: Postnatal changes in rat ventricular function. *Circ Res* 32:685–691, 1973.

15. Girard GR: Metabolic fuels of the fetus. *Isr J Med Sci* 11:591–600, 1975.

16. Clark CM, Jr: Characterization of glucose metabolism in the isolated rat heart during fetal and early neonatal development. *Diabetes* 22:41–49, 1973.

17. Bove EL, Stammers AH: Recovery of left ventricular function after hypothermic global ischemia: age related differences in the isolated working rabbit heart. *J Thorac Cardiovasc Surg* 91:115–122, 1986.

18. Opie LH: The glucose hypothesis: relation to acute myocardial ischemia. *J Mol Cell Cardiol* 1:107, 1970.

19. Latter DA, De Varennes B: Myocardial preservation for cardiac transplantation. In: Chiu RC-J (ed). *Cardioplegia, Current Concepts and Controversies.* Austin, TX: RG Landes, Co.; 65–72, 1993.

20. Rosenkranz ER, Okamoto F, Buckberg GD, et al: Studies of controlled reperfusion after ischemia. *J Thorac Cardiovasc Surg* 92:488–501, 1986.

21. Grosso MA, Banerjee A, St. Cyr JA, et al: Cardiac 5'nucleotidase activity increases with age and inversely relates to recovery from ischemia. *J Thorac Cardiovasc Surg* 103:206–209, 1992.

22. Mask WK, Abd-Elfattah AS, Jessen M, Brunsting LA, Lekven J, Wechsler AS: Embryonic versus adult myocardium: adenine nucleotide degradation during ischemia. *Ann Thorac Surg* 48:109–112, 1989.

23. Bolling SF, Olszanski DA, Bove EL, Childs KF: Enhanced myocardial protection during global ischemia with 5'-nucleotidase inhibitors. *J Thorac Cardiovasc Surg* 103:73–77, 1992.

24. Galinanes M, Hearse DJ: Exogenous adenosine accelerates recovery of cardiac function and improves coronary flow after long-term hypothermic storage and transplantation. *J Thorac Cardiovasc Surg* 104:151–158, 1992.

25. Kawauchi M, Gundry SR, Alonso deBegona J, Razzouk AJ, Bailey LL: Utilization of pediatric donors salvaged by cardiopulmonary resuscitation. *J Heart Lung Transplant* 12:185–188, 1993.

26. Pridjian AK, Levitsky S, Krukenkamp I, Silverman NA, Feinberg H: Developmental changes in reperfusion injury: a comparison of intracellular calcium accumulation in the new born, neonatal, and adult heart. *J Thorac Cardiovasc Surg* 93:428–433, 1987.

27. Zimmerman ANE, Hulsmann WC: Paradoxical influence of calcium ions on the permeability of the cell membranes of the isolated rat heart. *Nature* 2:646–647, 1966.

28. Yamamoto F, Braimbridge MV, Hearse DJ: Calcium and cardioplegia: the optimal calcium concentration for the St. Thomas Hospital, cardioplegic solution. *J Thorac Cardiovasc Surg* 87:908–912, 1984.

29. Caspi J, Herman SL, Coles JG, et al: Effect of low perfusate calcium concentration on new born myocardial function after ischemia. *Circulation* 82(suppl 4):4-371–4-379, 1990.
30. Teitel D, Chin T, Hayman MA: Developmental changes in myocardial contractility. *J Am Coll Cardiol* 1:1183, 1983.
31. Buckberg GD: Phases of myocardial protection during transplantation (invited letter). *J Thorac Cardiovasc Surg* 10:461, 1990.
32. Pallis C: Brainstem death: the evolution of a concept. *Sem Thorac Cardiovasc Surg* 2:135–152, 1990.
33. Yoshioka T, Sugimoto H, Uenishi M: Prolonged hemodynamic maintenance by the combined administration of vasopressin and epinephrine in brain death. *Neurosurgery* 8:565–567, 1986.
34. Blaine EM, Tallman RD, Frolicher D: Vasopressin supplementation in a porcine model of brain dead potential organ donors. *Transplantation* 83:459–464, 1984.
35. Luksza AR: Brain dead kidney donor: selection, care, and administration. *Br Med J* 1:1316–1319, 1979.
36. Dyke CM, Yeh T, Lehman JD, et al: T3-enhanced left ventricular function after ischemic injury. *Ann Thorac Surg* 52:14–19, 1991.
37. Chang MY, Kunos G: Short-term effects of T3 on rat heart receptors. *Biochem Biophys Res Commun* 100:313, 1981.
38. Novitsky D, Cooper DKC, Reichart B: Hemodynamic and metabolic responses to hormonal therapy in brain dead potential organ donors. *Transplantation* 43:852–854, 1987.
39. Notvitsky D: Triiodothyronine replacement, the euthyroid sick syndrome, and organ transplantation. *Transplant Proc* 23:2460–2462, 1991.
40. Jeevanandam V, Todd B, Regillo T, Hellman S, Eldridge C, McClurken J: Reversal of donor myocardial dysfunction by triiodothyronine replacement therapy. *J Heart Lung Transplant.* 13:681–687, 1994.
41. Drinkwater DC, Laks H, Buckberg GD: A new simplified method of optimizing cardioplegic delivery without right heart isolation. *J Thorac Cardiovasc Surg* 100:56–63, 1990.
42. Billingham ME, Baumgartner WA, Watson DC, et al: Distant heart procurement for human transplantation: ultrastructural studies. *Circulation* 62(Pt 2):111–119, 1980.
43. Breda MA, Drinkwater DC, Laks H, et al: Successful long-term preservation of the neonatal heart with a modified intracellular solution. *J Thorac Cardiovasc Surg* 104:139–150, 1992.
44. Jeevanandam V, Auteri JS, Sanchez JA, et al: Cardiac transplantation after prolonged graft preservation with the University of Wisconsin solution. *J Thorac Cardiovasc Surg* 104:224–228, 1992.
45. Jeevanandam V, Barr ML, Auteri JS, et al: University of Wisconsin solution versus crystalloid cardioplegia for human donor heart preservation. *J Thorac Cardiovasc Surg* 103:194–199, 1992.
46. Collins GM, Peterson T, Wiacomb WN, Halasz NA: Experimental observations on the mode of action of "intracellular" flush solutions. *J Surg Res* 1984;36:1–8, 1984.
47. Reitz BA, Brody WR, Hickey PR, Michaelis LL: Protection of the heart for 24 hours with intracellular (high K) solution and hypothermia. *Surg Forum* 25:149–151, 1974.
48. Griepp RB, Stinson ED, Angell WW, Dong E, Shumway NE: Hypothermic preservation of the canine heart. *Transplant Proc* 6:315–318, 1974.
49. Gay WA, Ebert PA: Functional, metabolic, and morphological effects of potassium-induced cardioplegia. *Surgery* 74:284–290, 1973.
50. Kinoshita K, Ehara T: Importance of sodium ions and the protective effects of high potassium, high glucose solutions, and electromechanical activities in the guinea pig's myocardium. *J Mol Cell Cardiol* 16:405–419, 1984.
51. Gharagozloo F, Buckley BH, Hutchings GM, et al: Potassium induced cardioplegia during normothermic cardiac arrest. *J Thorac Cardiovasc Surg* 77:602–607, 1979.
52. Kohno H, Shiki K, Ueno Y, Tokunaga K: Cold storage of the rat heart for transplantation: 2 types of solution required for optimal preservation. *J Thorac Cardiovasc Surg* 77:86–94, 1979.
53. Belzer FO, Southard JH: Principles of solid organ preservation by cold storage. *Transplantation* 45:673–676, 1988.

54. Wahlberg GA, Southard JH, Belzer FO: Development of a cold storage solution for pancreas preservation. *Cryobiology* 23:477–482, 1986.
55. Stein DG, Drinkwater DC, Laks H, et al: Cardiac preservation in patients undergoing transplantation. *J Thorac Cardiovasc Surg* 102:657–665, 1991.
56. Rosenkranz ER, Okamoto F, Buckberg GD, Robertson JM, Vinten-Johansen J, Bugy IH: Safety of prolonged aortic cross clamping with blood cardioplegia. *J Thorac Cardiovasc Surg* 91:428–435, 1986.
57. Allen BS, Okamoto F, Buckberg GD, et al: Studies of controlled reperfusion after ischemia. *J Thorac Cardiovasc Surg* 92:621–635, 1986.
58. Bigelow WG, Linday WK, Greenwood WF: Hypothermia: its possible role in cardiac surgery. *Ann Surg* 132:849–866, 1950.
59. Lower RR, Stofer RC, Horley EJ, Dong E, Cohn RB, Shumway NE: Successful homotransplantation of canine heart after anoxic preservation for seven hours. *Am J Surg* 104:302–306, 1962.
60. Takahashi A, Hearse DJ, Braimbridge WV, Chambers DJ: harvesting hearts for long-term preservation: detrimental effects of initial hypothermic infusion of cardioplegic solution. *J Thorac Cardiovasc Surg* 100:371–378, 1990.
61. Wicomb WN, Rose AG, Cooper DKC, Novitzky D: Hemodynamic and myocardial histologic and ultrastructural studies on baboons from 3–27 months following autotransplantation of hearts stored by hypothermic perfusion for 24–48 hours. *J Heart Transplant* 5:122–129, 1986.
62. Prieto M, Barren P, Andreone PA, et al: Multiple ex-vivo organ preservation with warm blood. *J Heart Transplant* 7:227–237, 1988.
63. Beeman SK, Shuman TA, Perna AM, et al: Intermittent reperfusion extends myocardial preservations for transplantation. *Ann Thorac Surg* 43:484–489, 1987.
64. Drinkwater DC, Laks H: Pediatric cardioplegia techniques. *Sem Thorac Cardiovasc Surg* 5:168–175, 1993.
65. Guarnierri C, Flamigi F, Caldarac N: Role of oxygen in the cellular damage induced by reoxygenation of hypoxic heart. *J Mol Cell Cardiol* 12:797–808, 1980.
66. Zweier JL, Flaherty JT, Weisfeldt ML: Direct measurements of free radical generation following reperfusion of ischemic myocardium. *Proc Natl Acad Sci USA* 84:1404–1407, 1987.
67. Stein DG, Bhuta SM, Drinkwater DC, et al: Ultrastructural evidence of damage in clinical transplantation despite modified reperfusion. *J Heart Lung Transplant* 10:1951–1957, 1991.

Chapter 6

Infant and Pediatric Cardiac Transplantation

Steven R. Gundry, MD

Introduction

Infant and pediatric cardiac transplantation represents effective therapy for children with severe forms of congenital or acquired heart disease. It is most commonly used for children who cannot undergo palliative and/or corrective operations. Recently, it has received attention as definitive therapy, whereas, the results of other surgical repairs have been unsatisfactory or are still evolving.

Cardiac transplantation was first performed on a 3-week-old infant by Kantrowitz et al[1] in December 1967. Pediatric heart transplantation as a systematic planned procedure was initiated by Shumway at Stanford in December 1980. The introduction of cyclosporine (CsA)[2] in 1980 as the principal immunosuppressant produced reversible preferential suppression of T-lymphocyte function, spared the nonspecific immune system, and consequently reduced the risk of infection in transplant patients.[3] Despite the advances attributed to this agent, pediatric heart transplantation was impeded by concerns about the long-term effects of immunosuppression in children, differences in myocardial preservation, lack of adequate animal experimentation, and ethical and philosophical concerns. Many of these concerns were lessened or eliminated after the first successful newborn heart transplantation was performed at Loma Linda University in 1985. Since then, such treatment has been offered at many centers to children with incurable heart disease.

This chapter reviews current management of pediatric heart transplantation, focusing on the recipient, the donor, operative and postoperative management, complications, results, and future trends.

From: Franco KL (ed). *Pediatric Cardiopulmonary Transplantation*. Armonk, NY: Futura Publishing Company, Inc.; © 1997.

The Recipient

Indications for Cardiac Transplantation

Most infant and pediatric patients considered for cardiac transplantation have either a cardiomyopathy, a congenital cardiac malformation, or both,[4] with congenital defects, such as hypoplastic left heart syndrome (HLHS) being the most frequent.

Patients with congenital heart disease who are candidates for transplantation may have a wide variety of lesions. Approximately 10% of infants born with congenital heart disease have complex abnormalities that preclude corrective surgery.[6] A more complete list of these conditions are presented in Table 1, but perhaps the most notable among them is the HLHS. HLHS can be palliated by the Norwood reconstruction, followed by a bidirectional Glenn shunt or "hemi'Fontan," and subsequent atriopulmonary connection. However, long-term results have been less than optimal, and have served as an impetus for developing heart transplantation as a potentially definitive procedure. Moreover, the Norwood procedure includes three operations, as opposed to one for transplantation.

Potential recipients should be evaluated by a team of specialized medical and surgical consultants. A blood work-up is performed for the assessment of renal and hepatic function, and screening for cytomegalovirus (CMV), toxoplasmosis, herpes simplex virus (HSV), rubella, Epstein-Barr virus (EBV), hepatitis B surface antigen, varicella-zoster virus, and the human immunodeficiency virus (HIV) antibody. Cardiac evaluation includes electrocardiogram (ECG), chest x-ray, echocardiography, and often cardiac catheterization. Neurologic evaluation may include head ultrasound (infants), electroencephalogram, and occasionally a computed tomographic (CT) scan of the head to exclude major central nervous system (CNS) disorders.

Contraindications to heart transplant may be absolute or relative and are listed in Table 2. Absolute contraindications include major CNS abnormalities, irreversible

---

Table 1.

Indications for Pediatric Cardiac Transplantation

Cardiomyopathy
Congenital heart lesions
  Hypoplastic left heart syndrome
  Critical variant of Shone's complex
  Complex single ventricle with systemic outflow obstruction
  Interrupted aortic arch and significant subaortic stenosis
  Critical aortic stenosis with severe endocardial fibroelastosis
  Pulmonary atresia, intact ventricular system plus sinusoids
  Severe intrauterine atrioventricular valve insufficiency with ventricular
    dysfunction
  Congenitally corrected transposition of the great arteries with single
    ventricle and heart block
  Transposition of the great arteries and straddling atrioventricular and
    tensor apparatus
  Unbalanced atrial ventricular septal defect variants
  Ebstein's anomaly in a symptomatic newborn
Unresectable symptomatic cardiac neoplasms

failure of other organ systems (excluding renal failure), uncontrolled infections, uncontrolled malignancy, and severe dysmorphism. Chronic unresolved infections or uncontrolled sources of recurrent sepsis contraindicate transplantation, unless they can be eliminated. Relative contraindications include marked prematurity (< 36 weeks gestational age), low birth weight (< 2 kg), positive drug screen, and a family structure unable to support the long-term medical needs of the recipient. Cardiac transplantation may be contraindicated in children with elevated pulmonary vascular resistance (> 4 to 5 Woods U/m^2) that is not reversible with vasodilator therapy or oxygen. Recipients with elevated, fixed pulmonary vascular disease are at a high risk for postoperative right ventricular failure. This feature may be especially common in children who have had previous palliative procedures, in whom the measurement of pulmonary vascular resistance is difficult. Heart-lung transplantation may be offered to children with severe combined cardiac and pulmonary vascular disease.[6,7] More recently, single-lung transplantation coupled with correction of congenital heart defects has been effective in managing patients with Eisenmenger's physiology.[8]

Hepatic and renal dysfunction may be present secondarily, due to congestive heart failure (CHF). Although their presence increases the perioperative risk, they usually resolve after transplantation and, therefore, do not form absolute contraindications. Indeed 10 out of 11 patients in our series on perioperative dialysis resolved their renal failure. Severe primary hepatic or renal dysfunction usually contraindicates isolated heart transplantation, although occasional heroic efforts of combined transplantation have been successful.

Preoperative Management

Specialized management is often required for infants awaiting heart transplantation. Continuous intravenous prostaglandin E_1 (PGE_1) reliably maintains patency of the ductus arteriosus in newborns and young infants with severe left heart abnormalities and a ductus-dependent circulation. Occasionally, mechanical ventilation and manipulations of $PaCO_2$ are necessary to control pulmonary arterial flow. Balloon atrial septostomy, reduction of FIO_2 to 16% to 18% by the addition of nitrogen, and ductus stenting[9] have been used for infants with ductus-dependent systemic circulation for up to 6 months, and have

---

Table 2.

Contraindications to Pediatric Heart Transplantation

Irreversible elevated pulmonary vascular resistance (>4–5 Woods U/m^2)*
Active systemic infection
Uncontrolled malignancy
Severe primary renal or hepatic dysfunction
Major central nervous system abnormality
Severe dysmorphism
Marked prematurity (gestational age <36 wk)
Low birth weight (<2 kg)
Positive drug screen
Lake of family support

*Unless "domino" or "preconditioned" donor heart available.

resulted in successful transplantation. Initial palliation for hypoplastic left heart syndrome using Norwood's operation is yet another option to gain time for the donor organ search.[10] Many centers use this philosophy as a standard approach, reserving transplantation for those infants who do poorly following the Norwood reconstruction. Occasionally, recipients with inadequate or excessive pulmonary blood flow may require a modified Blalock-Taussig shunt or pulmonary artery banding respectively.

Preoperative infectious disease screening consists of a chest x-ray, complete blood cell count (CBC), and bacterial and viral cultures of the nasopharynx, sputum, urine, and blood. Blood is screened for toxoplasmosis and viral antibodies. Similar maternal blood, urine, and vaginal cultures are recommended for screening of neonatal recipients.

The Donor

Pediatric heart donors are referred after brain death is declared. Selection criteria are much the same as those for an adult donor, but vary from state to state and even between hospitals. Donor and recipient are matched for blood group (ABO) compatibility, and the donor is assessed for freedom from serious chronic infection, including hepatitis and HIV.

The donor heart is evaluated by ECG and echocardiography. Acceptable echocardiographic criteria include normal structure (except atrial and ventricular septal defects that can be repaired after explantation), fiber shortening greater than 25% on inotropic support with appropriate volume preloading, and absence of ST-T wave changes. Donor hearts often have inadequate volume loading caused by diabetes insipidus, and if the echocardiographic function is poor, it may be repeated a few hours after appropriate volume replenishment and inotropes. Because of the scarcity of donor organs, oversize donor hearts can be accepted; the donor's body weight can be up to four times that of the recipient. Undersized donor hearts are more problematic, particularly for neonates and young infants, and may not support the circulation adequately if the donor's weight is less than 70% to 80% of the recipient's body weight. For recipients with elevated pulmonary vascular resistance, an oversized heart is best, perhaps even a "preconditioned" heart from an asthmatic donor or a "domino" heart[11] from a heart-lung recipient.

Neither the safe limits for donor heart ischemic times in children, nor the limits of long-distance procurement are known. Indeed, we have found no short- or long-term difference in hearts ischemic for longer than 6 hours versus those less than 6 hours. We have successfully transplanted hearts after cold ischemic times of up to 10 hours, and achieved good postimplant function.

Donor Harvesting

Donor procedures for children closely mimic the standardized methods set forth for adult cardiac transplantation. Multiorgan procurement is a standard practice. Immediately before harvest, the donor is heparinized, and given steroids, antibiotics, and dextrose. While the abdominal organs are prepared for removal, the heart and lungs are prepared for isolation and preservation, and a cardioplegia catheter is inserted into the ascending aorta. When all teams are ready, the inferior vena cava (IVC) is divided, and the donor exsanguinated into the right pleural space. The aorta is cross-clamped, and cardioplegia is infused into the ascending aorta. We use Roe's solution at 4°C administered by simple gravity infusion (the cardioplegia infusion is not pressurized). The heart is excised with as much aorta, pulmonary artery, and systemic veins as will be essential for reconstruction of the particular anatomy of the recipient (Figure 1). In patients who have had previous palliation, additional lengths of systemic vein and pulmonary arteries are taken to aide in reconstruction. For a HLHS transplant, because the recipient's aorta is hypoplastic, the donor aorta must be secured past the three arch vessels to permit sufficient length for recipient reconstruction. The arch vessels are ligated and divided before the aorta is cross-clamped, and the descending aorta is dissected down to the first intercostals. At harvest, the entire arch is taken with the heart.

After excision, the graft is placed in a plastic bag containing 500 mL of normal saline solution (approximately 4°C) with 10 mL of 50% dextrose. Any atrial or ventricular sep-

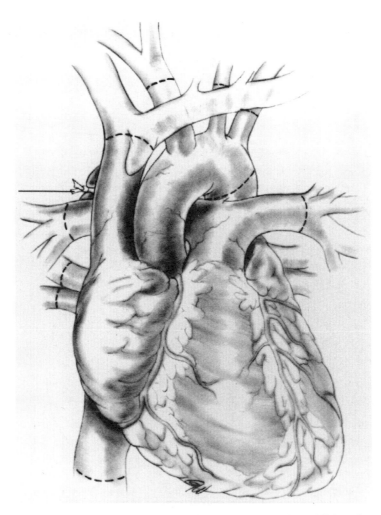

Figure 1. A donor heart removed at the time of procurement with additional great veins, pulmonary artery, and aortic arch. The removal of additional donor tissue at the time of organ removal is important for patients with congenital heart disease who have had previous operations. (Reproduced with permission from Kapoor AS, Lak H: *Atlas of Heart-Lung Transplantation.* New York: McGraw–Hill, Inc.; 1994.)

tal defects are closed, while the heart is kept cool in the saline solution. The outer bag is then surrounded with crushed ice in a thermal picnic container for convenient transport.

The Recipient Operation

General Conduct

Orthotopic heart transplantation for infants with cardiomyopathy or neoplasm is accomplished in the same fashion as that for adults. Graft implantation is performed with hypothermia and reduced systemic perfusion. If reconstruction of the ascending aorta is planned as part of the implantation, the aortic cannula is placed beyond the innominate artery in the transverse aorta. If there is complete ductal-dependent

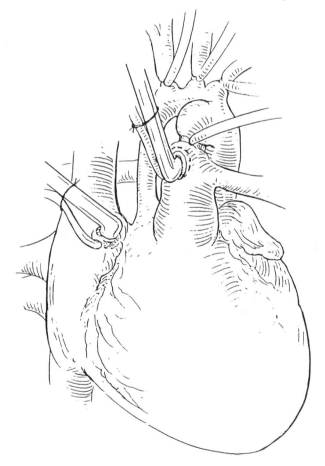

Figure 2. In patients with a ductal-dependent circulation, the systemic perfusion cannula is placed in the pulmonary artery and directed through the ductus arteriousus, which is snared as bypass is begun. Venous cannulation is via a cannula in the right atrial appendage. (Reproduced with permission from Baue AE, Geha AS, Hammond GL, Laks H, Naunheim KS: *Glenn's Thoracic and Cardiovascular Surgery.* Norwalk, CT: Appleton & Lange; 1991.)

systemic circulation, as in HLHS, the perfusion cannula is placed in the main pulmonary artery and directed through the ductus to the systemic circulation, and the ductus is then snared around the cannula, directing arterial blood flow into the aorta (Figure 2). In patients with both aortic and ductal dependency (e.g., a single ventricle and interrupted arch), a Y is placed in the aortic perfusion line, and both the ascending aorta and main pulmonary artery are cannulated and perfused.

Venous drainage is accomplished with separate cannulation of superior vena cava (SVC) and IVC, unless circulatory arrest is anticipated when only a single venous cannula is used. Infants and children with complex arch anomalies (HLHS), in whom complete arrest is anticipated, are cooled to approximately 18°C, rectally. After the recipient heart is excised, the atria and great vessels are attached by continuous suture technique (Figure 3). Transplantation for complex structural disease, alterations in situs, and those following serial palliative operations may be technically challenging (Figure 4). Utilization of extra donor tissue can usually accommodate any alteration in arterial or venous anatomy or situs. Aortic arch reconstruction is performed during circulatory arrest.[12,13]

Modifications with Complex Congenital Lesions

Atrial and Venous Return Anomalies

Several techniques have been described for correction of abnormal atrial and venous return, such as atrial septation, atrial enlargement, superior systemic venous return rerouting, inferior systemic venous return rerouting, double venous rerouting, and septal realignment.[14] Anomalies such as bilateral SVC can be successfully reconstructed by using donor SVC and innominate vein harvested en-bloc with the donor graft.

Situs Anomalies

Children with dextrocardia and atrial inversion present a complicated problem. Doty et al[15] reported systemic venous reconstruction with rerouting of the IVC using the right atrium as a conduit along the inferior surface of the pericardium. However, we have found it feasible to perform transplantation in infants with *situs inversus* using external reconstructive techniques. The superior caval connection is made with donor SVC and innominate vein. The inferior connection can be accomplished with minimal modification of the IVC and atrial free wall.

Pulmonary Artery Malformations

Prohibitive perioperataive mortality was previously described for pediatric heart transplantation after palliative operations for congenital heart disease involving the pulmonary arteries.[16,17] Cooper et al[18] described repair of pulmonary artery lesions in 7 of 46 children undergoing heart transplantation between 1984 and 1990. Individualized pulmonary arterial reconstruction was employed, including use of previously created pulmonary artery conduits, homografts, and angioplasty with and without

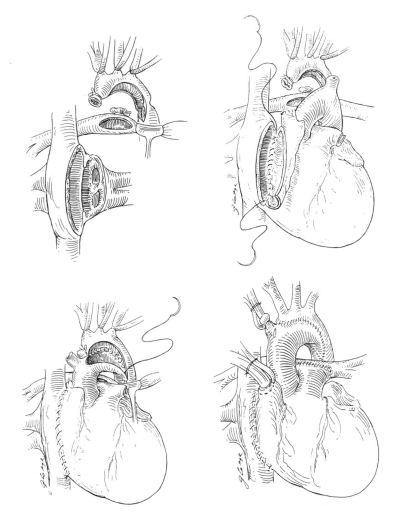

Figure 3. Transplantation for hypoplastic left heart syndrome (HLHS). Under profound cooling and circulatory arrest, the ascending aorta and the proximal ductus arteriosus are tied. The heart is excised, leaving as much left atrial tissue as possible, and the inner curvature of the recipient aorta is opened with an incision extending from the proximal transverse arch to the descending thoracic aorta, just beyond the junction of the ductus arteriosus. The donor heart is implanted starting with the atrial anastomoses. After the aortic anastomosis is completed, the arterial profusion cannula is placed in the donor innominate artery and the patient is rewarmed as the pulmonary artery anastomosis is completed. (Reproduced with permission from Baue AE, Geha AS, Hammond GL, Laks H, Naunheim KS: *Glenn's Thoracic and Cardiovascular Surgery.* Norwalk, CT: Appleton & Lange; 1991.)

pericardial patches. Transplantation was successful in all of these children, and posttransplant pulmonary artery pressure gradients were acceptable and tended to decrease with time. These investigators recommended that additional length of donor aorta and pulmonary artery be harvested for possible use and design in pulmonary artery connections where lesions such as this exist. Complex pulmonary arterial anatomy does not constitute an insurmountable obstacle to successful heart transplantation, provided the pulmonary arteries at the lung hila are of adequate size. It is occasionally necessary to reconstruct the pulmonary arteries at the hilum of each lung.

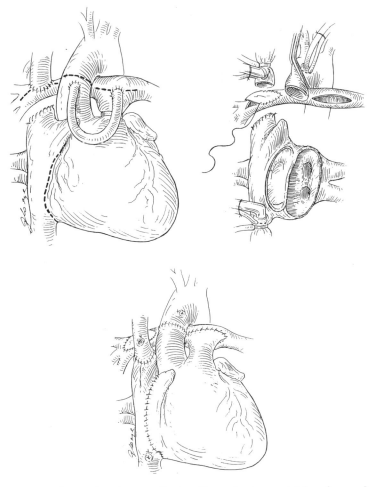

Figure 4. Heart transplantation in a patient with a single ventricle after pulmonary artery banding, a bidirectional Glenn shunt and a central shunt. An angled metal-tipped venous cannula is placed high in the superior vena cava (SVC). The SVC is separated from the right pulmonary artery, and the opening in the right pulmonary artery repaired with a pericardial patch. The atrial incision is carried in front of the atrial appendage and the recipient's pulmonary artery is transected at the bifurcation. The recipient's native atrial appendage is stretched and rotated superiorly, and then anastomosed to the superior vena cava. Donor implantation is then completed in a standard fashion with atrial, aortic, and pulmonary anastomoses. (Reproduced with permission from Baue AE, Geha AS, Hammond GL, Laks H, Naunheim KS: *Glenn's Thoracic and Cardiovascular Surgery*. Norwalk, CT: Appleton & Lange; 1991.)

We prefer to individually connect the left and right pulmonary arteries of the donor to the recipient's hilar vessels, provided sufficient length has been harvested at the time of explantation.

Aortic Arch Deficiencies

For reconstruction of the hypoplastic aortic arch, the donor aorta is prepared by incising along its distal outer curvature. During circulatory arrest, the recipient aortic arch is opened along its inner curvature just beyond the point at which the ductus has been excised. Backer et al[19] described a slight modification of the technique using bicaval cannulation to limit the duration of circulatory arrest to the aortic reconstruction phase only. The left atrial anastomosis is performed on bypass, followed by the arch reconstruction during circulatory arrest; then the right atrial and pulmonary anastomoses are performed on bypass again. However, even when all anastomoses are performed under circulatory arrest, the arrest times average 40 minutes.

Postoperative Management

Early Management

The same principles of postoperative care for children undergoing conventional open-heart surgery apply to post-transplant infants. Inotropic support in the form of dopamine (2 to 3 μg/kg/min) and isoproterenol (0.02 to 0.06 μg/kg/min) are routinely started and usually maintained for 2 or 3 days. Infants receiving PGE_1 before transplantation are weaned from the drug postoperatively over a period of 5 days.

Although no significant differences in infection rates have been attributed to differences in isolation techniques, some sort of protective isolation is used at most centers. We have abandoned the use of masks and gowns. Invasive lines are removed as soon as possible. All blood products given should be CMV-negative if the recipient is CMV-negative or a neonate. Radiation or leucocyte filtration of blood products for recipients is also recommended. Antibiotic therapy (cefazolin) is started preoperatively and continued until all intravascular catheters are removed. Additional antimicrobials are used to treat specific infections. Acyclovir or gancyclovir is given prophylactically for a period of 3 months, postoperatively.

Intravenous H2 antagonists are routinely used in the immediate postoperative period to reduce the risk of stress ulceration and whenever steroid therapy is required. Enteral feeding or intravenous (IV) hyperalimentation is begun early, with preference given to enteral feedings to reduce the incidence of systemic complications.

Recipients with oversized donor hearts present a unique challenge. A high heart rate is maintained with isoproterenol or atrial pacing to reduce ventricular diastolic volume. Excising the pericardium widely on both sides, anterior to the phrenic nerve, usually provides sufficient space for a large heart. Occasionally, the sternum may need to be left open with sternal closure delayed until after resolution of edema. Hypertension is aggressively controlled with nitroprusside, tolazoline, angiotensin-converting enzyme (ACE) inhibitors, calcium antagonists, and occasionally, beta-blocking agents. Infants with large donor hearts will often have respiratory difficulties after extubation; therefore, we often wait several days (until all edema is resolved) before extubation, so that pulmonary function is optimized. No untoward effects on early or late pulmonary function have been noted.

Immunosuppression

Semiselective immunosuppression is CsA-based at virtually all centers, except at the University of Pittsburgh, where FK-506 is used. Most centers use CsA in triple-drug regimens that include steroids and azathioprine. Other protocols using OKT3 or antithymocyte globulin (ATG) prophylactically are used, but less frequently. Triple-drug therapy allows effective immunosuppression by synergistic actions, while simultaneously allowing minimal doses to reduce associated side effects. However, there is much to suggest that such a practice is unwarranted.

The Loma Linda University protocol involves CsA and azathioprine. The routine use of steroids is avoided for several reasons. Avoidance of steroids may reduce the incidence of post-transplant infections, perhaps reduce the occurrence of chronic graft atherosclerosis, and hopefully avoid other common complications of chronic steroid use, especially abnormal growth and development. Steroids are administered for acute rejection and to children with abnormal endomyocardial biopsies (low-dose maintenance therapy) until the biopsy pattern normalizes. Rarely, recipients demonstrate chronic immune reactivity toward their hearts, which can be controlled by the addition of oral methotrexate or some other more extreme immune intervention such as total lymphoid irradiation.

CsA is administered intravenously in the initial perioperative period, and is started preoperatively in infant recipients at a dose of 0.1 mg/kg hourly, and maintained until blood levels are obtained. The appropriate dose varies greatly among patients, and levels must be monitored carefully on a daily basis. Optimum blood levels for children in the postoperative period are not known. We maintain the CsA trough level between 200 and 300 ng/mL initially (COBAS-EMIT method). When gastrointestinal function appears stable, oral CSA is begun at a dose of 10 to 20 mg/kg per day, administered in two or three equally divided doses. Beyond the first transplant year, CsA levels are maintained between 100 and 150 ng/mL. This chronic blood trough level is relatively free of undesirable side effects.

In most centers, a large dose of steroid is given at the time of surgery. In the Loma Linda protocol, methylprednisolone is administered (25 to 50 mg/kg/d every 12 hours for 2 days). Virtually all newborn and infant recipients of heart allografts in the Loma Linda series have been managed successfully without the need for maintenance corticosteroids or more exotic immunomanipulation.

Azathioprine (3 mg/kg/d) is administered IV once daily and later given orally. The dose is reduced if the white blood cell count is below 4×10^9/L. The dose is tapered toward 1 mg/kg per day after the first 3 months, and then discontinued after 1 year of follow-up for newborn recipients whose immunotherapy beyond the first post-transplant year is limited to CsA monotherapy. All other children are maintained on low-dose azathioprine indefinitely.

Intravenous immunoglobulin (Ig) at a dose of 400 mg/kg is administered for 3 to 5 days after transplantation to reduce the number of opportunistic viral infections. This dose is repeated during treatment of rejection episodes. Antithymocyte serum ATS (Nashville) is routinely administered for the first 5 days postoperatively for induction therapy in all infants and children older than 1 month of age.

Surveillance

Surveillance techniques are initially used twice a week. Clinical examination, ECG, echocardiography, and some assessment of immune response to follow the progress of transplanted children are included at our center.

Clinical signs of graft rejection include an unexplained persistent increase in the resting heart rate, presence of a third heart sound, arrhythmias, tachypnea, diaphoresis, and/or cool extremities. Fine crackles and hepatosplenomegaly may be found, as well as irritability, malaise, fever, and oliguria, or a persistent change in feeding, sleeping, and/or activity patterns.

Laboratory examination results may show elevated creatinine phosphokinase (CPK) and isoenzyme (CK-MB) levels, or increasing spontaneous blastogenesis but, to date, laboratory testing has yet to yield a reliable predictor of rejection. A chest x-ray may indicate advancing global cardiomegaly and pulmonary edema, or pleural effusion. ECG may demonstrate a >20% reduction in combined ECG voltage, significant change in the QRS axis, or significant new arrhythmias. The finding of a decrease in QRS voltage may imply cardiac rejection, but unfortunately this is nonspecific.[21]

In older children, as in adults, endomyocardial biopsy is performed weekly during the first 2 to 3 months after surgery, and then biopsy is guided by noninvasive assessment. In neonates and infants, biopsies are deferred unless essential. Canter et al[22] reported the safe use of echocardiographically guided biopsy in six children over 5 years of age, and seven infants transplanted between the ages of 2 weeks and 15 months, with only one incidence of increased tricuspid regurgitation in each group. They found it to be a reliable and safe means for surveillance in infants and young children.

Few echocardiographers would have difficulty in diagnosing established acute or chronic rejection of a cardiac graft. Global myocardiopathy and/or ventricular dilatation and dysfunction are easily observed, but are late findings. Earlier echocardiographic signs of acute graft rejection include rapidly increasing left ventricular (LV), posterior and septal wall thickness, decreasing posterior and septal ventricular function, pericardial effusion, new atrioventricular (AV) valve insufficiency, or decreasing LV fiber shortening fraction. Boucek et al[23] described digitalized echocardiography as a surveillance technique. This method uses a more sensitive multifunctional analysis, permitting diagnosis of rejection before systolic decompensation. M-mode tracings are digitized and analyzed for LV wall thickness, mass index, LV volume, shortening fractions, and endomyocardial thickening. AV valve dysfunction and pericardial effusion are also assessed. Loss of diastolic compliance occurs relatively early, and it appears that digitized analysis is sensitive to the early phases of depressed diastolic function. Increases in LV mass and LV wall mass may signify rejection episodes.[24] Predictive accuracy for the presence or absence of graft rejection using all of these indices was 93%. This technique has the advantage of being noninvasive, and can be repeated frequently and accomplished on an outpatient basis.

Complications

Graft rejection remains one of the primary concerns after cardiac transplantation. In an international survey by Pennington et al,[25] 72% of children experienced rejection, with an average of 1.7 rejections per patient. Acute rejection accounted for 19% of deaths, and chronic rejection for 12%. The incidence of rejection in the pediatric population averages approximately 1.5 to 2.5 episodes per patient, with the highest incidence in the 1 to 4 year old age group. In infants (<1 month of age) transplanted at Loma Linda University, the highest incidence of rejection occurred in the second week after transplantation (33%) and reached 78% by 1 month post-transplant.[26] This frequency has been reduced in half by ATS induction.

Acute rejection is treated most commonly with IV steroids; a much smaller percentage of patients receive ATS. We administer IV methylprednisolone (25 to 30 mg/kg per dose every 12 hours for 8 doses), depending on response. If the response is slow, or if evidence for rejection recurs after discontinuation of the steroids, a 7- to 10-day course of ATS is initiated and surveillance continued. Should the rejection pattern fail to respond, the graft my be rescued by a course of IV methotrexate.

Ventricular failure accounts for 26% of deaths after pediatric cardiac transplantation; rejecton and infection account for 31% and 18%, respectively. The three principal causes of allograft failure are accelerated graft atherosclerosis, rejection, and nonspecific graft failure.

Extracorporeal membrane oxygenation (ECMO) has been used in this setting. Galantowicz et al[27] reported its use in 10 patients in the perioperative period, with four survivors. They also used ECMO as treatment in six patients with acute rejection, with three survivors (one received another transplant).

Cardiac retransplantation remains an option for allograft failure. Karwande et al[28] reported on 449 cardiac retransplants. Uncontrolled rejection, short interval (<6 months) between transplantations, and the need for mechanical circulatory support were identified as risk factors. However, if these factors were not present, the short-term and long-term survival rates were similar to those for patients having a single transplant. Retransplantation within 6 months of the initial transplant was associated with a 1-year actuarial survival of 36%, compared with 61% for those whose retransplantation was more than 6 months later.

At Loma Linda, retransplantation has been performed in five children. Two of the procedures were performed within 1 day of the initial transplant, but neither child survived. The third procedure was performed 1 month after the initial transplant, and the patient survived. Two other procedures were performed late for chronic rejection and graft vasculopathy.

Infection is an important cause of postoperative morbidity and mortality in the transplant recipient.[29] In the recent survey by Pennington et al,[25] infections averaged one episode per patient and accounted for 18% of deaths. Surprisingly, almost half of the patients had no infections at all. Half of the documented infections were bacterial; viral and fungal infections accounted for most of the others.

The lungs are the most common site of infection. Bronchial washings, transbronchial biopsy, and open-lung biopsy are considered early on for patients with undiagnosed or progressive pulmonary infiltrates. Rapid and aggressive antimicrobial treatment can limit the associated morbidity and mortality.[30]

CMV infection has often been a lethal complication. Preoperative CMV-negative patients who become positive after transplantation have the worst outcome. When possible, CMV-positive donors are used in CMV-positive recipients. However, with current CMV prophylaxis and therapy, we do not hesitate to implant a CMV-positive graft in a CMV-negative recipient. Only CMV-negative or leukocyte-filtered blood should be given. Gancyclovir is administered to patients who have clinical signs of active CMV infection.[31]

Fungal infections tend to originate from the oropharynx and urinary tract, and occur most frequently during rejection therapy or during a course of antibiotics. Oral irrigation using nystatin suspension provides reasonable prophylaxis. Amphotericin B is recommended for suspected invasive fungal infections.

Prophylactic use of trimethoprim-sulfamethoxazole to avoid pneumocystis carinii pneumonia (PCP), and acyclovir to prevent HSV infections has been effective in adult heart transplant recipients and may have a role in the pediatric setting. Kramer et al[32] found that a 12-month period is a sufficient length of therapy if immunosuppressant treatment is stable. However, we do not use such therapy at Loma Linda.

Other Complications

Hypertension may occur early postoperatively because of CsA, steroids, volume overload, increased cardiac output, and a reactive vascular system. Treatment may require diuresis, afterload reduction, negative inotropic agents, and possibly, reduction of CsA levels. Careful control of hypertension is essential to prevent catastrophic neurologic decompensation.

Chronic hypertension, which is seen in the majority of adult patients, is rarely a problem in the pediatric patient.[33,34] In the survey by Pennington et al, 39% of patients had systemic hypertension and required antihypertensive medication; this finding was comparable to those of other studies.[25,35] Calcium channel blockers are the most effective blood pressure control.[36]

Focal or generalized post-transplantation seizures are occasionally observed. There are numerous causes, including toxic levels of CsA, use of deep hypothermia, circulatory arrest, cerebral edema, emboli, metabolic derangement, sudden onset of hypertension, increased cerebral perfusion pressure, electrolyte imbalance, infection, fever, or some other encephalopathy. These seizures are usually transient and are controlled with phenobarbital and/or benzodiazepines. Rarely do patients require chronic anticonvulsive therapy or suffer long-term sequelae.

Pennington et al noted that postoperative seizures occurred in 25% of pediatric patients.[25] It was believed that most of the seizures were caused by CsA therapy, and they were usually managed successfully by adjustment of CsA dosage. The seizures were not related predominantly to the use of hypothermic circulatory arrest, because they occurred least often in infants.

Other CNS problems include lethargy, confusion, behavioral disturbances, localized neurologic defects, and even coma. Investigations such as CT scan, spinal fluid analysis, and electroencephalography studies are indicated to define the nature of these disorders. Fortunately, the problems usually resolve completely.

Reduced postoperative renal function may be a result of preoperative renal insufficiency, poor cardiac function in the early postoperative period, and/or the toxic side effects of CsA. Acute renal failure usually resolves with supportive care and reduction of blood levels of CsA. Many infants experience a transient period of oliguria between 36 and 48 hours, which is typically self-limiting and requires no specific treatment. If severely compromised renal function occurs, the early institution of peritoneal dialysis is extremely effective.[37] Most patients can be salvaged with adequate resolution of their renal failure.

Hepatic dysfunction that is present preoperatively usually resolves after transplantation. Both CsA and azathioprine may become hepatotoxic. Adjustments in dosage levels are usually effective in reversing the toxicity. Cholestasis may develop in patients kept without feedings for long periods, but this typically resolves when enteral alimentation is begun. In our experience, even severe hepatic dysfunction resulting from low cardiac output, hepatotoxic drug use, and poor nutrition will be resolved after transplantation.

CsA may cause hyperplasia of the lining of the intestine, which may serve as a lead point for intussusception. Infants and small children are most vulnerable to this complication. In addition to stresses from transplantation, steroids may promote gastritis and ulceration. Children are usually given a prophylactic H2 antagonist to prevent stress ulceration in the immediate postoperative period.

Bone marrow toxicity includes neutropenia, thrombocytopenia, and lymphopenia. This may be secondary to viral infection (e.g., CMV), cytotoxic immunosuppressive agents, or antithymocyte antibodies. Successful treatment of the cause usually resolves the pattern of bone marrow suppression. We usually reduce the dose of imuran and/or methotrexate in such patients.

T cell lymphoma has been reported in children and adults after transplantation and was usually related to excessive immunosuppression or the presence of EBV. It is unclear whether this is a neoplastic or infectious process. Reduction of immunosuppression usually leads to regression if the disease is detected early. However, deaths have been reported in recipients presenting with greatly advanced disease. The malignancy rate in the survey by Pennington et al was only 3%. We have seen only one case of lymphoproliferative disease (LPD) in 200 infant heart transplants.

Accelerated Graft Atherosclerosis

Accelerated graft atherosclerosis is a serious problem for the cardiac transplant patient.[38] Pediatric heart transplant recipients will be at risk for many years, and the true incidence over time is not yet known. In the study by Pennington et al, the incidence of coronary artery disease (CAD) was only 8%, a number that agrees with our own results in 300 patients. However, in some centers, it has ranged between 14% and 29%. Braunlin et al[39] found angiographically identifiable coronary artery abnormalities in 6 of 17 patients (35%) receiving transplants between the ages of 6 months and 18 years. These children were maintained on triple-drug immunosuppression, including prednisone. None of these recipients died or underwent retransplantation because of CAD.

The cause of accelerated graft atherosclerosis is unclear. The possibilities include an antibody-mediated immune response, chronic CMV infection, steroid use, and hypercholesterolemia. The coronary lesions are diffuse; therefore, angioplasty or coronary bypass are rarely applicable. No effective therapy, short of retransplantation, has been found.[40]

At Loma Linda University, in a study of 157 transplants in infants (< 1 year of age), accelerated coronary artery occlusive disease was documented at autopsy in five children who died of unremitting rejection. Coronary artery occlusive disease was documented in only one other child.

Until December 1995, 301 children less than 18 years of age received cardiac transplants at Loma Linda University. The 1-year actuarial survival was 83% (n = 119), and the 5-year actuarial survival was 71% (n = 6). Children less than 1 year of age (n = 157) had a 1-year actuarial survival of 85% (n = 99), and a 5-year survival of 77% (n = 6). Patients who underwent transplantation at less than 1 month of age (n = 66) had a 1-year survival of 88% (n = 45), and a 5-year survival of 86% (n = 4).

The most common causes of death include ventricular failure and rejection. Infection and rejection are the most common complications. Nearly all survivors have excellent hemodynamics and functional results. Growth and development for the group as a whole approaches normal. Merrill et al[43] also reported normal linear growth in their children treated routinely with only CsA and azathioprine. Abnormal growth and development have been noted in a few children for whom chronic steroid therapy was required because of recurrent rejection.

In a significant number of children (28%), rejection does not occur; however, most children have one or two episodes during the first few post-transplant months. Half develop a significant infection within the first 6 months after transplantation. Backer et al[44] reported a hospital readmission rate of only 1.4 admisions per patient per year.

In Pennington's survey,[25] 85% of 190 patients were in the best functional category. They were able to attend school and participate in sports and recreational activities. Only 4% were bedridden, and 3% could not attend school. These data suggest that rehabilitation after cardiac transplantation is more successful in children than in adults. Psychomotor and mental development have been normal, and 89% of survivors are believed to be neurodevelopmentally normal.[45]

The Future

The single most important issue confronting the future of pediatric heart transplantation is donor organ supply. Donor organ resources under investigation include xenotransplantation,[46] reanimation of "dead" hearts,[47] and further assessment of anencephalic infants as possible organ donors.[48]

Improved immunoregulatory agents and techniques, coupled with newer surveillance methods for the detection of early graft rejection, will very likely enhance the durability and predictability of heart transplant therapy. In addition, further research into the etiology and treatment of post-transplant atherosclerosis should improve long-term results.

Conclusions

Cardiac transplantation in infants and children is an effective therapeutic modality with postoperative results comparable to those of adults. Adaptations to accommodate children with complex malformations remain a challenge to the pediatric heart surgeon. The most common causes of death include rejection and ventricular failure, but infection and rejection are the most frequent long-term complications. Other common problems include hypertension, seizures, and a small incidence of CAD. It is clear that cardiac transplantation is worthwhile and provides excellent functional lives for many children and their families.

References

1. Kantrowitz A, Haller JD, Joss H, et al: Transplantation of the heart in an infant and an adult. *Am J Cardiol* 22:782–790, 1968.
2. Borel JF: Immunosuppressive properties of cyclosporin A (CY-A). *Transplant Proc* 12:233, 1980.
3. Strom TB, Carpenter CB: Transplantation: immunogenetic and clinical aspects. Part II. *Hosp Pract* 1:135–150, 1983.
4. Griffin ML, Hernandez A, Martin TC, et al: Dilated cardiomyopathy in infants and children. *J Am Coll Cardiol* 11:139–144, 1988.
5. Lewis AB: Clinical profile and outcome of restrictive cardiomyopathy in children. *Am Heart J* 123:1589–1593, 1992.
6. Penkoske PA, Rowe RD, Freedom RM, et al: The future of heart and heart-lung transplantation in children. *J Heart Transplant* 3:233–238, 1984.
7. Griffith BP, Hardesty RL, Trento A, et al: Heart-lung transplantation: lessons learned and future hopes. *Ann Thorac Surg* 43:6–16, 1987.
8. Starnes VA, Lewiston NJ, Luikart H, et al: Current trends in lung transplantation: lobar transplantation and expanded use of single lungs. *J Thorac Cardiovasc Surg* 104:1060–1066, 1992.
9. Ruiz CE, Gamra H, Zhang HP, et al: Stenting of ductus arteriosus of infants with hypoplastic left heart syndrome—first human experience (abstr). *Eur Heart J* 13(suppl):329, 1992.
10. Starnes VA, Griffith ML, Pitlick PT, et al: Current approach to hypoplastic left heart syndrome: palliation, transplantation, or both? *J Thorac Cardiovasc Surg* 104:189–194, 1992.
11. Kells CM, Marshall S, Kramer M, et al: Cardiac function after domino-donor heart transplantation. *Am J Cardiol* 69:113–116, 1992.
12. Bailey L, Concepcion W, Shattuck H, et al: Method of heart transplantation for treatment of hypooplastic left heart syndrome. *J Thorac Cardiovasc Surg* 92:1–5, 1986.
13. Mavroudis C, Harrison H, Klein JB, et al: Infant orthotopic cardiac transplantation. *J Thorac Cardiovasc Surg* 96:912–924, 1988.
14. Chartrand C: Pediatric cardiac transplantation despite atrial and venous return anomalies. *Ann Thorac Surg* 52:716–721, 1991.
15. Doty DB, Renlund DG, Caputo GR, et al: Cardiac transplantation in situs inversus. *J Thorac Cardiovasc Surg* 99:493–499, 1990.
16. Trento A, Griffith BP, Fricker FJ, et al: Lessons learned in pediatric heart transplantation. *Ann Thorac Surg* 48:617–623, 1989.
17. Mayer JE Jr, Perry S, O'Brien P, et al: Orthotopic heart transplantation for complex congenital heart disease. *J Thorac Cardiovasc Surg* 99:484–492, 1990.
18. Cooper MM, Fuzesi L, Addonizio LJ, et al: Pediatric heart transplantation after operations involving the pulmonary arteries. *J Thorac Cardiovasc Surg* 102:386–395, 1991.
19. Backer CL, Idriss FS, Zales VR, et al: Cardiac transplantation for hypoplastic left heart syndrome: a modified technique. *Ann Thorac Surg* 1990;50:894–498, 1990.
20. Bailey L: The Loma Linda drug protocol for infant heart transplantation. *J Heart Lung Transplant* 10(suppl):836–837, 1991.
21. Baughman KL: Monitoring of allograft rejection, in heart and heart-lung transplantation. In: Baumgartner WA, Reitz BA, Achuff SC (eds). 157–164, 1990.
22. Canter CE, Appleton RS, Saffitz JE, et al: Surveillance for rejection by echocardiographically guides biopsy in the infant heart transplant recipient. *Circulation* 84(suppl):310–315, 1991.
23. Boucek MM, Mathis CM, Kanakriyeh MS, et al: Noninvasive cardiac rejection surveillance in infant transplantation (abstr). *Pediatr Res* 25:21, 1989.
24. Kawauchi M, Boucek MM, Gundry SR, et al: Changes in left ventricular mass with rejection after heart transplantation in infants. *J Heart Lung Transplant* 11:99–102, 1992.
25. Pennington DG, Noedel N, McBride LR, et al: Heart transplantation in children: an international survey. *Ann Thorac Surg* 52:710–715, 1991.
26. Chiavarelli M, Boucek MM, Nehlsen-Cannarella SL, et al: Neonatal cardiac transplantation: intermediate-term results and incidence of rejection. *Arch Surg* 127:1072–1076, 1992.

27. Galantowicz ME, Stolar CJH: Extracorporeal membrane oxygenation for perioperative support in pediatric heart transplantation. *J Thorac Cardiovasc Surg* 102:148–152, 1991.
28. Karwande SV, Ensley RD, Renlund DG, et al: Cardiac retransplantation: a viable option? *Ann Thorac Surg* 54:840–845, 1992.
29. Hofflin JM, Potasman I, Baldwin JC, et al: Infectious complications in heart transplant recipients receiving cyclosporine and corticosteroids. *Ann Intern Med* 106:209–216, 1987.
30. Andreone PA, Olivari MT, Elick B, et al: Reduction of infectious complications following heart transplantation with triple drug immunotherapy. *J Heart Transplant* 5:13–19, 1986.
31. Onorato IM, Morens DM, Martone WJ, et al: Epidemiology of cytomegaloviral infections: recommendations for prevention and control. *Rev Infect Dis* 7:4, 1985.
32. Kramer MR, Stoehr C, Lewiston NJ, et al: Trimethoprimsulfamethoxazole prophylaxis for pneumocystis carinii infections in heart-lung and lung transplantation: how effective and for how long? *Transplantation* 53:586–589, 1992.
33. Addonizio LJ, Rose EA: Cardiac transplantations in children and adolescents. *J Pediatr* 111: 1034–1038, 1987.
34. Starnes VA, Bernstein D, Oyer PE, et al: Heart transplantation in children. *J Heart Transplant* 8:20–26, 1989.
35. Addonizio LJ, Hsu DT, Smith CR, et al: Late complications in pediatric cardiac transplant recipients. *Circulation* 82(suppl):295–301, 1990.
36. Dunn JM, Cavarocchi NC, Balsra RK: Pediatric heart transplantation at St. Christopher's Hospital for Children. *J Heart Transplant* 6:334–342, 1987.
37. Vricella L, Alonso de Begona J, Gundry S, et al: Aggressive peritoneal dialysis for treatment of renal failure after neonatal cardiac transplant (abstr). *J Heart Lung Transplant* 10:183, 1991.
38. Pahl E, Fricker FJ, Armitage J, et al: Coronary arteriosclerosis in pediatric heart transplant survivors: limitation of long-term survival. *J Pediatr* 116:177–183, 1990.
39. Braunlin EA, Hunter DW, Canter CE, et al: Coronary artery disease in pediatric cardiac transplantl recipients receiving triple-drug immunosuppression. *Circulation* 84:303–309, 1991.
40. Fricker FJ, Griffith BP, Hardesty RL, et al: Experience with heart transplantation in children. *Pediatrics* 79:138–146, 1987.
41. Uzark K, Crowley D, Callow L, et al: Hypercholesterolemia after cardiac transplantation in children. *Am J Cardiol* 66:1385–1387, 1990.
42. Kottke TE, Pesch DG, Frye RL, et al: The potential contribution of cardiac replacement to the control of cardiovascular diseases: a population-based estimate. *Arch Surg* 125:1148–1151, 1990.
43. Merrill WH, Frist WH, Stewart JR, et al: Heart transplantation in children. *Ann Surg* 213: 393–400, 1991.
44. Backer CL, Zales VR, Harrison HL, et al: Intermediate term results of infant orthotopic cardiac transplantation from two centers. *J Thorac Cardiovasc Surg* 101:826–832, 1991.
45. Baum MF, Cutler DC, Fricker FJ, et al: Physiologic and psychologic growth and development in pediatric heart transplant recipients. *J Heart Lung Transplant* 10(suppl):848–855, 1991.
46. Bailey LL: Another look at cardiac xenotransplantation. *J Cardiac Surg* 5:210–218, 1990.
47. Gundry SR, Kawauchi M, Liu H, et al: Successful heart transplantation in lambs using asystolic, pulseless, "dead" donors (abstr). *J Am Coll Cardiol* 15:224, 1990.
48. Bailey LL: Donor organs from human anencephalics: a salutory resource for infant heart transplantation. *Transplant Proc* 20(suppl):35–38, 1988.

Chapter 7

Benefits and Pitfalls of Transplantation for Patients With Congenital Heart Disease

Linda J. Addonizio, MD; Marianne R. Kichuk, MD,
Jonathan M. Chen, MD; Robert E. Michler, MD

Introduction

In almost 30 years since the first successful human cardiac transplant, the outlook for the transplant patient has improved dramatically. The International Society for Heart and Lung Transplantation (ISHLT) has recorded over 30,000 cardiac transplants since 1980. Although the procedure is an accepted therapy for end-stage heart disease in adults, the evolution and acceptance of cardiac transplantation as a standard of care in children remains elusive. It has only been in the last decade that a rapid expansion of the worldwide experience in pediatric cardiac transplantation has occurred, with children now comprising about 10% of the total cardiac transplants performed annually. Currently, the 5-year actuarial survival is 70% in children.[1] Although long-term survival can be considered excellent, and equivalent to adult series, the ultimate outlook for extended survival remains unknown, and will be affected by the management of late complications that occur either as a result of side effects of the immunosuppressive drugs, or from ineffective immunosuppressive protection of the graft. Additionally, further expansion of cardiac transplantation to accommodate the growing number of children now surviving with palliative repairs of complex congenital heart lesions continues to emphasize the limited supply of donor organs. It is this on-going donor organ demand that provides the impetus for research expansion to find alternative donor sources and therapies for children with end-stage heart disease.

From: Franco KL (ed). *Pediatric Cardiopulmonary Transplantation.* Armonk, NY: Futura Publishing Company, Inc.; © 1997.

Historical Perspective

The first reports of cardiac transplantation in the pediatric age group were by Kantrowitz et al in 1967[2] and Cooley et al in 1968[3] that occurred at the same time as the pioneering efforts in adult patients by Shumway and Barnard. Although both these infants died perioperatively, the early adult experience was equally discouraging, because the available immunosuppressive therapy was nonspecific and inadequate. The lifestyles of the few survivors was difficult, with recurrent rejection episodes and multiple, serious infections often leading to death. Few children were transplanted thereafter until the advent of cyclosporine (CsA) immunosuppression. CsA's more selective immunosuppressive properties led to greatly improved survival in adult series. As it became clear that transplant patients could lead active and productive lives using CsA-based immunosuppression, a rapid increase in the number of pediatric cardiac transplants soon followed. Whereas, prior to 1980, less than five children (all adolescents) received cardiac transplants each year, a rapid increase in early childhood transplantations began in 1984. Thirty-seven children were transplanted in 1984 as reported by the ISHLT Registry, with 25% being less than 10 years of age. By January 1994, the ISHLT Registry had recorded over 2100 heart transplants that were performed in children between birth and 18 years. In addition, the mean age of the children receiving transplants had decreased notably. For the past 5 years, over half of the recipients each year have been less than 5 years of age.[1]

Diagnostic Indications for Transplantation

Cardiac transplantation is indicated in any patient with end-stage heart disease who is refractory to maximal medical therapy, and for whom there is no available surgical procedure that could reasonably restore them to a productive life. The two main diagnostic indications for heart transplant in the pediatric age group are diseases of the heart muscle and complex congenital heart disease. Over 90% of pediatric recipients fall into either of these diagnostic categories: cardiomyopathy in 57% of children, and congenital heart disease in 35%.[4] Although there are still a greater total number of pediatric patients who have received transplants for cardiomyopathic processes, over the past 10 years, there has been a gradual and steady increase in the number of patients with complex congenital heart lesions coming to transplant as a primary or salvage procedure. Whereas, in the early 1980s, cardiomyopathy was the most common diagnosis in the young transplant recipient, accounting for 80% of the patients, according to the ISHLT Registry, the proportion of children with congenital heart disease who were transplanted increased from 16% in 1984 to 46% in 1993. In addition, there has been a growing number of pediatric cardiac recipients les than 1 year of age that can be explained by the advocacy of many centers for transplantation as the primary procedure for infants with hypoplastic left heart syndrome (HLHS). Retransplantation in pediatric patients accounts for only 3% of the cardiac transplants performed yearly.

The cardiomyopathies represent a diverse number of diseases affecting the myocardial muscle (Table 1). The most common type to require cardiac transplantation is

Table 1.

Diagnostic Indications for Heart Transplantation in Children

Cardiomyopathy

Dilated
  Idiopathic
  Familial
  Postviral (Myocarditis)
  Adriamycin toxicity
  Endocardial fibroelastosis
Restrictive
  Idiopathic
  Endocardial fibroelastosis
Hypertrophic
  Nonobstructive
  Obstructive

Congenital Heart Disease

Complex defects when repair unfeasible
  Pulmonary atresia with coronary sinusoids
  Complex single ventricle with AV valve insufficiency
Ventricular failure following previous surgery
Failed physiology (failed Fontan)

Ischemic Disease

Anomalous left coronary artery (postrepair)
Kawasaki's disease

This list of diagnostic indications for cardiac transplantation is not exhaustive, but is meant to give the general types of disease which may eventually come to transplantation. AV=atrioventricular.

dilated cardiomyopathy. The majority of these cases are of the idiopathic subtype. However, there are a substantial number of children with dilated cardiomyopathy who have been transplanted for endocardial fibroelastosis, adriamycin toxicity, postmyocarditis myopathy, and familial dilated cardiomyopathy. Hypertrophic and restrictive cardiomyopathies represent a small number of the cases. A multi-institutional study was performed by the Pediatric Heart Lung Transplant Study Group, evaluating the outcome of children listed for transplantation in 1993.[5] In 33% of the children over 6 months of age at listing the diagnosis was idiopathic dilated cardiomyopathy, myocarditis in 8%, hypertrophic cardiomyopathy in 8%, and restrictive cardiomyopathy in 3%, whereas 47% had congenital heart disease. In contrast, 86% of the infants less than 6 months of age at listing had congenital heart disease (59% alone had HLHS), and only 5% had idiopathic cardiomyopathy.[6] It is estimated that perhaps 10% to 20% of children with congenital heart disease might benefit from transplantation in their lifetimes. Since the outcome from complex congenital heart repairs has improved dramatically over the years, with the ability of these children to have long-term quality survival, most children who come to transplant with congenital heart disease have undergone one or more attempts at palliative or corrective cardiac surgery (Table 1). Heart transplantation in these children presents a number of special problems.

Clinical Indications

The general clinical indications for referral to a transplant program include increasing congestive heart failure (CHF) despite maximal oral anticongestive medications, and afterload reduction with an angiotensin-converting enzyme (ACE) inhibitor, or deteriorating left ventricular (LV) function despite the above measures. A patient with end-stage heart disease should be evaluated if they are being hospitalized frequently, or if an estimate of their life expectancy is less than 12 months. Malignant arrhythmias that cannot be well controlled with medications, devices, or ablations, are an indication for transplant if the risk of sudden death is considered high. In these patients, an implantable defibrillator may be used as a bridge to transplantation. In addition, patients with end-stage heart disease who have growth failure, protein-losing enteropathy, cardiac cachexia, severe cyanosis from arteriovenous malformations following surgical repair, and/or an unacceptably poor quality of life should be referred for transplant evaluation, even when their "failure" appears to be in "control," because their margin of safety is very narrow, and the wait for a suitable donor can be prolonged.

Although the majority of patients who require transplant have severe systemic ventricular dysfunction, there are many children with congenital heart lesions in whom the basis for referral is not LV failure. The clinical indications for transplant are less easily determined in these patients, and the diagnosis of "CHF" very much depends on the normal physiology of their specific congenital lesion. A child may be a candidate for transplant with severe right ventricular (RV) failure and multivalvar insufficiency where the surgical risk for repair is deemed too high, even though systemic ventricular dysfunction is only mildly depressed. This is seen most often in the context of ventricular inversion where the systemic ventricle is a morphologic right ventricle. In a patient with a Fontan repair, there is no pulmonary ventricle and, therefore, the cardiac output from the LV is dependent on passive pulmonary blood flow. In these patients, only a mild decrease in LV function or a decrease in diastolic compliance, particularly in combination with an abnormality in lung function or perfusion could be responsible for low cardiac output (failure of forward flow), and make transplantation the only option for survival. However, sometimes in this lesion, other reasons such as bronchopulmonary collaterals may be responsible for competing with the passive pulmonary flow, and embolization may obviate the need for a transplant. Children with complex congenital heart disease, especially those with Fontan physiology, who may require a transplant should be evaluated at an experienced congenital heart surgery center to ensure that other operative alternatives are not indicated, and that all necessary preoperative questions are answered.

Recipient Selection

Because cardiac transplantation is a cure of last resort, the evaluation and selection process must initially be directed toward determining the existence of other treatment options for palliation or cure, as well as toward appropriateness of the candidate for transplantation. Each child referred for transplantation should be evaluated by members of the transplant team, including a pediatric cardiologist, cardiothoracic surgeon, transplant nurse specialist, pediatric neurologist, pediatric psychiatrist, social worker, physical therapist, and beyond the infant stage, a pediatric dentist. The patient is assessed for the presence of other diseases of the major organ systems, or permanent underlying organ dysfunction, which would affect post-transplant management, or make transplantation dangerous or unsuitable. In addition, the psychosocial preparedness of the child and family are considered, and plans are formulated for care and support.

Contraindications to transplantation have decreased dramatically since the early transplant series, as surgical techniques have excelled and myocardial protection has improved. In addition, we have learned more about postoperative care of these patients, and immunosuppression has become more specific. The consequence of these improvements is that there are now few absolute contraindications to orthotopic cardiac transplantation. Anatomically, orthotopic cardiac transplantation is feasible in even the most complex of congenital heart lesions if the pulmonary arteries are of a reasonable size; the patient with "string-like" pulmonary arteries would not be a candidate for an orthotopic transplant, and would need to be considered for a heart-lung transplant. However, orthotopic transplantation has been performed in cases where there is only one pulmonary artery, and the other lung is fed by collaterals or relatively unperfused.[7-10] The type of reconstructive surgery of extracardiac defects required at implantation must be carefully considered. Pulmonary artery reconstruction both for kinking or stenoses following systemic to pulmonary shunts or bands, can be performed successfully at the time of transplantation.[11] Previous studies have detailed the many unique and creative technical approaches to cardiac transplantation in patients with systemic and venous anomalies, heterotaxy syndromes, HLHS, dextrocardia, and transposition of the great arteries.[7-20]

Prior to transplantation, the child must have a complete cardiac catheterization to rule out other operative alternatives and to delineate the extent of the accompanying defects that will affect not only the transplant surgery, but also the postoperative care. For example, the child with the single ventricle complex who has been cyanotic in the past or after Fontan, should be evaluated for the presence of bronchial collateral vessels and pulmonary arteriovenous malformations. Knowledge of the systemic and pulmonary venous anatomy is also important to plan appropriate surgical repair. Additionally, it is necessary to know the condition of the femoral system in those children who have had multiple, previous operations, where the institution of groin bypass might be preferable before entering the chest. The catheterization must also include evaluation of the pulmonary vascular resistance. High pulmonary vascular resistance has always been an absolute contraindication for orthotopic cardiac transplantation, because the donor RV is not functionally able to pump against this instantaneous workload. However, the physiologic upper limit of resistance beyond which orthotopic transplantation cannot be successful has not been determined. It is a continuum of risk. An early analysis of pulmonary vascular resistance and transplantation in 82 adult patients at our institution showed the necessity of indexing pulmonary resistance to body surface area, hence the term pulmonary vascular resistance index (PVRI).[21] Although accepted by pediatric cardiologists, indexing is no less pertinent in the adult patient, especially in cases where the cardiac outputs are low. No patient developed right heart failure after transplantation in our study, if the PVRI was less than six indexed units. Whereas we observed four deaths secondary to acute right heart failure in adult patients with preoperative PVR less than five Wood units (nonindexed). Indexing PVR identified a subpopulation of 25 out of the 73 patients previously known to have acceptably low PVR by Wood criteria, who were at risk for developing right heart failure. In the patients with PVRI >6, 30% developed right heart failure with a 15% mortality. Pediatric patients referred for transplantation often have a higher incidence of elevated pulmonary vascular resistance, whether secondary to unoperated congenital heart lesions, or long-term CHF. In 1993, we reported on our experience with cardiac transplantation in children with markedly elevated pulmonary vascular resistance.[22] Of 72 pediatric recipients, 40% had PVRI >6 with a mean of 10 indexed units (range from 6 to 16). The mean transpulmonary gradient (TPG) in these patients was 20 mm Hg, with 80% of the patients having TPG >15. With maximal vasodilator testing, there were 12 patients whose resistance remained >6, with 8 patients developing right heart failure perioperatively, with two deaths. Two of the eight required temporary right ventricular assist devices (RVAD) and survived. From this extensive experience, we developed the following recommendations for preoperative evaluation of PVRI. If the PVRI is <6 indexed units initially, then the patient may be listed. At the same time, the medical regimen should be optimized either by the addition of intravenous inotropes, and vasodilator therapy, when the cardiac index is extremely low or alteration of their oral regime, if the patient is stable. If the PVRI >6 and the cardiac index is near normal, then the patient is given a graded nitroprusside infusion to test acute vasoreactivity. If unsuccessful, a 1-week course of tailored inotropes and vasodilators including dobutamine, amrinone, and nitroprusside will be given and a repeat hemodynamic study is performed. In selected patients, prostacyclin or nitric oxide, if available, can be used for testing and therapy. Our purpose for these multiple studies is not only to determine transplantability, but also to find the optimal postoperative regimen. If the resistance remains in the 6 to 9 range, despite all these measures, then the patient could still receive an orthotopic transplant, but at a greatly increased risk, with the knowledge that the severity of the postoperative right heart failure will be unknown, and that an assist device may be necessary. If the resistance stays >9, despite maximal care, then the patient should be evaluated for either a heart-lung, heart-single lung, or heterotopic transplantation, unless longer-term vasodilator and inotrope therapy might be deemed useful. Patients with PVRI >9 have successfully been transplanted with a higher risk for RV (40%), however, with only a 10% to 15% mortality.[21,22]

Other testing that should be performed pretransplant on children, especially with congenital heart disease, include pulmonary function studies and quantitative ventilation perfusion scans. These studies provide important physiologic information that can aid in post-transplant management, and add to the understanding of the cardiac dysfunction preoperatively in these patients. In addition, patients with poor ventricular function are also at risk for the development of atrial and ventricular thrombi in these low-flow states, with the attendant complications that could preclude transplantation. Hsu et al reported that 39% of our pediatric patients had either experienced an embolic event such as a stroke, or pulmonary embolus, or were at risk for such an occurrence on the basis of known intracardiac thrombus by the time they were referred for heart transplant evaluation.[23] Preoperative brain imaging should be considered at the request of the neurologist, particularly in those patients with previous events, or who are very cyanotic.

Serologic and immunologic screening is also performed during the evaluation process. Serologies are obtained for cytomegalovirus (CMV), toxoplasmosis, Ebstein-

Barr virus (EBV), hepatitis A, B and non-A, non-B, human immunodeficiency virus (HIV), varicella, and herpes simplex virus (HSV). Skin testing for tuberculosis and anergy screening are performed. CMV and toxoplasmosis screening are important because of the potential for transmission of these infections via the donor organs, and the high morbidity and mortality associated with them in transplant recipients who are seronegative. Since approximately 40% of the population is positive for CMV virus, screening is essential. Prophylactic use of hyperimmune globulin and antiviral agents, such as acyclovir, is advocated in patients who are CMV-negative, who receive hearts from CMV-positive donors. CMV-negative blood products are used at the time of transplant, even in seropostive recipients, because of the chance for exposure to a different strain of CMV. Exposure to EBV has been associated with the development of post-transplant lymphoproliferative disease (PTLD), a form of lymphoma that can occur in transplant recipients. It has been shown that transplant patients who acquire the virus soon after transplant (or from their donor) seem to have an increased risk for developing an early and severe form of PTLD, therefore, preoperative screening and donor screening are important.[24,25] Varicella status is important in the pediatric population because of the high exposure to active cases. The remainder of the immunologic work-up consists of ABO blood typing for donor matching, human lymphocyte antigen (HLA) typing for retrospective use, and measurement of percent reactive antibody (PRA) against a donor panel. If the PRA is high, attempts are made to effect a donor-recipient cytotoxic screen prior to transplantation. Likewise, if prominent sensitivity to a specific HLA type is demonstrated, donor HLA typing will be carried out prior to transplantation. Unlike the adult population, in our pediatric series, there is a high incidence of elevated PRA greater than 25% pretransplant that did not correlate with poor outcome post-transplant.[26]

Optimal Timing for Referral

The natural history of adults with heart failure secondary to idiopathic cardiomyopathy and ischemic disease has been well documented. Multiple risk factors for poor survival and sudden death have been isolated for adults, such as low ejection fraction, persistent high-filling pressures despite maximal medical therapy, ventricular and atrial arrhythmias, low serum sodium, and a history of previous cardiac arrest.[27-30] These parameters are felt to be reliable predictors of early mortality and, therefore, are used to identify patients in need of transplantation. In contrast, for the pediatric patient, the natural history of heart failure syndromes is not precisely defined. Although it is obvious that a child with end-stage heart failure who requires inotropic support should be evaluated for transplant, the progression of disease in children with cardiomyopathy who are not yet hospital bound can be very unpredictable. In many children with significant ventricular dysfunction, the symptoms of heart failure may or may not be present, and clinical parameters alone are deceptive. Therefore, it is often more difficult to determine the timing for referral for transplant evaluation of the pediatric outpatient whose heart failure seems compensated.

In a large pediatric series, Lewis and Michelle reviewed the clinical and laboratory features of 81 infants and children with dilated cardiomyopathy (mean age 3.6 years), in order to identify patients who should be referred for transplantation.[31] They found that nonsurvivors were more likely to have significant arrhythmias, and higher left ventricular end diastolic pressure (LVEDP) (mean 29.5 mm Hg), than survivors over a mean follow-up of 3.5 years. The left ventricular ejection fraction (LVEF) by echocardiography and the age at presentation was not predictive of mortality. The actuarial survival revealed that the mortality was highest during the first 6 months after presentation (19%). From these data, they concluded that markedly elevated LVEDP is a significant risk factor for early death, as all but one patient with an LVEDP greater than 25 mm Hg had either died or undergone transplantation. The 1- and 5-year survival in these children was 64% and 32%, respectively. Therefore, this subgroup would appear to benefit from urgent transplantation. Data from two pediatric studies in our own institution show that children who are extremely ill, requiring maximal medical support at the time of presentation for evaluation, have a decreased chance of surviving to transplantation, as well as surviving after transplantation.[32,33] A retrospective analysis of our early series of pediatric cardiac transplant recipients showed that only 23% of them were considered normal risk; 77% were high-risk candidates that had developed significant pulmonary hypertension or hemodynamic decompensation requiring inotropic support, and mechanical ventilation prior to transplantation. We studied the effects of preoperative factors on postoperative mortality to try to identify those future patients who might have the most successful outcome following transplantation.[32] These preoperative variables included: pulmonary hypertension; inotrope dependency; age; need for hospitalization; congenital heart disease; surgical pulmonary artery reconstruction; prior stroke; cardiac arrest(s); and mechanical ventilator dependence. None of the individual potential risk factors was a significant predictor of risk, although pulmonary hypertension approached significance. However, the combined presence of pulmonary hypertension and inotrope dependency was a highly significant predictor of post-transplant mortality (relative risk 4 to 1). The 1-year actuarial survival following transplantation of patients with this combination was 30% versus 84% without these risk factors. Although long-term survival was possible in our population with these high-risk factors, clearly, the best results and survival in pediatric transplantation are obtained when candidates do not have pulmonary hypertension or inotrope dependency. We next examined the outcome of over 60 children with cardiomyopathy who were listed for transplantation, in order to determine specific risk factors for death pretransplant. Children with a combination of LV fractional shortening of less than 10% who also require mechanical ventilation as a therapy for heart failure, had a greater than tenfold risk of dying prior to cardiac transplantation.[33] This finding has been substantiated by data collected from a multi-institutional study from the Pediatric Heart and Lung Transplant Study Group on outcome of listing of pediatric patients for cardiac transplantation.[5] By multivariable analysis, two risk factors were identified for death, while waiting, in the 146 children over 6 months of age listed during a 1-year period: status 1 at listing (patients in ICU on inotropic support) and ventilator support at listing. Among status 1 patients at listing, ventilatory support was the single risk factor identified for earlier death. In addition, recipients who were blood group O had a significantly longer wait until transplant. Since a high percentage of status 1 patients belonged to blood group O, it was clear that extremely ill children with O blood type had a high risk of dying pretransplant.

These studies confirm the world experience that many children referred for transplantation already have severe hemodynamic decompensation and inotrope dependency prior to referral, and may also have developed pulmonary hypertension with increased pulmonary vascular resistance from years of LV dysfunction. Although children can survive transplantation and thrive despite extreme debilitation and multiorgan failure preoperatively, it is clear that these risk factors affect their chance for survival and their postoperative morbidity. In addition, with the increasing demands for donor hearts, as well as the unpredictable waiting time for a donor organ, many more children will die prior to transplantation, or will develop complications that would make them ineligible for the procedure. This preoperative mortality can be as high as 30%, even in patients who have medical regimens optimally tailored using hemodynamic studies. It is critical to evaluate these children earlier in the course of their disease, even though transplant may be postponed for an extended period. Knowledge of future therapeutic options is helpful to a family facing these decisions, and having the evaluation completed means that the child could be listed urgently, should a rapid deterioration in clinical status occur.

As pretransplant waiting times become prolonged and the competition for a limited donor supply also increases, mechanical devices should also be considered as a bridge to transplant when maximal medical support becomes ineffective. Depending upon the degree of cardiac dysfunction and anatomy of the patient, right, left, or biventricular support may be necessary. Left ventricular assist devices (LVAD) and RVAD can be used in all age groups. Because of the size limitations of the totally implantable battery driven devices, only external forms of support can be used in most small children and infants. Some examples include extracorporeal membrane oxygenation (ECMO), biomedicus pumps, Abiomed pulsatile devices, and TCI (Thermo Cardiosystems Incorporated heartmate LV assist device. Circulation of blood is maintained via either pneumatically driven drive chambers, pusher plate action, or centrifugal pumps similar to those incorporated into routine cardiopulmonary bypass. With these types of circuits, the cannulae are implanted into the venous (inflow) and arterial (outflow) sides of the system, usually directly into the heart through a median sternotomy. If isolated LV support is required, an LVAD can be used with inflow cannulation of the left atrium and outflow cannulation of the ascending aorta. This, however, presumes adequate pulmonary blood flow and oxygenation, though an oxygenator can be added to the circuit. LV support is effective in patients in whom low systemic output is the major concern, however, in many patients RV function is not adequate enough to handle the normal flow provided by the LVAD, and a biventricular device (BVAD) must be used. Additionally, all devices with the exception of the implantable Heartmate require heparinization to prevent clot formation. The advantage of using assist devices as a bridge to transplant is that once normal cardiac output is restored, end-organ dysfunction may be halted and improved prior to transplant. However, when the choice for devices involve only the external pumps secondary to pediatric size limitations, a donor heart must be identified quickly to prevent the occurrence of infection, uncontrolled coagulopathy, or embolic events that can occur with lengthy dependence on external mechanical support.[34]

RVADs and ECMO cannulation can be placed through the internal jugular and carotid artery, an effective, short-term management for certain patients with lung damage in whom transplantation is being considered. Patients who do well with this type of management include those with temporary pulmonary dysfunction secondary to a transient and treatable event, such as aspiration pneumonia, postoperative complications, or respiratory distress syndrome ("shock lung"). We have not limited the use of mechanical assist devices to patients who are awaiting cardiac transplant, and in fact have successfully used right heart assist devices after transplantation in patients with persistent pulmonary hypertension and right heart failure.[35]

Donor Selection and Operation

As with adult transplant recipients, there are several criteria used in the pediatric population for identifying an appropriate donor heart. Hearts are matched by blood type, body size, degree of recipient illness (status), and length of time on the waiting list. HLA matching occurs only in retrospect with the exception of patients in whom it is felt a direct cross-match is necessary because of preformed antibodies. ABO blood type compatability is of primary importance. Hearts from donors with type O blood can be transplanted successfully into recipients of any blood type; however, type O recipients can only receive type O donor hearts. Since patients are listed nationally not only by blood type, but also by length of time on the list, recipients with type O blood necessarily wait longer for donors, because same-sized A and B recipients who have been listed longer will receive a type O heart before them. Pediatric organ donors must fulfill the criteria for brain death, and have no active infections or disseminated malignancies. However, because of the severe organ shortage, especially in the infant weight range, every effort is made to utilize marginal donors, including repair of small structural defects (e.g., atrial or ventricular septal defects).

Size mismatch of the donor and recipient is common in the pediatric population. It is unusual to find an exact size match for an infant or child, and the acceptable weight range for a donor can be quite broad, up to triple the body weight of a recipient. Cardiomegaly in the recipient affords this greater potential pericardial space to accommodate the larger donor organ. In the recipient with a normal-sized heart, as in restrictive cardiomyopathy or certain congenital lesions, care must be taken to more precisely match donor body size to prevent postoperative restriction and tamponade. Echocardiographic measurements of cardiac size can be used to determine if a heart is too big or too small, when compared to standard nomograms for the "normal" size heart for that recipient. Radiographic estimates of heart size, taken from plain chest films, are not as exact and may lead to donor-recipient mismatch.

Ischemic time of the donor heart must be considered. Most hearts can tolerate up to 4 to 5 hours of ischemic time, with relatively normal function after transplantation. The current use of improved forms of myocardial preservation, such as UW (University of Wisconsin) cardioplegia solution, has diminished the damaging effects of long periods of cold ischemia. This advantage is afforded by the biochemical composition of the preservative solution; precursors of oxidative metabolism, antioxidants, and mediators of endothelial cell function are contained in a viscous vehicle that further decreases myocardial edema. It has been suggested that pediatric donor hearts are more able to tolerate longer ischemic times. While these newer forms of myocardial preservation are beneficial, and successful preservation times of up to 9 hours have been reported, it is still not clear whether or not these extraordinary ischemic times postoperatively result in more myocardial edema, diminished contractility, and increased myocardial hypertrophy.

Beyond the newborn age, most children with congenital heart disease who ultimately undergo transplantation have previously sustained one or more attempts at palliative or corrective heart surgery. Thus, heart transplantation in these children presents a number of potential problems unique to this predicament. The indications and optimal timing of transplantation (as discussed previously) can be difficult to determine in patients with complex heart disease. The type of reconstructive surgery for extracardiac defects must be considered carefully by the surgical team prior to transplantation. Previous studies have reported many innovative technical approaches to cardiac transplantation in patients with systemic and venous anomalies, pulmonary artery stenosis, HLHS, dextrocardia, and transposition of the great arteries.

Preparation and Conduct of the Operation

The goal of heart transplantation in complex congenital heart disease is twofold: it represents both replacement and reparative surgery. While intracardiac congenital malformations are replaced, and, therefore, pose few obstacles to the transplant surgeon, extracardiac malformations, whether they are congenital or iatrogenic in origin (from prior palliative reconstructive procedures), present a major challenge to the operative team.

Understanding the operative plan for managing each lesion is essential for the donor team in order to harvest sufficient additional donor tissue to allow for adequate anastomoses and for the creation of potential conduits. Thus, since time is often limited at operation, preparation for the procedure requires a thorough discussion of the options well in advance of the date of surgery.

Following the placement of intravenous lines, a central venous line, and when possible, a Swan-Ganz catheter, the patient is put to sleep after confirming the acceptability of the donor heart with the donor team. It is at this time that estimated times of cross-clamping of the donor heart and travel time are calculated, permitting the procedure to begin. However, it is not infrequent that the recipient team must commence its procedure prior to visualization of the donor heart in order to limit the amount of donor heart cold ischemic time. These decisions are based upon the time estimate for reentry into the patient who has undergone prior corrective or palliative open-heart procedures, and is intended to minimize the duration of donor ischemia as well as recipient cardiopulmonary bypass time.

In patients with multiple prior reoperative procedures, as well as in all patients who have undergone previous Fontan procedures, peripheral cardiopulmonary bypass is uniformly instituted through cannulation of the femoral artery and vein. When recipient size permits, a Biomedicus centrifugal pump is used for the venous cannulation. Once entry into the chest has been accomplished, and the great vessels and atria have been dissected, it is not uncommon to recannulate the patient centrally in order to ensure sufficient flow at low-line pressure.

Of note, the aortic cannula may be inserted in the distal ascending aorta. However, for those patients in whom reconstruction and/or replacement of the ascending aorta is an anticipated potential procedure, the cannula may be placed beyond the innominate artery. Further, those patients with ductal-dependent circulation may benefit additionally from a cannula placed in the main pulmonary artery directed through the ductus.[36] Similarly, although venous drainage is generally achieved through separate cannulation of the venae cavae, patients with previous procedures involving the superior vena cava (SVC)(such as a Glenn shunt) may require cannulation proximal to the anastomosis. Other venous anomalies will be discussed below.

The recipient is cooled to 32°C if a relatively straightforward procedure and short ischemic time are anticipated. However, for complex procedures in which either more extensive dissection and reconstruction or increased bronchial venous return is anticipated, patients are cooled to 24°C. The aorta is cross-clamped and the recipient heart is excised using standard excision lines as previously described by other authors.

For those patients with particular anomalies of either congenital or iatrogenic origin, these lines of excision and anastomosis must be altered, and these variations will be discussed in the sections that follow.

Anomalies of the Atria

There are essentially two types of anomalies of the atria—those involving size discrepancies between the donor and recipient atria, and those created by iatrogenic surgical distortion. The most frequently encountered size discrepancy is that between the donor and recipient atria. In this situation, we have employed two techniques (often in concert) to better size-match for atrial size.

First, the recipient right atrium may be reduced in size by over-sewing the cephalic atrium, thus extending the length of the recipient SVC (Figure 1). Second, the donor right atrial incision may be performed in the sinus venosus region of the right atrium posterior to the sinoatrial node (Figure 2). This paraseptal incision may then be extended through the ligature on the donor SVC, thereby significantly increasing the size of the donor right atrium available for subsequent anastomosis. Interestingly, in our experience, this second technique has not resulted in an increased incidence of atrial arrhythmias.

Patients who have undergone prior Mustard or Senning atrial inversion procedures often develop significant distortion of the atria. First, in such patients, the right atrium may be abnormally large, and the left atrium abnormally small. We have additionally observed in these patients that both venae cavae tend to be drawn to the left side. Because of this, following baffle excision, the orifices of the venae cavae then tend to be aligned in close proximity to the orifices of the pulmonary veins (Figure 3). The size discrepancies of donor and recipient atria may be addressed with the two techniques previously described. Further, the intra-atrial septum of the donor heart may be used to fashion a new atrial septum in the common atrium of the recipient (Figures 4A, 4B, and 4C), or, as others have suggested, the inclusion of a "tongue" of left atrial wall on the right side may allow for the creation of atrial septation by anchoring either to the posterior atrial wall (common atrium) or to a septal remnant.[37]

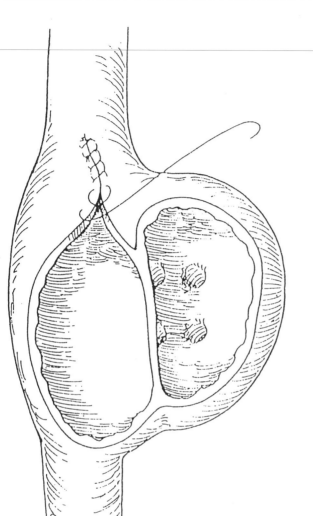

Figure 1. Over-sewing of the cephalad aspect of the recipient right atrium extends the length of the superior vena cava (SVC) and reduces the size of the right atrial orifice.

Anomalies of Systemic and Pulmonary Venous Return

We have encountered two types of anomalies of systemic and pulmonary venous connections: 1) left SVC, and 2) viscero-atrial situs inversus in which the donor and recipient atria are spacially inverted.

For the patient with a left SVC, in which the vena cava drains into a coronary sinus *not* in communication with the left atrium, we have found that the recipient

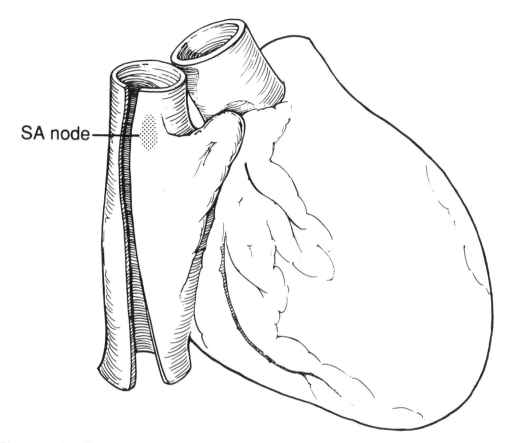

Figure 2. An alternative donor right atrial incision posterior to the sinoatrial (SA) node increases the amount of tissue available for the right atrial anastomosis.

cardiectomy may be performed by leaving the coronary sinus intact. However, in this scenario, the middle cardiac vein must be transected and over-sewn prior to the completion of the left atrial anastomosis (Figure 5). In contrast, for the patient in whom the coronary sinus is unroofed, and a sinoatrial septal defect is present, the left SVC may be ligated, divided, and subsequently anastomosed directly to the donor innominate vein (Figure 6).

Viscero-atrial situs inversus represents an anatomic variant for which several complicated techniques have previously been described for successful transplantation. We have developed a simple and reproducible technique for the management of this predicament.[9] The presence of bilateral SVC, with the left SVC and IVC entering to the left of the pulmonary veins, allows for the excision of the intra-atrial septum and the subsequent application of a lateral "T" incision in the left atrium (Figure 7). Two baffles may then be created along the back wall of the common atrium to bring the vena caval return rightward, and thus to allow for standard left atrial and right atrial anastomoses (Figure 8 and Figure 9). Alternatively, a baffle may be used to shunt flow from the left SVC to the right atrium with autologous atrial tissue (Figure 10).

Additionally, patients with a single ventricle who have either previously undergone procedures creating venopulmonary arterial flow, or who have bilateral SVC,

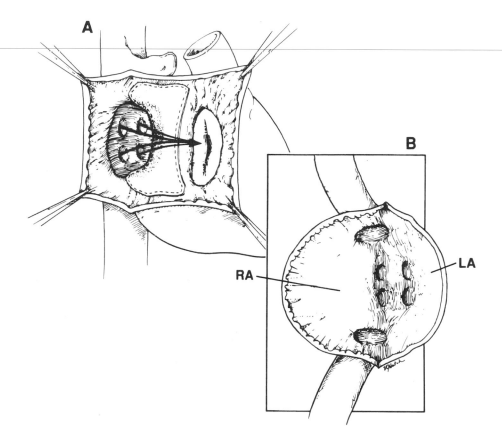

Figure 3. A. Mustard operation. Vena caval blood is baffled through the mitral valve and pulmonary venous blood flows through the tricuspid valve. **B.** The configuration of the atria and venae cavae following recipient cardiectomy and removal of the intra-atrial baffle. Note the large right atrium, small left atrium, and the deviation of the venae cavae toward the pulmonary vein orifices.

have been reported to have reconstruction using donor SVC and innominate vein for anastomoses to the left and right venae cavae, respectively.[36]

Anomalies of the Great Arteries

These anatomic variants represent anomalies of malposition, size, and surgical distortion, in addition to those anomalies produced by aortopulmonary collateral arteries. Great arterial malposition may readily be managed by complete separation of the recipient aorta and pulmonary artery, as well as by harvesting additional donor great vessel. The most common size discrepancy is that seen with HLHS. Here, several techniques for management have been described that involve the harvesting of additional aortic arch that may be used to reconstruct the arch below the ductus to which the brachiocephalic vessels may be anastomosed as a single Carrel patch. Patients with interruption of the aortic arch similarly may be repaired using additional transverse and proximal descending aorta harvested from the donor.[36,38]

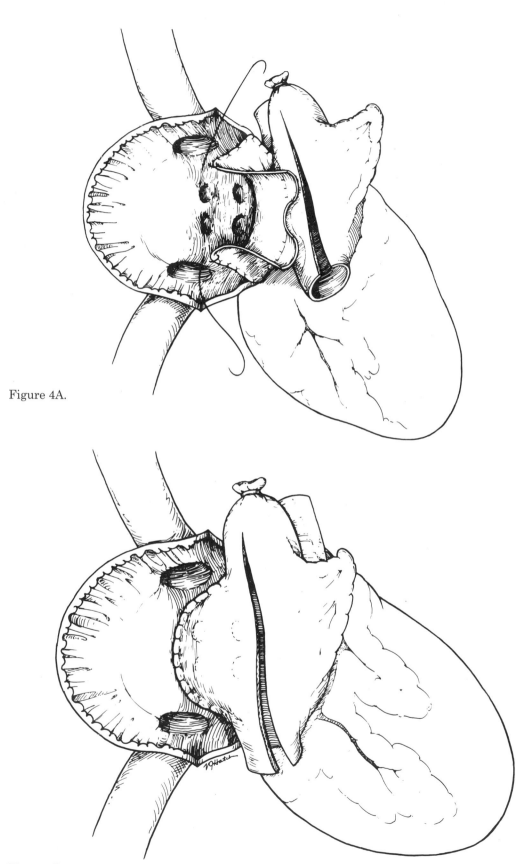

Figure 4A.

Figure 4B.

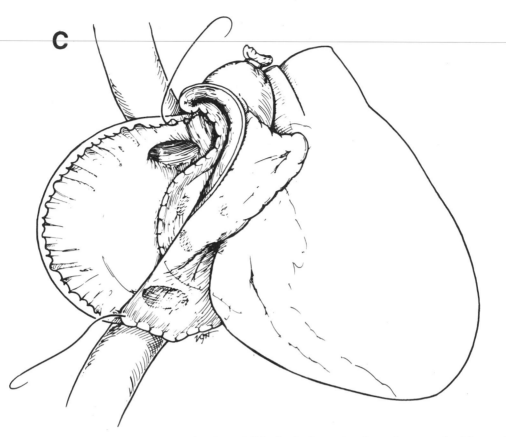

Figure 4. A and B. Donor implantation in a child who had previously undergone the Mustard Operation. The left atrial anastomosis is carefully woven between the orifices of the venae cavae and right pulmonary veins. **C.** The donor paraseptal right atrial incision provides additional donor tissue for suturing around the leftward deviated venae cavae.

We have previously reported our techniques for the surgical reconstruction of the pulmonary artery.[11] Here, we identified three categories of pulmonary artery anatomy necessitating different approaches to reconstruction: abnormalities of position; pulmonary outflow obstruction; and previous systemic-pulmonary or atrial-pulmonary connections. For those patients in our series with levo-transposition of the great arteries, and who additionally had undergone previous reconstructions with ventricular-pulmonary artery conduits or homografts, or with modified Blalock-Taussig shunts, and subsequent reconstruction with a right ventricular-pulmonary artery valved homograft, the valved conduits were transected distal to the valve prosthesis, and the donor pulmonary artery was anastomosed end-to-end directly to the remaining portion of homograft, either anterior or posterior to the aortic anastomosis.

For those patients with pulmonary outflow obstruction who have received Waterson shunts, or pulmonary artery banding, reconstruction of the pulmonary arteries may be performed with pericardial patching and with band removal and partial pulmonary arterioplasty (Figure 11). Others have described repair of the Waterson shunts

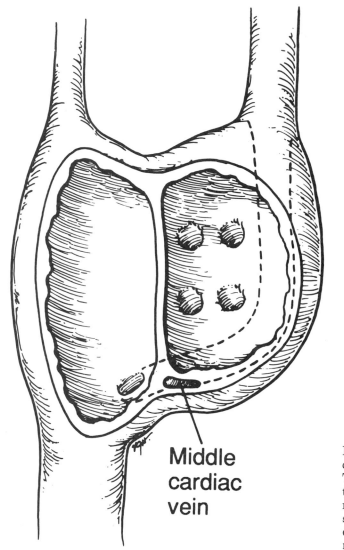

Middle cardiac vein

Figure 5. Left superior vena cava (SVC) to coronary sinus. There is no sino-septal atrial septal defect. Therefore, following recipient cardiectomy and over-sewing of the divided middle cardiac vein, standard atrial anastomosis can be performed.

from within the aorta, and of pulmonary artery bands by anastomosis to the pulmonary artery bifurcation, distal to the banding site when anatomically allowed. Blalock-Taussig shunts typically may be over-sewn from within the pulmonary artery following cardiectomy soon after circulatory arrest, and Glenn shunts may be taken down bilaterally, the pulmonary arteries repaired, and the venae cavae reconstructed end-to-end with the donor SVC and/or innominate vein.[18,19]

Our experience at The Columbia-Presbyterian Medical Center confirms the feasibility of heart transplantation in patients with complex congenital heart disease. Patients with intracardiac malformations pose few technical difficulties for the transplant surgeon. However, extracardiac malformations, whether congenital or those resulting

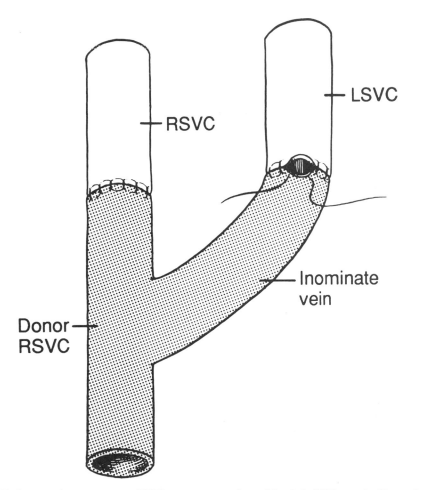

Figure 6. Left superior vena cava (SVC) to coronary sinus. The left SVC may be ligated, divided, and subsequently anastomosed to the donor innominate vein.

from prior palliative or corrective procedures, must be considered thoughtfully, and an appropriate surgical plan developed by the transplant team.

Postoperative Management

The intraoperative and immediate postoperative management of transplant patients is directed at optimizing allograft function in the face of three variables: acute denervation, the effects of cold preservation and the ischemic time, as well as acclamation to the recipient's hemodynamic environment. With acute denervation, the allograft's stroke volume (assuming adequate preload) is relatively fixed in the first few postoperative days. Alteration of the cardiac output can be aided by pharmacologically maintaining the heart rate between 100 to 120 for the infant and young child. Using

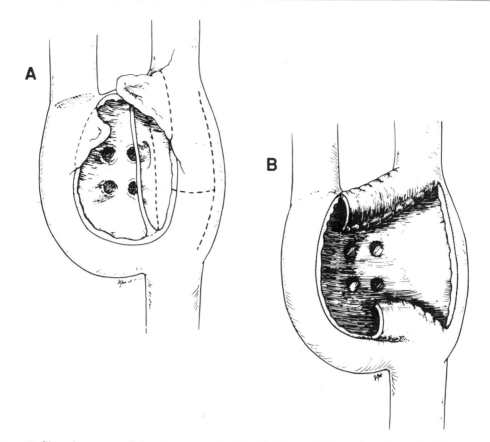

Figure 7. Situs inversus of the viscera and atria. **A. Dotted lines** show intended lines of incision for excision of the atrial septum and creation of caval baffles from the recipient left atrium. **B.** Intracardiac baffles fashioned from left-sided atrial tissue reroute systemic venous return from the left superior vena cava (SVC) and inferior vena cava (IVC) to the right of the pulmonary vein orifices.

low-dose isoproterenol to accomplish this additionally gives added inotropy, and a margin of safety for the allograft which is usually catecholamine depleted. Inotropic support and heart rate control is usually only necessary for 1 to 2 days. Since the patient is given a functionally normal heart, the recovery is rapid, and the children are extubated and mobilized as quickly as possible for rehabilitation.

In patients with high PVRI, it is crucial to begin specific vasodilators intraoperatively. The preoperative hemodynamic testing helps to tailor the choice of postoperative vasodilators. RV failure post-transplant can be acute and devastating at the point of separation from cardiopulmonary bypass, or as is more usual, it can be occult and insidious, manifesting itself as low output 6 to 24 hours later. As myocardial edema becomes maximal, and mediators released from bypass and transfusions affect the microvascular tone in the lungs, the normal RV myocardium cannot generate adequate systolic pressure. In this type of RV failure, the central venous pressure is not extraordinarily high, there is simply no flow. The RV becomes increasingly dilated on echocardiogram, with a relatively empty, snappy LV. Usually the heart tones are soft,

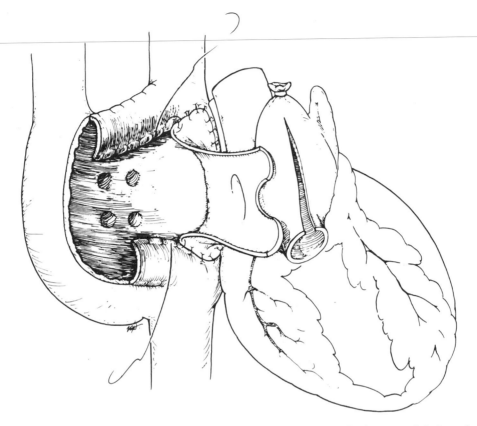

Figure 8. Left atrial anastomosis is being completed in a child with visceroatrial sinus inversus. The donor left atrium is sutured to the recipient's free left atrial margin and the intracardiac baffles. The remaining atrial cuff is anastomosed to the recipient atrium to the right of the pulmonary veins.

but a RV gallop is often heard. Efforts should be directed at minimizing the pulmonary resistance including continued intubation and deep sedation, arterial $pCO_2 \leq 40$, and $pO_2 > 100$ with no acidosis, and maintenance of adequate preload with maximal vasodilation. The RV usually responds in 2 to 3 days first with recovery, and then hypertrophy with resultant adequate systolic function. If the resistance is very high, or if the RV fails completely before these measures are taken, an RVAD may be necessary, however, the recovery of the ventricle can still occur within 2 to 5 days.

Complications after Transplant

Most of the complications that occur following cardiac transplantation are a result of the immunosuppressive therapy. Each cardiac transplant recipient must remain on life long immunosuppression to prevent rejection of the donor heart. It is a delicate balancing act between under immunosuppression with resultant acute rejection, or

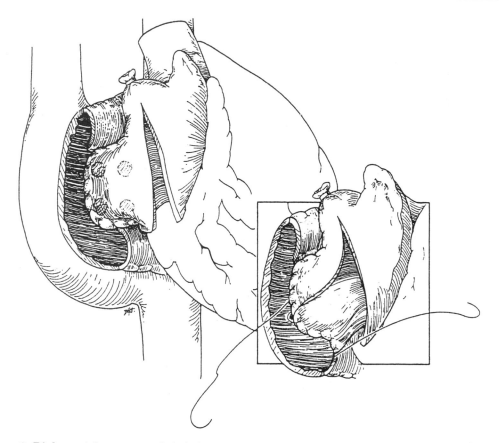

Figure 9. Right atrial anastomosis is being completed in a child with visceroatrial situs inversus. The donor atrial septum is sutured to the newly created recipient atrial septum, and remaining right atrial cuff is anastomosed to the recipient right atrial free wall.

chronic rejection (graft coronary disease), and over immunosuppression predisposing to infections and PTLDs. The "optimal immunosuppressive regimen" is the constantly changing, elusive goal for which we strive, consisting of precise allograft protection and minimal side effects.

There are several types of immunosuppressive regimens currently in use world wide, and individual transplant programs tailor them to fit their needs and patient populations and complications (Table 2). Patients are usually given their first doses of immunosuppressants before going to the operating room, and in some programs, a perioperative course of induction therapy is given in addition to the maintenance immunosuppression with either an antilymphocyte serum (ALS or ATG) or a monoclonal antibody preparation directed against activated T cells (OKT3). The mainstay of one type of maintenance regimen is CsA which is either used in the common "triple drug therapy" in combination with azathioprine and prednisone, or with azathioprine alone.[39] The group in Loma Linda have a small number of children transplanted as neonates who are on CsA monotherapy.[40,41] The action of CsA is to inhibit the production of the lymphokine, interleukin-2 (IL-2), which is necessary for helper T cells to

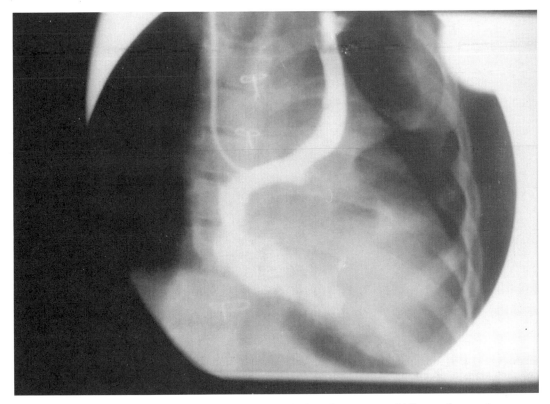

Figure 10. Angiogram of a 7-year-old patient with situs inversus and bilateral superior venae cavae (SVC), demonstrating flow from the left SVC to the right atrium through a baffle of autologous atrial tissue.

signal clonal expansion of undifferentiated cytotoxic T lymphocytes. The second type of regimen uses FK506 either as monotherapy or in combination with prednisone and sometimes azathioprine. This drug has only recently become available for general use, although the group in Pittsburgh have been testing it exclusively for the past 6 years in their pediatric heart transplant recipients.[42] FK506 is a macrolide compound that inhibits the formation of IL-2 by T lymphocytes, as well as IL-3 and gamma interferon. Ultimately, T cell proliferation is blocked. CsA and FK506 are metabolized in the liver and have both similar and disparate side effects. Rejection therapy is usually centered on steroid pulses, with OKT3, ALG, methotrexate, and total lymphoid irradiation reserved for resistant rejection. Specific details of immunosuppressive regimens are to be found in the immunology chapter.

Incidence and Diagnosis of Rejection

Rejection of the cardiac allograft is responsible for about 30% of deaths following transplantation in children.[43] Most patients will have at least one rejection episode early after transplantation during the period of adjustment of immunosuppressive drugs. The incidence of rejection among 332 pediatric cardiac transplant patients in a

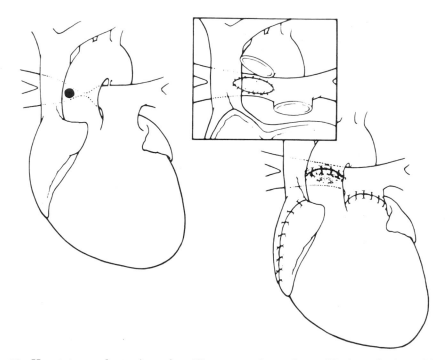

Figure 11. Heart transplantation after Waterston shunt for palliation of tricuspid and pulmonary atresia. "Kinking" of the right pulmonary artery was present at the site of the Waterston shunt with minimal flow to the left pulmonary artery, thus reconstruction after take down of the Waterston shunt employed a long pericardial patch at the shunt site.

prospective multi-institutional study was one episode per patient by 6 months and 1.5 per patient at 12 months following transplantation.[44] In this study, only rejection episodes that received increased immunosuppression were recognized. The actuarial freedom from rejection was 61% at 1 month, and only 37% by 6 months following transplant. The peak hazard for first rejection was at 2 months after transplant. The rejection detection method in this study was endomyocardial biopsy in 71% of the cases, echocardiography in 23%, and clinical criteria in 6% of the cases. By multivariable analysis, older recipient age and gender mismatch predicted earlier rejection. Induction therapy made no difference in rejection rates. The incidence of death from rejection in this series was low in infants less than 6 months at transplant (6%) and rose to between 23% to 30% in older children.

The introduction of CsA immunosuppression mollified the intensity and form of rejection episodes, which resulted in the inability to rely on noninvasive markers for rejection. However, in the newborn and young child, rejection seems to have manifest more symptoms while in the less aggressive stage. Symptoms of irritability, loss of appetite, fever, tachycardia, and gallop rhythm on physical examination are signs of early rejection in this age group that respond promptly to treatment. In the older child, often clinical parameters are insensitive indicators of rejection until it is so severe that myocardial performance is compromised. When present, clinical signs of rejection may include the appearance of a gallop rhythm, tachycardia, atrial arrhythmias, enlarged heart on chest x-ray, or change in echocardiographic function. Symptoms, when pres-

Table 2.

Evolution of Immunosuppressive Regimens

Early Regimen

• Azathioprine and Prednisone

Early 1980s

• *Cyclosporine and Prednisone*

Current Regimens

• Cyclosporine, Prednisone, and Azathioprine
• Cyclosporine and Azathioprine
• FK506 and Prednisone
• FK506 alone

Induction Agents

• ATG/ALS
• OKT3

Rejection Therapy

• Oral or IV Steroid boost
• OKT3
• ATG/ALS
• Methotrexate
• Total lymphoid irradiation (TLI)

This table depicts the evolution of immunosuppressive regimens since the first human heart transplantation. Although there are probably more variations, these are the regimens most commonly used. ATG = antithymocyte globulin; ALS = antilymphocyte globulin.

ent, usually center on fatigue and abdominal complaints instead of the classic heart failure signs of respiratory distress and edema.

Currently, the most reliable method for detection of acute rejection remains the topic of debate among transplant cardiologists. The "gold standard" of rejection surveillance has been endomyocardial biopsy, which is usually performed in the cardiac catheterization laboratory under fluoroscopic guidance. This procedure can be safely accomplished in the smallest of children. Obviously, pathologic detection is limited by the size and number of biopsy specimens. Rejection may be a focal occurrence, and may even be a mosaic: some areas of myocardium may exhibit a lower or higher grade of rejection than others. Despite this, endomyocardial biopsy remains the only direct method of detection of early rejection, as well as an important means for determining the adequacy of treatment of rejection episodes. Echocardiographic indices have been investigated for rejection detection. In adult studies with concomitant biopsies, the results have been conflicting and less reliable.[45] This in part may be related to increased interobserver variability, patient to patient differences, and the ventricular remodeling and healing that occur early after transplant. For these reasons, echocardiography has been less sensitive early after transplant, a time when the chance for rejection is highest. The original reports of the efficacy of echocardiography for rejection detection by Boucek et al describe an increase in LV mass with rejection in infants after transplantation.[46] A recent study from St. Louis compared the use of echocardiographic indices with endomyocardial biopsy for the detection of acute rejection in infants.[47] The study found that indexed LV mass increases significantly in acute rejection. However, these increases were not apparent early after transplant (within the first month). In addition, there was a wide scatter of data points such that no threshold value could be determined, and the inter- and intraobserver variability ranged from 7% to 80% depending on the value measured. One could speculate that this technique may be more applicable to infants, because rejection in them has more associated edema, as well as more pronounced clinical signs at an earlier stage than in older children.

However, it is important to continue to explore other methods of rejection detection. There has been some recent success in using radiolabeled monoclonal antibodies.[48] This method makes use of antibodies specific for cardiac myosin, which have been labeled with ^{111}In, a radioisotope that possesses good imaging properties. [111]In labeled monoclonal anticardiac myosin antibody Fab fragments will localize only to irreversibly damaged myocardial cells. This is certainly an advantage of this method, as it provides information regarding the entire heart. Early studies using ^{111}In labeled Fab fragments in humans have been encouraging, with an overall accuracy of 80%.[49] The pivotal human studies have been performed by Ballester et al in Barcelona, who attempted a quantitative approach to evaluate antimyosin uptake.[50] They performed 247 planar studies in 52 patients from 1 to 71 months following transplantation and correlated the results with endomyocardial biopsy. In all patients with rejection, the scans showed a diffuse pattern of uptake. There was significant correlation between increasing antimyosin uptake and severity of rejection. Based on this data, the center in Barcelona currently uses antimyosin scans for clinical rejection surveillance. The disadvantages to ^{111}In labeled Fab imaging include the long half-life and high energy of ^{111}In, which increases the radiation burden on the target organ and the kidney. Improved antimyosin labeling using radionuclides with shorter half-lives must be developed before serial studies can be safely performed in children. As discussed above, endomyocardial biopsy can occasionally be unreliable in verifying a rejection episode thought to be clinically present. In cases such as this, clinical judgment and intuition must be used with other noninvasive tests in order to make a diagnosis.

Graft Coronary Artery Disease

Graft coronary artery disease (GCAD) is thought to be the single most important limitation to longevity in cardiac transplant recipients, accounting for the majority of deaths after the first postoperative year.[51] The occurrence of this "accelerated CAD" has been reported to affect from 30% to 50% of the allografts of adult recipients by 5 years after transplant, with a similar incidence reported in the early pediatric transplant literature.[52,53] The pathophysiologic mechanisms leading to graft arteriopathy appear to be immune mediated. This disease is not an accelerated form of native coronary atherosclerosis, but rather an obliterative vasculopathy that has been seen in every type of solid organ transplant, and that selectively involves only vessels of the allograft, sparing all the native vessels.[54] The incidence of graft arteriopathy in the adult literature has not changed over the years, despite improved patient survival using triple drug immunosuppression. However, the overall incidence of CAD in the pediatric transplant population may be changing. A detailed review of this complication is contained in the separate chapter on graft vasculopathy.

Post-Transplant Lymphoproliferative Disorders

The long-term use of immunosuppressive medications is also associated with an increased risk for malignancy, predominantly post-transplant lymphoproliferative disorders (PTLDs). The incidence of tumors in the adult cardiac transplant population has ranged from 4% to 13%, with some authors finding a higher incidence in patients receiving monoclonal antibody therapy (OKT3). The majority of the tumors following transplant are classified as PTLDs that represent a spectrum of diseases ranging from infectious mononucleosis and polyclonal B cell hyperplasia to aggressive monoclonal B cell lymphoma. EBV has been found to play a role in the initiation of many of these tumors, and particularly those that occur early after transplant. Since most young children are EBV-negative and acquire the disease during early childhood and adolescence, the potential for acquisition of this disease after transplantation in young children is high.

Bernstein et al recently reported on a series of 80 pediatric cardiac transplant recipients in whom the overall incidence of tumors was 12.5%.[55] The tumor incidence was greatest in those patients transplanted in the pre-CsA era (44%). In contrast, the incidence of tumor formation in CsA-treated children was 8.5%. They found an increased risk in children who received antithymocyte globulin, but not in those who received OKT3. The time to detection of the tumor ranged from as early as 3 months to 10 years after transplantation. Eight of 10 of these patients had PTLD; one had hepatocellular carcinoma, and one had squamous cell carcinoma. Half of these patients died, however, only two died from their lymphoma. Zangwill et al reported on our experience with serial follow-up of EBV infections in our pediatric transplants, and the relationship to the development of PTLD.[24] Of 30 EBV-negative children pretransplant, 20 acquired EBV infection post-transplant (67%), with 12 developing PTLD. Neither the children who remained negative nor the children who had acquired their infection pretransplant developed PTLD. One of the 12 children with PTLD died from a rapidly progressive lymphoma that included 24 separate, distinct primary neoplasms arising from his colon.

The treatment of PTLD has been evolving and requires an individualized approach, because the character of the tumor may change over time. One unique feature of PTLD that is different from other malignancies, is the relationship to the intensity of immunosuppression. Treatment involves a decrease in immunosuppression and the use of acyclovir for suppression of EBV proliferation. The majority of the less aggressive tumors respond to this type of management and the prognosis is good. Even large tumors in extranodal sites with local tissue invasion have responded to decreased immunosuppression. However, chemotherapy is indicated when there is disseminated disease or malignant morphology.[25] Care should be taken for close follow-up of all children who convert their EBV serology, and if they have an acute mononucleosis presentation, their immunosuppression should be decreased slightly until they are clinically improved and acyclovir should be continued for at least 6 months. Thereafter, clinicians should have a high index of suspicion for occult tumor formation. It is encouraging that the overall incidence of this disease seems to be decreasing as we learn more about immunosuppression. Further research into the role of EBV in this disease and its management will help decrease the morbidity and mortality from this complication.

Complications of Immunosuppressive Agents

The previous sections have discussed the general complications resulting from over- or underimmunosuppression. In addition, there are unique side effects from the immunosuppressive agents themselves which can have consequences requiring long-term management.

CsA has many side effects, which include hypertension, and at high doses, nephrotoxicity. CsA-induced hypertension, which is almost universal in the adult population, occurs in approximately 60% of adolescent pediatric patients, but appears to occur much less frequently in the small infant and child. Patients have a loss of the normal diurnal variation in blood pressure, in that they have higher blood pressures at night than during the day. The mechanism is felt to be related to volume expansion and increased sympathetic tone, and seems to be independent of renal toxicity. It usually begins early within the first month after transplant, and in most cases is easily treated with either calcium channel blockers, ACE inhibitors, or beta blockers.

Renal dysfunction from chronic CsA administration can also occur. CsA causes renal vasoconstriction, principally of the afferent arterioles and, therefore, a decrease in renal blood flow. Most of the decrement in renal function occurs in the first 6 months after transplant. However, the effect of years of CsA usage may cause some further deterioration in renal function, necessitating a decreased dosage. Renal failure requiring dialysis or renal transplantation is rare, and usually is related to poor renal function or damage pretransplant. The use of nonsteroidal anti-inflammatory medications should be avoided, as they potentiate the nephrotoxic effects of CsA.

The cosmetic effects of CsA are striking, including a coarsening of the facial features, gingival hyperplasia, and hirsutism. The degree of cosmetic change that occurs varies greatly. Children with lighter hair and features tend to have less hirsutism than the child, who pretransplant, already has significant facial and body hair, and whose family tends to be hirsute. Pediatric patients may require multiple gingivectomies over time. In particular, calcium channel blocker therapy for treatment of their hypertension potentiates the gingival hyperplasia that occurs with CsA. Additionally, CsA causes increased nasal mucosal congestion and nasopharyngeal secretions that can hinder sinus drainage, leading to recurrent sinusitis and otitis media, infections that are particularly troublesome in toddlers and school-age children. In cases where the infections are recurrent, unusual organisms must be considered. The use of myringotomy tubes can play an important role in these children to prevent recurrent infections.[56] Another side effect of CsA usage is an increased incidence of cholelithiasis in the pediatric patients, probably on the basis of its influence on bile flow and bile salt secretion. The incidence of cholelithiasis in the general pediatric population is estimated to be less than 1%. Weinstein et al reported an incidence in our pediatric cardiac transplant population of 6.7%.[57]

The new immunosuppressant drug FK506, which has similar actions to CsA, has very different side effects. Pittsburgh reported the toxicity profile in using FK506 in 49 pediatric heart transplant recipients.[42] In contrast to CsA, FK506 does not cause gingival hyperplasia or hirsutism. In fact, children switched from CsA to FK506 for rejection rescue therapy have a dramatic change in appearance. FK506 also rarely causes hypertension, however, it appears to be equally nephrotoxic, with two children requiring kidney transplants in their series. The other major side effects of this new therapy include severe anemia, eosinophilia with allergic symptoms, gastrointestinal symptoms (chronic diarrhea and recurrent abdominal pain), and hyperactivity.

Institutions that use steroid therapy as part of their regimen begin at an induction level at the time of transplantation, and then taper the dose to a minimal daily amount over the next 3 to 6 months. The side effects of steroids are well known and include sodium and water retention, enhanced appetite, weight gain, abnormal fat deposition in the face and suprascapular areas, growth retardation, and, occasionally, steroid-induced diabetes. As the steroid dose is tapered to very low levels (or stopped), most of these side effects become less apparent. Indeed, in our pediatric experience at Columbia, since our maintenance dose of steroids is only 0.1 mg/kg/d to a maximum of 10 mg/d, growth retardation and serious steroid side effects have not been significant. Azathioprine, the third drug administered as part of the daily regimen, is an antimetabolite that inhibits cell-mediated hypersensitivity and suppresses T cell effects and antibody production to a variable degree. Side effects can include leukopenia, thrombocytopenia, macrocytic anemia, liver toxicity (especially cholestatic jaundice), and pancreatitis. These disorders abate with decreasing or temporarily stopping the azathioprine. All children at our institution receive additional folate therapy to counteract some of these effects.

Noncompliance

An important late complication seen in pediatric cardiac transplant recipients is noncompliance with medications, particularly immunosuppressive therapy. It usually occurs late after transplant when their lifestyles return to normal and they feel well. Families become less vigilant as children become apparently more self-reliant. This problem, which has been seen in other chronic illnesses, is much more lethal in the cardiac transplant patient. Renal transplant patients have dialysis to return to, and diabetics can be rescued from ketoacidosis. However, the cardiac transplant patient with acute graft failure has few alternatives. Noncompliance has been found to occur in at least 20% of our pediatric cardiac transplant experience. Douglas et al reported that it was significantly associated with adolescent age and was heralded by the appearance of late acute rejections (over 1-year post-transplant).[58] The 5-year actuarial survival in patients with documented noncompliance was 30% compared to 80% in compliant patients. Previous history and the psychosocial evaluation are imperfect for predicting which patients will become noncompliant. The impact of noncompliance on not only survival, but also on the morbidity associated with treatment of severe late rejections and/or the development of CAD is not fully known. An increased awareness of this potential problem not only at transplant centers, but with the family physicians, along with intensive patient and family education, may help decrease the incidence of this tragic complication.

Results of Transplantation

According to the 1993 statistics of the ISHLT, survival for all patients (pediatric and adult) after cardiac transplantation is approximately 80% at 1 year and 70% at 5 years. Survival for children transplanted between 1 year to 18 years is the same as the adult experience; 78% at 1 year and 75% at 5 years. However, the survival in infants transplanted under 1 year of age is slightly less, 70% at 1 year and 68% at 5 years post-transplantation.[1] Advancements in surgical technique, including enhanced myocardial preservation of the donor and technically better preoperative and postoperative care of extremely ill patients, contribute to excellent survival early after transplantation. An improved immunosuppressive regimen and experience developed in managing the late complications such as infections and CAD, account for similar survival after transplantation in both adult and pediatric age groups.

Between June 1984 and February 1996, we have performed 120 transplants in 115 children ranging in age from 5 days to 19 years at Babies Hospital, Columbia Presbyterian Medical Center. Thirty-seven percent of the children had congenital heart disease, and 60% had cardiomyopathies, with five children requiring retransplantation for CAD. The overall survival rate of the entire experience was 76% at 1 year and 63% at 5 years. However, for the past 9 years, we have been using a triple drug immunosuppressive protocol with CsA, low-dose prednisone, and azathioprine. Since that time, the 1-year survival has been 80%, and the 5-year survival has been 78%, which is much improved over our early experience with double drug immunosuppression (CsA and prednisone). It has been reported that the mortality following transplantation among children with congenital heart disease is higher than that of patients transplanted for other reasons. In our experience, there was no difference in 1- and 5-year survival (70% versus 77%, and 64% versus 65%), rejection frequency, or length of hospital stay between children with congenital heart disease and those without.[20] Cardiopulmonary bypass and donor ischemia time were significantly longer in patients with congenital heart disease. Serious infections within 3 months of transplant were more common in children with congenital heart disease (13/37 versus 6/47 patients, P=0.01). In spite of the more complex cardiac surgery required at implantation and longer donor ischemic time, heart transplantation can be performed in children with complex congenital heart disease, with similar success when compared with patients with other cardiac diseases.

Previous reports have always focused on results of short-term follow-up in children. Sigfusson et al presented the results of a multicenter report from Pittsburgh, Columbia, and Stanford of 68 children who have survived for greater than 5 years after transplantation.[59] The longest pediatric survivor is now 17 years after transplant. The probability of survival to 10 years in this population is 80%, and 67% at 15 years. All survivors are in New York Heart Association class I, with 45 in full-time education, and 10 engaged in full-time employment. One survivor is married with two children. Growth, as described by various centers series of pediatric cardiac transplant recipients, has shown growth and development in small children and adolescents to be normal.[60,61] Two recent reports from centers who specialize in infant transplantation have shown that the growth velocity in children transplanted as neonates is near normal, but the children generally are less than the 30th percentile for height.[62,63]

Future Goals and Controversies

The improvement in survival following pediatric cardiac transplantation over the last decade has advanced this once rare procedure to an accepted form of therapy in pediatrics. With longer survival, late complications such as GCAD or PTLDs, have emerged to challenge the clinician caring for these patients. New noninvasive methods for detecting rejection and CAD are necessary. Continued progress and advances in immunologic strategies for more selective immunosuppression should reduce the frequency of these late complications, prolong graft survival, and enhance the quality of life for these children.

The critical donor shortage brings into focus, controversies about current donor allocation, and issues of mechanical or biologic bridging to transplantation. In pediatrics, the donor scarcity is most severe in the infant size range. Presently, 30% to 40% of neonates waiting for transplantation die prior to the location of a suitable donor.[6] Attempts at maximizing the donor pool by using donor organs that previously would have been rejected has made little difference in decreasing the shortage. The efforts to obtain anencephalic heart donors has been hopelessly stalled in legal battle. Research into xeno transplantation as a bridge to transplant is also continuing.[64] Mechanical device development has blossomed, and currently there are excellent implantable battery operated assist devices that allow a total recovery and discharge for the adult-size patient. These, however, are not available for the infant. The only mechanical assist that is currently available for infant bridging, is ECMO from which the complication rate is high, and the length of time that it can be used is short. When the adult transplant groups were faced with similar critical shortages for their patients, they reexamined their recipient pool to remove patients who were too well, or for whom other alternatives could be found to maximize their quality of life without taking undue risk for death.[65] With improved neonatal surgical experience, it is time to reexamine our protocols regarding the optimal treatment for infants with HLHS, who comprise 60% of the infants listed for cardiac transplantation.

Infants born with HLHS, a previously lethal congenital defect, can currently be extended the option of surgical correction or cardiac transplantation. Cardiac transplantation has been proven to be successful in infants born with HLHS, as reported by Boucek et al.[41] However, the staged Norwood procedure has become a reasonable alternative when performed by an experienced center that routinely performs this surgery. The overall survival after the first stage Norwood procedure in our institution is 68%, which is equivalent to ISHLT survival after infant transplantation.[66] When faced with the decision of which procedure to choose, a parent must be informed that the true survival rate of an infant listed for transplant is only 40% to 45% because of an obligatory 30% to 40% pretransplant loss of infants from lack of donors. Since there is no difference in survival rates after surgery, the child with the Norwood who does not need lifelong immunosuppression with all the complications that have been discussed, will have the better quality of life. We have also shown that the length of stay in hospital for the entire three stages of repair is significantly shorter than the length of stay for a transplanted infant. Should the results from the Norwood 1 operation prove unsatisfactory, the child could still be transplanted, now that the infant will be stable enough to wait for a donor, most probably at home. Although the operative survival following infant transplantation is comparable to that after Norwood procedure, it is clear from the marked differences in overall survival, cumulative hospitalizations, and quality of life, that the Norwood procedure, performed in an experienced center, should be the initial therapy advocated for infants with HLHS. If this would occur, there would be a large number of infant donors to be offered to children who have no other alternative for life.

Conclusions

Cardiac transplantation clearly has evolved rapidly over the past 25 years to the point at which it now represents the best therapy available to many children with end-stage heart failure. Although the ultimate extended survival for the transplanted hearts in these children is only now being elucidated, the immediate limitation to the expansion of pediatric cardiac transplantation is the current availability of donor organs. The further extension of cardiac transplantation to accommodate the growing number of children both with complex congenital heart lesions, as well as those who have had palliative repairs, continues to emphasize this need, and it is this perpetual donor organ demand that provides the impetus for on-going investigations in search of alternative donor sources and therapies for children with end-stage heart disease.

References

1. Miller W, Kaye M, Baum D: Pediatric heart, heart-lung and lung transplantation: the world experience from 1984 to 1993. *Progr Pediatr Cardiol* 2:4–8, 1993.
2. Cooley D, Bloodwell R, Hallman G, et al: Organ transplantation for advanced cardiopulmonary disease. *Ann Thorac Surg* 8:30–46, 1969.
3. Kantrowitz A, Haller S, Joos H, et al: Transplantation of the heart in an infant and an adult. *Am J Cardiol* 22:782–790, 1968.
4. Hosenpud J, Novick R, Breen T, Daily O: The Registry of the International Society for Heart and Lung Transplantation: Eleventh Official Report—1994. *J Heart Lung Tranplant* 13:561–570, 1994.
5. Addonizio LJ, Naftel D, Fricker J, et al: Risk factors for pretransplant outcome in children listed for cardiac transplantation: a multiinstitutional study. *J Heart Lung Transplant* 14(Part 2):S48, 1995.
6. Morrow R, Naftel D, Chinnock R, et al: Outcome of listing for cardiac transplantation in infants (age<6 mos): predictors of death and interval to transplant. *J Heart Lung Transplant* 14(Part 2):S63, 1995.
7. Michler RE, Edwards NM, Hsu D, et al: Pediatric retransplantation. *J Heart Lung Transplant* 12:S319-S327, 1993.
8. Michler RE, Rose EA: Pediatric heart and heart-lung transplantation. *Ann Thorac Surg* 52:708–709, 1991.
9. Michler RE, Sandhu AA: Novel approach for orthotopic heart transplantation in visceroatrial situs inversus. *Ann Thorac Surg* 60:194–197, 1995.
10. Shah AS, Michler RE: Successful heart transplantation for acquired pulmonary arteria atresia. *Ann Thorac Surg* 59:1557–1559, 1995.
11. Cooper MM, Fuzesi L, Addonizio LJ, et al: Pediatric heart transplantation after operations involving the pulmonary arteries. *J Thorac Cardiovasc Surg* 102(3):386–394, 1991.
12. Chartrand C, Guerin R, Kangah M, Stanley P: Pediatric heart transplantation: surgical considerations for congenital heart diseases. *J Heart Transplant* 9:608–617, 1990.
13. Chartrand C: Pediatric cardiac transplantation despite atrial and venous return anomalies. *Ann Thorac Surg* 52:716–721, 1991.
14. Bailey LL, Concepcion W, Shattuck H, Huang L: Method of heart transplantation for treatment of hypoplastic left heart syndrome. *J Thorac Cardiovasc Surg* 92:1–5, 1986.
15. Doty DB, Renlund DG, Caputo GR, Burton NA, Jones KW: Cardiac transplantation in situs inversus. *J Thorac Cardiovasc Surg* 99:493–499, 1990.
16. Harjula ALJ, Heikkila LJ, Neiminen MS, et al: Heart transplantation in repaired transposition of the great arteries. *Ann Thorac Surg* 46:611–614, 1988.
17. Hehrlein FW, Netz H, Moosdorf R, et al: Pediatric heart transplantation for congenital heart disease and cardiomyopathy. *Ann Thorac Surg* 52(1):112–117, 1991.

18. Menkis AH, McKenzie FN, Novick RJ, et al: Expanding applicability of transplantation after multiple prior palliative procedures. *Ann Thorac Surg* 52(3):722–726, 1991.
19. Menkis AH, McKenzie N, Novick RJ, et al: Special considerations for heart transplantation in congenital heart disease. *J Heart Transplant* 9:602–607, 1990.
20. Hsu DT, Addonizio LJ, Smith C, et al: Cardiac transplantation in children with congenital heart disease. *J Am Coll Cardiol* 26(3):743–749, 1995.
21. Addonizio LJ, Welton G, Robins M, et al: Elevated pulmonary vascular resistance and cardiac transplantation. *Circulation* 76 (suppl)(5):52–55, 1987.
22. Addonizio LJ, Hsu DT, Douglas JR, et al: Cardiac transplant in children with markedly elevated pulmonary vascular resistance. *J Heart Lung Transplant* 12(1):S93, 1993.
23. Hsu DT, Addonizio LJ, Hordof A, Gersony W: Acute pulmonary embolism in pediatric patients awaiting heart transplantation. *J Am Coll Cardiol* 17:1621–1625, 1991.
24. Zangwill S, Hsu D, Kichuk M, et al: The incidence and outcome of primary Epstein-Barr virus infection and lymphoproliferative disease in pediatric heart transplant recipients. *J Heart Lung Transplant* 14(Part 2))(1):S63, 1995.
25. Chen L, Barr M, Chadburn A, et al: Management of lymphoproliferative disorders after cardiac transplantation. *Ann Thorac Surg* 56:527–538, 1993.
26. Hsu DT, Addonizio LJ, Reed E, Rose EA, Suciu-Foca N: Anti-HLA antibody formation in pediatric heart allograft recipients. *J Heart Lung Transplant* 11(Part 2)(1):205, 1992.
27. Keren A, Gottlieb S, Tzivoni D, et al: Mildly dilated congestive cardiomyopathy *f* use of prospective diagnostic criteria and description of the clinical course without heart transplantation. *Circulation* 81:506–517, 1990.
28. Keogh A, Baron D, Hickie J: Prognostic guides in patients with idiopathic or ischemic dilated cardiomyopathy assessed for cardiac transplantation. *Am J Cardiol* 65:903–908, 1990.
29. Keogh A, Baron D, Hickie J: Timing of cardiac transplantation in idiopathic dilated cardiomyopathy. *Am J Cardiol* 61:418–422, 1988.
30. Romeo R, Pelliccia F, Cianfrocca C, et al: Determinants of end-stage idiopathic dilated cardiomyopathy: a multivariate analysis of 104 patients. *Clin Cardiol* 12:387–392, 1989.
31. Lewis AB, Michelle C: Outcome in infants and children with dilated caridomyopathy. *Am J Cardiol* 68:365–369, 1990.
32. Addonizio LJ, Daphne H, Fuzesi T, et al: Optimal timing of pediatric heart transplantation. *Circulation* 80(suppl III)(5):84–89, 1989.
33. Kichuk M, Hsu DT, Douglas J, Gersony W, Addonizio LJ: Outcome in children with cardiomyopathy awaiting cardiac transplantation. *Circulation* 88(4):195, 1993.
34. Pennington DG: Mechanical circulatory support prior to cardiac transplantation. *Sem Thorac Cardiovasc Surg* 2(2):125–134, 1990.
35. Chen JM, Levin HR, Rose EA, et al: Experience with right ventricular assist devices for perioperative right-sided circulatory failure. *Ann Thorac Surg* 61(1):305–313, 1996.
36. Haas G, Laks H: Techniques of cardiac transplantation. In: Kapoor AS, Laks H, Schroeder JS, Yacoub MH (eds). *Cardiomyopathies and Heart-Lung Transplantation*. New York: McGraw Hill; 197–220, 1991.
37. Hasan A, Au J, Hamilton RL, et al: Orthotopic heart transplantation for congenital heart disease. *Eur J Cardiothorac Surg* 7:65–70, 1993.
38. Haas G, Bailey L, Pennington DG: Pediatric cardiac transplantation. In: Baue AE (ed). *Glenn's Thoracic and Cardiovascular Surgery*. 5th Ed. Norwalk, CT: Appleton & Lange; 1297–1317, 1991.
39. Addonizio LJ, Hsu DT, Douglas J, et al: Incidence of coronary disease in pediatric cardiac transplant recipients using increased immunosuppression. *Circulation* 88(Part 2):224–229, 1993.
40. Bailey LL, Wood M, Razzouk A, Van Arsdell G, Gundry S: Heart transplantation during the first 12 years of life. *Arch Surg* 124:1221–1226, 1989.
41. Boucek M, Kanakriyeh M, Mathic C, Timm R, Bailey LL: Cardiac transplantation in infancy: donors and recipients. *J Pediatr* 116:171–176, 1990.
42. Korang A, Boyle G, Webber S, et al: Experience of FK506 immunosupression in pediatric cardiac transplantation. *J Heart Lung Transplant* 14(Part 2)(1):S61, 1995.

43. Pennington DG, Noedel N, McBride LR, Naunheim KS, Ring WS: Heart transplantation in children: an international study. *Ann Thorac Surg* 52(3):710–715, 1991.

44. Rotondo K, Naftel D, Boucek R, et al: Allograft rejection following cardiac transplantation in infants and children: a multiinstitutional study. *J Heart Lung Transplant* 15(Part 2) (1):S80, 1996.

45. Dodd D, Brady L, Carden K, et al: Echocardiographic abnormalities with acute cardiac allograft rejection in adults: correlation with endomyocardial biopsy.*J Heart Lung Transplant* 12:1009–1019, 1993.

46. Boucek M, Mathis C, Kanakriyeh M, et al: Echocardiographic evaluation of cardiac graft rejection after infant heart transplantation. *J Heart Lung Transplant* 12:824–831, 1993.

47. Santos-Ocampo S, Sekarski T, Saffitz J, et al: Echocardiographic characteristics of biopsy-proven cellular rejection in infant heart transplant recipients. *J Heart Lung Transplant* 15:25–34, 1996.

48. Addonizio LJ: Detection of cardiac allograft rejection using radionuclide techniques. *Pro Cardiovasc Dis* 23(2):73–83, 1990.

49. Ballester-Rodes M, Cario-Gasset I, Abadal-Berini L, et al: Patterns of evolution of myocyte damage after human heart transplantation detected by indium-111 monoclonal antimyosin. *Am J Cardiol* 62:623–627, 1988.

50. Ballester M, Obrador D, Carrio I, et al: Early postoperative reduction of monoclonal antimyosin antibody uptake is associated with absent rejection related complications after heart transplantation. *Circulation* 85:61–68, 1992.

51. Gao SZ, Schroeder JS, Alderman EL, et al: Clinical and laboratory correlates of accelerated coronary artery disease in the cardiac transplant patient. *Circulation* 76(suppl V):V56-V61, 1987.

52. Pahl E, Fricker FJ, Armitage J, et al: Coronary arteriosclerosis in pediatric heart transplant survivors: limitation of long-term survival. *J Pediatr* 116:177–183, 1990.

53. Addonizio LJ, Hsu DT, Smith C, Gersony W, Rose E: Late complications in pediatric cardiac transplant recipients. *Circulation* 82(IV):IV295-IV301, 1990.

54. Miller LW: Allograft vascular disease: a disease not limited to hearts. *J Heart Lung Transplant* 11(Part 3):S32-S37, 1992.

55. Bernstein D, Baum D, Berry G, et al: Neoplastic disorders after pediatric heart transplantation. *Circulation* 88(Part 2):230–237, 1993.

56. Haddad J, Inglesby T, Addonizio LJ: Head and neck infections in pediatric cardiac transplant patients. *ENT Journal* 74(6):4–8, 1995.

57. Weinstein S, Lipsitz E, Addonizio LJ, Stolar C: Cholelithiasis in pediatric cardiac transplant patients on cyclosporine. *J Pediatr Surg* 30(1):61–64, 1995.

58. Douglas J, Hsu DT, Addonizio LJ: Noncompliance in pediatric heart transplant patients. *J Heart Lung Transplant* 12:S92, 1993.

59. Sigfusson G, Fricker F, Bernstein D, et al: Long-term survivors of pediatric heart transplantation: a multicenter report of 68 children who have survived greater than 5 years. *Circulation* 1994.

60. Addonizio LJ, Hsu DT, Gersony W: Linear growth in pediatric cardiac transplant patients. *J Am Coll Cardiol* 13(2):134A, 1989.

61. Uzark K, Crowley D, Callow L, Bove E: Linear growth after pediatric heart transplantation. *Circulation* 78(II):II-492, 1988.

62. Baum M, Chinnock R, Larsen R, et al: Intermediate follow-up of somatic growth of infant heart transplant recipients.*J Heart Lung Transplant* 15(Part 2)(1):S82, 1996.

63. Huddleston C, Mendeloff E, Canter C: Growth following heart transplantation in neonates. *J Heart Lung Transplant* 15(Part 2)(1):S82, 1996.

64. Chen JM, Michler RE: Heart xenotransplantation: lessons learned and future prospects. *J Heart Lung Transplant* 12(5):869–875, 1993.

65. Stevenson L, Warner S, Kobashigawa J, Drinkwater D, Laks H: All donor hearts will soon be required for urgent candidates. *J Heart Lung Transplant* 11(Part 2)(1):191, 1992.

66. Addonizio LJ, Hayes C, Gersony W, et al: Management of hypoplastic left heart syndrome: norwood procedure versus transplantation. *J Heart Lung Transplant* 14(Part 2)(1):S47, 1995.

Chapter 8

Graft Vasculopathy in Pediatric Cardiac Transplantation

Linda J. Addonizio, MD

Introduction

In the nearly 30 years since the first successful human cardiac transplant, the outlook for transplant recipients has dramatically improved. It has only been over the last decade that cardiac transplantation has become a common and rapidly expanding surgical option for the child with end-stage heart disease. Children now comprise about 10% of the total cardiac transplants performed annually, with 30% occurring in patients less than 1 year of age. It is unequivocal that heart transplantation is successful, with excellent survival in those children with end-stage heart disease for which there is no other option. Currently, the 5-year actuarial survival is 70% for these patients. Rejection, infection, and nonspecific graft failure are the major causes of death during the early postoperative period.[1] However, the ultimate outlook for extended survival remains unknown, and will be affected by the management of late complications that occur either as a result of side effects of the immunosuppressive drugs, or from ineffective immunosuppressive protection of the graft. Cardiac allograft coronary artery disease (CAD) is thought to be the single most important limitation to longevity in transplant recipients accounting for the majority of deaths after the first postoperative year.[2,3]

Incidence

The occurrence of this "accelerated CAD" or graft vasculopathy has been reported to currently affect from 30% to 50% of the allografts of adult recipients by 5 years following transplant, with a similar incidence reported in the early pediatric transplant literature.[4,5] Historically, this disease entity was first described by Thompson[6] in 1969 and

---

From: Franco KL (ed). *Pediatric Cardiopulmonary Transplantation*. Armonk, NY: Futura Publishing Company, Inc.; © 1997.

in a pathologic study by Bieber in 1970.[7] However, the full significance of the scope of graft vasculopathy was not realized in the early years of transplantation, because long-term survival was infrequent. Survival rates between 1968 to 1974, as reported by the Stanford group, were 48% at 1 year and 18% at 5 years, using the rudimentary immunosuppressive regimens that were available at that time.[8] The prevalence of allograft vasculopathy in the small number of *living* recipients in this early series was 42% after 5 years of follow-up. With the introduction of cyclosporine immunosuppression, the early deaths from rejection and infection were prevented, and CAD came to the front as the leading cause of death after the first postoperative year. Significant numbers of recipients were now available to be studied using serial coronary angiograms and, therefore, more accurate estimates of the incidence of CAD could be ascertained. Gao and Schroeder reported a 33% incidence of transplant vasculopathy, as detected by angiography, in their follow-up study on adult recipients using cyclosporine-based therapy at Stanford, with 60% of retransplantations secondary to severe CAD.[2] It became clear that because of enhanced survival, the numbers of recipients with significant CAD continued to increase yearly. Uretsky et al [9] published a life-table analysis of the Pittsburgh adult series which emphasized the progressive nature of graft vasculopathy. Even using cyclosporine and prednisone immunosuppression, their incidence by angiogram was 18% at 1 year, 27% at 2 years, and 44% at 3 years.[9] With further refinement of the immunosuppressive regimens to the current common combination of cyclosporine, prednisone, and azathioprine (triple drug therapy), it was anticipated that less CAD would occur. However, researchers at the University of Minnesota documented essentially the same incidence of vasculopathy at 2 years in adult recipients on triple therapy as the Pittsburgh double therapy group (24%).[5] More recent manuscripts have also failed to show an alteration in the prevalence of this disease in the adult transplant population.[10,11]

Although the incidence of graft arteriopathy in the adult literature has not decreased over the years despite improved patient survival, the overall incidence of CAD in the pediatric transplant population may be changing. In a recent study of 55 pediatric transplant survivors, our group at Columbia reported a 2% incidence of CAD using an augmented triple immunosuppressive regimen, which is significantly lower than the 30% incidence we reported in 1989 in patients on double therapy.[12,13] In earlier reports of pediatric heart transplant series, most centers, like ours, reported a similar prevalence of transplant vasculopathy (Table 1). Pahl et al, in 1990, showed 30% of the 21 pediatric operative survivors in Pittsburgh developed CAD which was identical to our early experience at Columbia.[4] In 1991, Braunlin et al detailed the pediatric experience at the University of Minnesota which showed a very high incidence of angiographically detected CAD (43%) by 3 years following transplantation.[14] This was, however, data from a small number of operative survivors (n=17) which may not prove accurate in larger cohorts. Also in 1991, Baum et al[15] reported on the 15-year experience with pediatric cardiac transplantation at Stanford. Of 53 patients transplanted, 42 who survived to hospital discharge in this series were at risk for CAD. Eight of the 42 survivors (19%) had coronary vasculopathy.[15] Radley-Smith published in 1992 that 3 of 59 (5%) surviving pediatric patients at Harefield Hospital developed CAD.[16] More recently, during the Second Symposium on Cardiac Allograft Vasculopathy held in 1995, she reported that there were 139 children who had been transplanted at Harefield Hospital, with 90 having follow-up $\geq$ 1 year. There were seven patients (8%) in this group that developed CAD.

No single institution had sufficient numbers of long-term survivors in the pedi-

Table 1.

Incidence of Coronary Vasculopathy in Pediatric Heart Transplant Recipients

Author/Year	# of Patients	Immunosuppression	% CAD
Pahl/1990	21	T	30%
Addonizio/1990	29	D,T	30%
Braunlin/1991	17	T	35%
Baum/1991	42	C,D,T	19%
Radley-Smith/1992	59	Cyclo & Aza	5%
Addonizio/1993	55	D,T	18% (2% T)
Pahl/1994 (MultiCenter)	560	D,T,FK506,C,M	7%
Addonizio/1995	87	T	2%

Table 1. The incidence of coronary vasculopathy in pediatric heart transplant series in the literature is shown. The number of patients in each series represent the operative survivors who had been discharged from the hospital.
C = conventional therapy: azathioprine, prednisone; D = double therapy: cyclosporine, prednisone; T = triple therapy: cyclosporine, prednisone, azathioprine; Multicenter study: M = monotherapy with cyclosporine, FK506 with and without steroids.

atric age range, to give an accurate incidence of allograft vasculopathy in children. Therefore, Pahl et al, in 1993, organized a multicenter national survey to evaluate coronary transplant vasculopathy in children.[17] The survey involved data on 815 children (including 188 neonates) transplanted between August 1974 and March 1993 from 17 pediatric cardiac transplant centers nationwide. Overall, there were 560 survivors (69%) including 132 neonates. Transplant CAD was identified by either angio-graphy or autopsy in 7.3% of this population with children of all ages that were affected. Despite speculation that neonates may be immunologically privileged, seven infants transplanted under 1 month of age developed CAD. The age at transplantation for the 58 patients with CAD ranged from 1 day to 18 years (mean 7.6 years). The age at diagnosis of CAD ranged from 2 months to 26 years. The CAD was first detected at postmortem in 13 of the 46 children. These recipients died with rapidly progressive obliteration of the coronary vessels prior to the first screening angiogram. This important multicenter study, which includes all patients transplanted over a 19-year period of variable immunosuppression, confirms that the incidence of coronary vasculopathy in the pediatric population may indeed be less than reported for adults. Although the present incidence seems greatly reduced, transplant CAD represented 37% of the late deaths in these children, with only 9 of the 58 patients with CAD still alive.

Pathology

The pathophysiologic mechanisms leading to graft arteriopathy appear to be immune mediated. This obliterative vasculopathy has been seen in nearly every type of solid organ transplant, and selectively involves vessels of the allograft, sparing all the native vesels.[18] The rapidity with which it can develop is also consistent with an immune-mediated process; severe coronary lesions have been found at autopsy as early as 2 to 5 months following transplantation.

Histology

There are a number of histologic differences between native coronary atherosclerosis and allograft coronary vasculopathy which have been well described by Billingham in a 1987 review of her 19-year experience at Stanford (Table 2).[19] Transplant vasculopathy is generally a diffuse process affecting the entire length of the epicardial vessel, but also including the intramyocardial and distal small vessels. There can be a mixture of proximal focal obstructions with the distal disease as well, especially in long-term survivors. In contrast, native CAD is made up largely of asymmetric focal lesions predominately in the proximal vessels sparing the branches and intramyocardial vessels, the classic atheroma. Morphologically, the classic lesion in transplant CAD is a concentric intimal proliferation of smooth muscle cells (SMCs) and macrophages which gradually and completely obstructs the lumen of the vessel (Figure 1). In most cases, the internal elastic lamina of the coronary vessels remains intact, as does the endothelium. There can be lipid accumulation and cholesterol crystals may be seen, however, grumous atheroma and calcification are rare in transplant disease. Although we primarily focus on the disease process involving the coronary arteries and arterioles, the donor aorta and coronary veins also display myointimal thickening.[20,21] This further substantiates the designation of transplant CAD as a true vasculopathy with an immunopathologic etiology.

As the disease progresses, the myocardium histopathologically displays multiple small infarctions with coagulation necrosis, granulation tissue, and subsequent fibrosis. These myocardial changes represent ongoing ischemia on a microvascular level at first, with progression to larger areas as the intimal proliferation chokes off the larger epicardial vessels. Numerous studies have reported transplant patients with apparently normal coronary studies, being victims of sudden death or returning *in extremis* in severe heart failure with obliterative CAD (Figure 2). Since this type of vessel disease causes a subtle and gradual disappearance of the microvasculature, the myocardium

---

Table 2.

Morphologic Comparison of Allograft Coronary Disease and Native Coronary Disease

Allograft Coronary Disease	*Native Coronary Disease*
• Cocentric intimal lesion	• Asymmetric lesion
• Elastica mostly intact	• Elastica damaged
• Affects length of vessel	• Focal lesions
• Branches involved	• Spares branches
• Intramyocardial vessels	• Spares intramyocardial vessels
• Calcification rare	• Calcification frequent
• Grumous atheroma rare	• Atheroma frequent

Table 2. This table compares the histopathologic differences between transplant vasculopathy and native coronary disease.

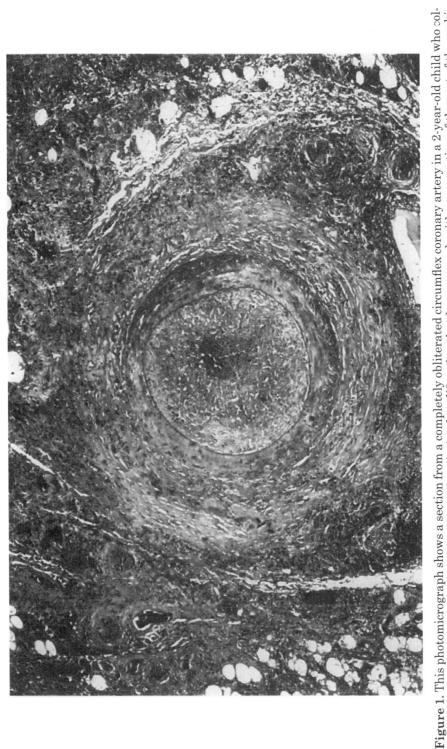
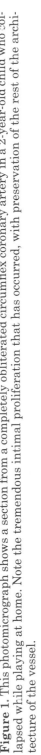

Figure 1. This photomicrograph shows a section from a completely obliterated circumflex coronary artery in a 2-year-old child who collapsed while playing at home. Note the tremendous intimal proliferation that has occurred, with preservation of the rest of the architecture of the vessel.

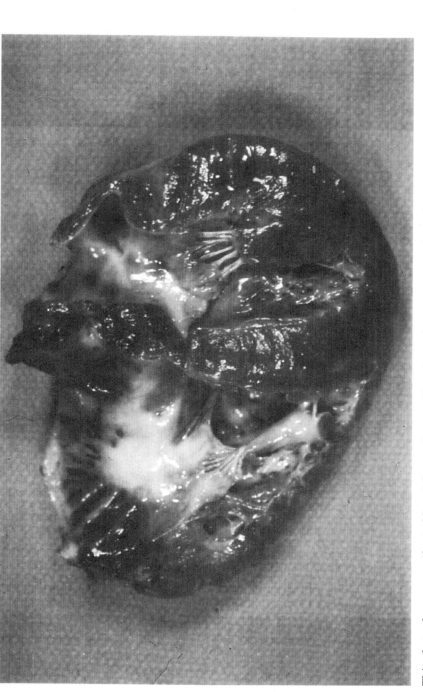

Figure 2. This photo shows an explanted heart from a 9-year-old patient who was retransplanted 5 years after initial transplant for coronary disease and chronic rejection. There is edema, multiple areas of infarction and fibrosis, and organizing clots in the right atrium. The child is thriving 6 years following retransplant.

adjusts and compensates in ways that it cannot when a large area of muscle is infarcted. Diffuse fibrosis and replacement of the myocardium with collagen occurs.

Pathophysiology

It is clear that damage to the vascular endothelium is the primary event in transplant CAD. The damage may result from one or more causes and may be propagated by others. It can begin as early as the day of implantation from suboptimal graft preservation, or result from cellular or humoral rejection, or alternatively viral triggers, such as cytomegalovirus (CMV) may begin the cycle and play a role in its chronicity. Once this initial insult occurs, the potential cascade of pathology that can follow has been well documented. Over the past several years, research has burgeoned in dissecting the cellular and molecular events that occur with endothelial injury and healing. This fascinating and exciting area of knowlege has become a separate subspecialty, and is beyond the scope of this discussion.[22-24]

The role of the vascular endothelium in initiating the "accelerated CAD" seen in transplant recipients can be discussed in a very simplified way. The cascade of events can be designated as "a response to injury," which is not unlike what is described with restenosis after coronary angioplasty. With injury to the vascular endothelium, cytokines are released and growth factors secreted which activate healing reactions in the endothelium. Adhesion molecules are then expressed on the endothelial surface (ICAM, VCAM, E-selectin and P-selectin) with resultant macrophage and fibroblast migration to the area of injury. Platelets also drawn to the area of injury release some of the growth factors and cytokines that promote proliferation and migration of these cells, including platelet-derived growth factor (PDGF). T lymphocytes, responding to the increased expression of donor human leukocyte antigen (HLA) antigens on the endothelium, can maintain a continuing pattern of injury to fuel this process by clonal expansion of the various T cell subpopulations. The recruited macrophages and lymphocytes, once inside the intima, emit additional cytokines that include SMC mitogens. Proliferation of SMCs in the vessel media occurs next, with subsequent migration of them into the intima, where they continue to proliferate and secrete extracellular matrix. Thus, the lesion begins as an intimal thickening, which depending on the amount of immunologic reactivity of the host, can either progress rapidly, or with the modification and removal of the continuing source of stimulation, the process can proceed more slowly.

Continued investigations and discoveries in this area of endothelial biology are of the utmost importance, and may allow the development of eventual therapies to ameliorate not only allograft vasculopathy, but native CAD. One can imagine a series of endothelial protectants to be added to cardioplegia solutions, and more accurate immunologic therapies to target specific host responses, and thereby prevent subsequent injurious events.

Recipient Risk Factors

The recipient risk factors for the development of graft vasculopathy which have been examined over the years have included the incidence of rejection, the degree of

HLA mismatch, donor-specific antibody production, CMV, donor age, recipient age and pretransplant diagnosis, and the presence of the traditional nonimmunologic risk factors for native CAD. In reality, when you review the diverse group of individuals who develop graft vasculopathy, it is clear that this process is a disease of multifactorial origin. Although certain risk factors are more strongly correlated with the development of disease, the cause in any one individual remains a combination of events.

Rejection

There is no question that graft vasculopathy is immune mediated, and the strong relationship between rejection episodes and this process is consistent with the term *chronic rejection*. Historically, investigators believed that cellular rejection was directly linked to the development of graft vasculopathy, but it was difficult to consistently prove by clinical studies. The early retrospective adult studies by Uretsky et al,[9] Olivari et al,[5] and Narrod et al,[25] which encompassed a total of 348 patients at three different institutions, all emphasized that the only consistent risk factor associated with the development of CAD was cellular rejection episodes. A few later reports which included small series of patients, did not show this relationship.[11,26] However, in a much larger single institutional experience of over 300 patients described by Zerbe et al, life-table and logistic regression analyses identified cellular rejection as having the only significant effect on the development of angiogram-evident graft coronary artery disease (GCAD).[27]

The evidence for a correlation between rejection and CAD is no less compelling in the pediatric population. Pahl et al, in 1990, showed that in Pittsburgh their pediatric patients who developed CAD had a linearized rejection rate twice as high as in patients without CAD.[4] In the multi-institutional survey she published in 1993, cellular rejection was present in 72% of the autopsies in this study, and was also associated with the development of CAD. In our first report from Columbia on late complications in pediatric recipients, we noted a 30% incidence of CAD.[12] The etiology of the graft loss in eight of the nine cases was acute rejection, however, extensive CAD was found as well. Therefore, we modified our immunosuppressive protocol to triple drug therapy, with tight control of cyclosporine levels at a higher trough, and aggressive rejection management. We saw a dramatic decrease in number and virulence of rejection episodes and similarly a decrease in CAD. To further test these inferences, we examined the association of eight potential risk factors with the development of CAD in our 55 long-term pediatric survivors by univariate and multivariate analyses.[13] The potential risk factors included the type of immunosuppression (double therapy with cyclosporine and prednisone, or triple therapy with cyclosporine, prednisone, and azathioprine), rejection frequency, total rejection number, timing of rejections from 0 to 3 months, 3 to 12 months, and over 12 months following transplant, age, and CMV status. The univariate analysis showed that double immunosuppression, rejection frequency, total rejection episodes, and rejection episodes occurring from 3 to 12 months, and after 1 year of follow-up were significantly associated with CAD. Early rejections, age, and CMV infection or disease were not significantly related to the development of CAD in our population. The multivariate analysis revealed only the type of immunosuppression and rejection frequency were independently predictive of the development of GCAD in this population, with a P value of 0.0001. The mean total rejection episodes for the patients on double therapy was 3.5+2.3 which was significantly higher than the mean of 1.6+1.6 episodes in the patients on triple therapy. There were 10 patients or 24% on triple therapy who never had any rejection episodes. The rejection frequency, which controls the length of time of patient survival, was 0.19+0.16 episodes/patient month in the patients receiving double immunosuppression which was similarly and significantly higher than the frequency in patients receiving triple immunosuppression (0.07+0.11 episodes/patient month). The strongest predictor of CAD in our pediatric patients was the type of immunosuppressive regimen they were receiving. Of the 13 patients on double therapy, 9 developed significant GCAD. However, of 42 patients receiving triple immunosuppression, only 1 patient developed coronary disease, $P<0.001$. There was no difference between the length of follow-up of the two groups: 34 versus 36 months, respectively. The incidence of CAD using our augmented triple immunosuppression decreased to 2%. Since that report was published in 1993, we have continued using this immunosuppressive regimen, and now have 87 children who have had a least one angiogram and the incidence of CAD remains 2%. We have found a markedly decreased incidence of GCAD in our pediatric recipients by aggressively treating rejection and tightly controlling immunosuppressant levels at our institution with up to 9 years of follow-up. There was no increase in side effects using the higher doses of cyclosporine. One could argue that we are missing significant disease by relying on angiographic methods of diagnosis; however, this is not likely, as patients on our previous double drug immunosuppressive regimen who had CAD, clinically declared themselves usually by sudden death. These results indicate that underimmunosuppression is a major component in the development of GCAD. However, increased immunosuppression may only serve to delay the onset of significant CAD. New advances toward more specific prevention of endothelial injury may obviate the need for higher immunosuppression.

Finally, Hosenpud et al in a recent, elegantly designed prospective study, confirmed that cell-mediated, not humoral alloimmunity to donor-specific vascular endothelium was significantly related to cardiac allograft vasculopathy.[28] Using donor aortic endothelial cells grown in culture and the corresponding recipient blood lymphocytes collected over time, they showed that recipient blood lymphocytes from patients who developed graft vasculopathy exhibited a proliferative response to exposure to the donor-specific human aortic endothelial cells significantly greater than recipients who did not have CAD. Humoral immunity did not seem to be significantly involved, as measured by donor alloantibody detection which was extremely low. In addition, there were greater HLA-DR mismatch (the target for CD4+ T lymphocytes), a higher incidence of late acute rejection, and lower maintenance doses of prednisone and azathioprine in the CAD patients. This superb work confirms the link between the classic cell-mediated rejection and coronary vasculopathy in transplant recipients, and challenges the clinician to closely monitor and tailor the individual patient's immunosuppressive regimen to their immunologic reactivity.

Human Leukocyte Antigen Matching

The relationship between histocompatibility mismatching and the development of CAD is poorly understood. A review article by Costanzo-Nordin details the numerous studies providing evidence for and against this association.[29] She emphasizes the difficulties of assessing the impact of HLA incompatibility because most cardiac allografts are poorly matched. No HLA matching of donors occurs in cardiac transplantation, and since the HLA system is extraordinarily polymorphic, the random allocation of organs allows few patients who have more than one or two matches in a particular locus. In renal transplantation where the majority of organs *are* HLA matched, it is easier to get a large number of patients with multiple matches for comparative study. In fact, Opelz reported a strong favorable association between the combination of matching HLA-A, B, and HLA-DR loci and graft survival in kidney recipients.[30] In a later study, Opelz and Wujciak[31] reviewed the outcome of 8331 heart transplant recipients from 104 transplant centers around the world and compared survival curves with the number of HLA mismatches. They found that the survival in patients with zero, one, or two mismatches was better than for three to six mismatches.[31] We must be cautious in interpreting this data, however, as there were only 128 donors out of over 8000 that had zero to one mismatches, and the difference in survival over 3 years was maximally 10%. The Cardiac Transplant Research Database Group analyzed the HLA information from 1190 donor and recipient pairs for the A, B, and DR loci that were singled out as significant in the renal transplant literature.[32] Patients with zero, one, or two mismatches had a 54% freedom from rejection at 1 year ,compared to a 34% freedom from rejection in patients with three or more mismatches. Although statistically significant, the difference in probability for a rejection death or retransplantion was 0% for zero, one, or two mismatches and only 5% for three to six mismatches. Some have advocated HLA matching donors for hearts because of the difference in long-term survival that is seen in the kidney experience. With the majority of heart recipients being very sick status 1 patients, it would not seem practical or judicial to pass a heart along to someone else who may be a better match but not as ill, when the maximal increase in survival would be only 5% to 10% over a 3-year period.

There has been no convincing evidence that HLA mismatches are related to CAD. You might suspect a correlation because of the strong association between rejection and vasculopathy. In fact, we may ultimately find no correlation between HLA incompatibility and vasculopathy, because recent experimental evidence points to non-HLA endothelial antigens as being the target for immunologic attack and the development of CAD.[33] In this study, specific antiendothelial antibody production was identified in multiple samples from cardiac transplant recipients. These antibodies persisted over 12 months after transplant in only those patients who developed coronary vasculopathy.

Other Risk Factors

There have been numerous studies evaluating the effect of traditional nonimmunologic risk factors for the development of transplant vasculopathy. Recipient characteristics such as age, sex, obesity, smoking, pretransplant diagnosis, hypertension, diabetes mellitus, and hyperlipidemia have been scrutinized, and comparative studies have been performed to assess their contribution to the development of graft vasculopathy. Johnson, in a review of the literature, compared the variable results of studies for each factor and determined that hyperlipidemia had the most consistently described relationship to graft vasculopathy.[34] Hyperlipidemia is common after cardiac transplantation and exacerbated by both cyclosporine and prednisone. Experimental evidence in the rabbit transplant model showed that added cholesterol in the diet increased the number of coronary lesions and SMC proliferation.[35] Eich and coworkers found hypercholesterolemia in the high-risk level after 6 months post-transplant to have strong predictive value for the development of CAD by 3 years.[36] In a study of 120 patients from Harefield Hospital,[37] elevated levels of total cholesterol and low-density lipoprotein (LDL) were significantly higher in patients who developed graft vasculopathy. They found no difference in triglycerides or high-density lipoprotein (HDL).[37] In the pediatric literature, Braunlin et al found no correlation between cholesterol and triglycerides and the development of CAD.[14]

CMV infection has been implicated in the development of graft vasculopathy. Multiple centers have shown that CMV infection is an independent risk factor for CAD. Stanford, in one of the largest series, analyzed data from 301 recipients and found the incidence of CAD in patients without evidence of CMV infection was 10%, compared to 30% in patients with CMV infection.[38] Since there was also a higher incidence of rejection in the CMV-positive patients, one could speculate that the rejection, not the infection was the causal factor. CMV, as a member of the herpes simplex virus (HSV) family, has the ability to establish latent infection. It has been shown to be an immunologic stimulant, able to up-regulate the expression of class I HLA antigens on the surface of vascular smooth muscle and able to destroy vascular endothelium. By these mechanisms and inferences, CMV can be considered a trigger for the development of CAD in the transplant recipient.[39] Another study of 129 patients provided more insight on this association. They divided the patients according to the type of CMV infection (i.e., primary, reactivation, or a persistent infection), and compared these groups for the development of vasculopathy. The only patients with an increased incidence of vasculopathy were those with persistent infection for over 4 months.[40] In our own pediatric series, CMV did not correlate with coronary vasculopathy, except in one case of a 4 year old who was infected just prior to transplant. The child had persistent CMV disease with thrombocytopenia and anemia, despite a course of gancyclovir and continued acyclovir for 9 months after transplant. An angiogram at 9 months and again at 12 months showed, at first, ectatic coronaries followed by diffuse obliterative disease. He was subsequently retransplanted.

Diagnosis

A major impediment to the development of strategies for prevention and treatment of GCAD, is determining the best method for early diagnosis, and how to evaluate the significance of the lesions. Since the heart is denervated, the transplant recipient has no premonotory or recurrent angina to alert the clinician to the development of significant CAD. Therefore, although the use of angiography can lack diagnostic sensitivity for this disease, it is currently the only method able to make the diagnosis prior to graft loss. The angiographic appearance of transplant coronary vasculopathy has been classified by Gao and colleagues, who described three major types of lesions after reviewing serial angiograms on 221 heart transplant recipients and comparing them to 32 patients with native CAD (Figure 3).[41] Type A disease consists of discrete stenosis, tubular stenosis, and multiple stenoses in the proximal or middle epicardial vessels, or

Anatomic Types of Transplant Vasculopathy

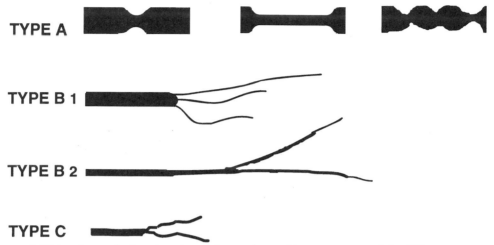

Figure 3. This schematic drawing shows the angiographic appearance of the different anatomic types of coronary disease after transplant.(Adapted with permission from Reference 3.)

distal segment branches. Type B disease usually has preserved proximal vessels with either abrupt onset of distal concentric narrowing and obliteration (type B_1), or gradual concentric tapering and obliteration distally (type B_2). In type C disease, the vessels are diffusely irregular with abrupt nontapered terminations and loss of tertiary and smaller branch vessels. Both types B and C obliterative lesions are seen exclusively in transplant vasculopathy, whereas type A focal narrowings are found with equal frequency in patients with native CAD and transplant vasculopathy. Another important feature of transplant CAD is the surprising absence of collateral blood supply as delineated by angiography in the majority of the cases with totally occluded vessels. This may be related to the rapidity of the disease process, or that in most cases, both the distal small arteries and veins are involved in this obliterative process so that no collaterals can form.

Since the majority of these coronary lesions cause a subtle, gradual, and often symmetrical disappearance of the microvasculature, it is understandable how a single angiogram might appear normal. In addition, histologic and angiographic comparisons of degree of disease revealed that angiograms often underestimated the degree of obstruction.[42] It is crucial that angiograms be examined serially to pick up this form of transplant vasculopathy prior to sudden death or cardiogenic shock. There is evidence that serial quantitative coronary studies following intracoronary vasodilation are more sensitive in identifying small arterial lumenal changes. Using this technique in adult recipients, Mills et al reported significant loss in arterial segment diameters between 2 to 3 years after transplant in angiograms that were visually passed as normal.[43] Many centers also utilize a predischarge angiogram as the "gold standard" for follow-up comparisons, instead of the first annual study, because CAD can occur as early as 2 months after transplant. Using this protocol, Everett et al,[44] determined the specificity of normal *qualitative* angiography in predicting the absence of graft vasculopathy to be 81%. This would mean that 15% to 20% of patients will have diffuse disease not detected by a qualitatively normal study, and advocate for more quantitative evaluation of the films.[44]

The use of noninvasive techniques such as nuclear scans, echocardiography, and ECGs have not previously been sensitive in detecting GCAD.[45,46] However, intravascular ultrasound is now being evaluated which allows assessment of the entire cross-section of the coronary vessel segment. This technique may prove to be the best test for early detection of CAD, when intimal hyperplasia is increasing the thickness of the vessel wall, but has not yet begun to narrow the lumen. Just as angiography may be an insensitive diagnostic tool for transplant vasculopathy, so intravascular ultrasound may be too sensitive; the majority of adult recipients over 1 year after transplant have evidence of intimal thickening by ultrasound that is not apparent by angiography.[47] In this initial study, only the proximal two thirds of the left anterior descending coronary artery (LAD) was examined which was a limitation to this technique, because one must assume this area of the LAD to be representative of all other areas of the coronary tree. As serial follow-up studies of patients with this new technique are accumulating, clinical end points are now being determined and new definitions of significant coronary involvement are emerging. Patients with moderate, angiographically silent, intimal thickening by ultrasound may never have any clinical consequence from this abnormality, and some may rapidly progress. Early detection could allow treatment protocols to begin prior to the development of severe end-stage disease. For example, when rapid thickening of the arterial intima is observed, alterations may be made to the immunosuppressive regimen.

Some of the newest studies have used intravascular ultrasound to examine multiple arteries and branches, and chronicle the rate of progression of intimal thickening and its correlation to outcome. Mayer et al reported that the natural history of intimal thickening was to linearly increase each year post-transplant in their studies of 178 adult recipients.[48] Wiedermann et al reported that severe intimal thickening revealed by ultrasound (> 1 mm for $> 180°$ of arc) was highly predictive of cardiac death or need for retransplantation within 1 year.[49] Rickenbacher and the group from Stanford further refined the prognostic importance of early intimal thickening in these patients.[50] They found that an intimal thickening of greater than 0.3 mm was associated with significantly lower survival and increased cardiac events, irrespective of the absence of angiographic disease. Further, they stated that this early degree of thickening was predictive of subsequent development of disease on angiogram. In an attempt to determine the functional consequences of these ultrasound findings, Heroux et al combined the intracoronary ultrasound assessment of the vessel wall morphology, with the evaluation of the vascular response to endothelium-dependent vasodilators.[51] They found that the vasodilator response to papaverine was blunted in the patients with intimal thickening and angiographically apparent coronary abnormalities. In the future, continued serial follow-up with this highly sensitive technique of intravascular ultrasound, combined with a type of functional assessment, may help to plan early treatment strategies for transplant vasculopathy.

Intravascular ultrasound of the coronaries has been used in children as young as 8 years; in the Kawasaki's experience, however, no data is available on imaging the degree of intimal thickening in the younger grafts of transplanted children.[52] This will be an important study to perform in children, since occult atherosclerotic CAD has been found in adult recipients to be frequently transmitted with the donor heart.[53] Tuzcu et al[53] found atherosclerotic plaques and intimal thickening in 56% of the recipients by 4 weeks after transplant. This finding was significantly associated with donor age and gender. In the multifactorial basis for the development of transplant-associated CAD, preexisting donor disease would provide an excellent foundation for further immunologic destruction of the endothelium. Perhaps the decreased incidence of CAD in the pediatric population compared to the adult population is on the basis of the younger-aged donors not having significant preexisting CAD. Only further serial studies and comparisons of risk factors will help to solve these inconsistencies.

There is a continued search for a noninvasive method to detect CAD in these patients. Heretofore, the false-negative rates have been prohibitive, and the sensitivity too low. Exercise echocardiography was found to have a high false-negative rate for patients with moderate stenosis.[54] Dobutamine stress echocardiography is now beginning to be tested for the detection of significant transplant vasculopathy. Preliminary studies show an overall sensitivity of 86% and a specificity of 91%.[55] No studies are available in transplanted children.

Treatment

The options for treatment are currently limited. We look first to strategies to prevent the occurrence of graft vasculopathy in these patients. The group at Stanford have advocated the use of the calcium channel blocker, diltiazem, to prevent the development of CAD. This recommendation was based on experimental evidence that it may prevent or retard the injury-induced atherosclerotic process including platelet adhesion and activation. Schroeder et al reported on a randomized prospective trial comparing the effects of diltiazem to no diltiazem in 134 cardiac transplant recipients.[56] The patients not on diltiazem had a significant decrement in coronary diameter 2 years after transplantation. Continued follow-up will determine if this is a long-term effect that is protective. A related trial currently in progress with native CAD is testing the ability of nifedipine, another calcium channel blocker, to prevent atherosclerosis (IN-TACT trial). This drug may be preferential in transplant recipients if the same protective effect is observed, because it has better antihypertensive properties. Newer immunosuppressants which may help prevent this disease have completed animal trials and are beginning to be used in clinical trials. The new immunosuppressants, rapamycin and leflunomide, were found to prevent the progression of intimal thickening in rat femoral grafts, whereas cyclosporine and mycophenolate mofetil did not. Leflunomide and rapamycin have a direct antiproliferative effect on the SMC, and may prove to help prevent coronary vasculopathy clinically.[57] There have also been animal studies comparing the effects of 15-deoxyspergualin to cyclosporine, in which they observed a significantly lower amount of graft arteriopathy in the animals given 15-deoxyspergualin.[58] The data from these active clinical trials is eagerly awaited so that these new targeted immunosuppressive drugs, that may help prevent graft vasculopathy, will become available.

Once CAD is established, there are few options for these patients. Some investigators have used percutaneous transluminal coronary angioplasty with varying success in the adult transplant patient. This can be tried when there are proximal focal obstructive lesions, but restenosis may occur at a faster rate, and the ultimate benefit from this procedure is unknown. The collective experience of 13 institutions performing angioplasty, atherectomy, and bypass surgery in cardiac transplant recipients was just reported by Halle et al.[59] Sixty-six patients underwent coronary angioplasty. Angiographic success ($\leq$ 50% residual stenosis) occurred in 94% of 162 lesions. Forty patients (61%) are alive without retransplantation at a mean of 19 months after the procedure. Two patients died periprocedure, and restenosis occurred in 55% of lesions within 8 months. Distal angiographic arteriopathy adversely affected survival. Eleven patients underwent atherectomy with success in 82% of lesions. However, two periprocedural deaths occurred with nine patients surviving without retransplanatation at 7 months. Coronary artery bypass was performed in 12 patients in this collective experience; four patients died perioperatively, and seven are alive without retransplantation at a mean of 9 months postoperatively. Revascularization might be considered as *palliative* therapy in selected recipients, but the experience is limited and mortality is high.

When graft GCAD is severe, retransplantation is the only alternative. Since the number of pediatric retransplantations at any one center is small, Michler et al from our institution, compiled the combined experience of four centers specializing in pediatric heart transplantation and reported the results of 17 children that were retransplanted.[60] The actuarial survival after pediatric retransplantation was 71% at 1 year and 47% at 3 years. Sixty-five percent of the procedures were performed for either CAD, or CAD combined with chronic rejection. Three of the 16 survivors undergoing retransplantation developed CAD in the second graft between 3 and 16 months after surgery. Since that study, we now have five children at our center who have been retransplanted. We have had excellent long-term success with this procedure, with survival as long as 6 years. There has been one death due to CAD from continued noncompliance. All pediatric retransplant patients at Columbia are given a perioperative course of total lymphoid irradiation to try to "erase" immunologic reactivity and possible sensitization. Severe rejections have not been seen, and all four surviving patients are New York Heart Association class I.

With the present donor shortage, it is a debatable issue if retransplantation should be performed at all, and there is no consensus among transplant clinicians who are faced with the dilemma of being their patient's advocate. Medical treatment aimed at the prevention of transplant CAD, either with improved selective immunosuppression, or with the use of new endothelial protectants, will be the only viable long-term solution for this problem.

References

1. Miller WW, Kaye M, Baum D: Pediatric heart, heart-lung, and lung transplantation: the world experience from 1984 to 1993. *Prog Pediatr Cardiol* 2:4–8, 1993.
2. Gao S-Z, Schroeder JS, Hunt S, Stinson EB: Retransplantation for severe accelerated coronary artery disease in heart transplant recipients. *Am J Cardiol* 62:876–881, 1988.
3. Gao S Z, Schroeder JS, Alderman EL, et al: Clinical and laboratory correlates of accelerated coronary artery disease in the cardiac transplant patient. *Circulation* 76:V56–V61, 1987.
4. Pahl E, Fricker FJ, Armitage J, et al: Coronary arteriosclerosis in pediatric heart transplant survivors: limitation of long-term survival. *J Pediatr* 116:177–183, 1990.

5. Olivari MT, Homans DC, Wilson RF, Kubo SH, Ring WS: Coronary artery disease in cardiac transplant patients receiving triple-drug immunosuppressive therapy. *Circulation* 80:III-111–III-115, 1989.

6. Thomson JG: Production of severe atheroma in a transplanted human heart. *Lancet* 2:1088–1092, 1969.

7. Bieber CP: Cardiac transplantation in man. *Circulation* 41:753–772, 1970.

8. Gao S-Z, Hunt SA, Schroeder JS: Accelerated transplant coronary artery disease. *Sem Thorac Cardiovasc Surg* 2:241–249, 1990.

9. Uretsky BF, Murali S, Reddy S, et al: Development of coronary artery disease in cardiac transplant patients receiving immunosuppressive therapy with cyclosporine and prednisone. *Circulation* 76:827–834, 1987.

10. Kobashigawa JA, Gleeson MP, Stevenson LW, et al: Benefit of steroid weaning late after cardiac transplant: relationship to transplant coronary artery disease (abstr). *JACC* 23(3): 230A, 1994.

11. Ratkovec RM, Wray RB, Renlund DG, et al: Influence of corticosteroid-free maintenance immunosuppression on allograft coronary artery disease after cardiac transplant. *J Thorac Cardiovasc Surg* 100:6–12, 1990.

12. Addonizio LJ, Hsu DT, Smith CR, Gersony WM, Rose EA: Late complications in pediatric cardiac transplant recipients. *Circulation* 82:IV295–IV301, 1990.

13. Addonizio LJ, Hsu DT, Douglas JF, et al: Decreasing incidence of coronary disease in pediatric cardiac transplant recipients using increased immunosuppression. *Circulation* 88:224–229, 1993.

14. Braunlin EA, Hunter DW, Canter CE, et al: Coronary artery disease in pediatric cardiac transplant recipients receiving triple-drug immunosuppression. *Circulation* 84:III-303–III-309, 1991.

15. Baum D, Bernstein D, Starnes VA, et al: Pediatric heart transplantation at Stanford: results of a 15-year experience. *Pediatrics* 88:203–214, 1991.

16. Radley-Smith RC: Long-term results of pediatric heart transplantation. *J Heart Lung Transplant* 11:S277–S281, 1992.

17. Pahl E, Zales VR, Fricker FJ, Addonizio LJ: Post-transplant coronary artery disease in children: a multicenter national survey. *Circulation* 90(5):56–60, 1994.

18. Miller LW: Allograft vascular disease: a disease not limited to hearts. *J Heart Lung Transplant* 11:S32–S37, 1992.

19. Billingham ME: Cardiac transplant atherosclerosis. *Transplant Proc* 19:19–25, 1987.

20. Ventura HO, Mehra MR, Stapleton DD, et al: An intravascular comparison of allograft and native aortic disease in cardiac transplantation. *J Heart Lung Transplant* 14:S58, 1995.

21. Oni AA, Ray J, Hosenpud JD: Coronary venous intimal thickening in explanted cardiac allografts. *Transplantation* 53:1247–1251, 1992.

22. Ip JH, Fuster V, Badimon L, Badimon J, Taubman MB, Chesebro J: Syndromes of accelerated atherosclerosis: role of vascular injury and smooth muscle cell proliferation. *J Am Coll Cardiol* 15:1667–1687, 1990.

23. Jang Y, Lincoff M, Plow EF, Topol EJ: Cell adhesion molecules in coronary artery disease. *J Am Coll Cardiol* 24:1591–1601, 1994.

24. Libby P: Do vascular wall cytokines promote atherogenesis. *Hosp Pract* 15:51–58, 1992.

25. Narrod J, Kormos R, Armitage J, Hardesty R, Ladowski J, Griffith B: Acute rejection and coronary artery disease in long-term survivors of cardiac transplantation. *J Heart Lung Transplant* 5:418–421, 1989.

26. Stovin PGI, Sharples L, Hutter JA, Wallwork J, English TAH: Some prognostic factors for the development of transplant-related coronary artery disease in human cardiac allografts. *J Heart Lung Transplant* 10:38–44, 1991.

27. Zerbe T, Uretsky B, Kormos R: Graft atherosclerosis: effects of cellular rejection and human lymphocyte antigen. *J Heart Lung Transplant* 11:S104–S110, 1992.

28. Hosenpud JD, Everett JP, Morris TE, Mauck KA, Shipley GD, Wagner CR: Cardiac allograft vasculopathy association with cell-mediated but not humoral alloimmunity to donor-specific vascular endothelium. *Circulation* 92:205–211, 1995.

29. Costanzo-Nordin MR: Cardiac allograft vasculopathy: relationship with acute cellular rejection and histocompatibility. *J Heart Lung Transplant* 11:S90–S103, 1992.

30. Opelz G: Strength of HLA-A, HLA-B, and HLA-DR mismatches in relation to short and long-term kidney graft survival. *Transplant Int* 5:621–624, 1992.
31. Opelz G, Wujciak T: The influence of HLA compatibility on graft survival after heart transplantation. *N Engl J Med* 330:816–819, 1994.
32. Jarcho J, Naftel DC, Shroyer TW, et al: Influence of HLA mismatch on rejection after heart transplantation: a multiinstitutional study. *J Heart Lung Transplant* 13:583–596, 1994.
33. Crisp SJ, Dunn MJ, Rose ML, Barbir M, Yacoub MH: Antiendothelial antibodies after heart transplantation: the accelerating factor in transplant-associated coronary artery disease? *J Heart Lung Transplant* 13:81–92, 1994.
34. Johnson MR: Transplant coronary disease: nonimmunologic risk factors. *J Heart Lung Transplant* 11:S124–S132, 1992.
35. Sasaguri S, Eishi Y, Tsukada T, et al: Role of smooth-muscle cells and macrophages in cardiac allograft arteriosclerosis in rabbits. *J Heart Lung Transplant* 9:18–24, 1990.
36. Eich D, Thompson JA, Ko D, et al: Hypercholesterolemia in long-term survivors of heart transplantation: an early marker of accelerated coronary artery disease. *J Heart Lung Transplant* 10:45–49, 1991.
37. Barbir M, Kushwaha S, Hunt B, et al: Lipoprotein (a) and accelerated coronary arterial disease in cardiac transplant recipients. *Lancet* 340:1500–1502, 1992.
38. Grattan MT, Moreno-Cabral CE, Starnes VA, Oyer PE, Stinson HB, Shumway NE: Cytomegalovirus infection is associated with cardiac allograft rejection and atherosclerosis. *JAMA* 261:3561–3566, 1989.
39. Kendall TJ, Wilson JE, Radio S, et al: Cytomegalovirus and other herpes viruses: do they have a role in the development of accelerated coronary arterial disease in human heart allografts? *J Heart Lung Transplant* 11:S14–S20, 1992.
40. Everett JP, Hershberger RE, Norman DJ, et al: Prolonged cytomegalovirus infection with viremia is associated with development of cardiac allograft vasculopathy. *J Heart Lung Transplant* 11:S133–S137, 1992.
41. Gao S-Z, Alderman EL, Schroeder JS, Silverman JF, Hunt SA: Accelerated coronary vascular disease in the heart transplant patient: coronary arteriographic findings. *J Am Coll Cardiol* 12:334–340, 1988.
42. Johnson DE, Alderman EL, Schroeder JS, et al: Transplant coronary artery disease: histopathologic correlations with angiographic morphology. *J Am Coll Cardiol* 17:449–457, 1991.
43. Mills RM, Hill JA, Theron HT, Gonzales JI, Pepine CJ, Conti CR: Serial quantitative coronary angiography in the assessment of coronary disease in the transplanted heart. *J Heart Lung Transplant* 11:S52–S55, 1992.
44. Everett JP, Hershberger RE, Ratkovec RM, et al: The specificity of normal qualitative angiography in excluding cardiac allograft vasculopathy. *J Heart Lung Transplant* 13:142–149, 1994.
45. Smart FW, Ballantyne CM, Cocanougher B, et al: Insensitivity of noninvasive tests to detect coronary artery vasculopathy after heart transplant. *Am J Cardiol* 67:243–247, 1991.
46. Gao S-Z, Schroeder JS, Hunt SA, Billingham ME, Valantine HA, Stinson EB: Acute myocardial infarction in cardiac transplant recipients. *Am J Cardiol* 64:1093–1097, 1989.
47. St. Goar FG, Pinto FJ, Alderman EL, et al: Intracoronary ultrasound in cardiac transplant recipients: in vivo evidence of "angiographically silent" intimal thickening.*Circulation* 85:979–987, 1992.
48. Mayer EL, De Franco AC, James KB, et al: Cardiac allograft vasculopathy is a continuous linear process: a natural history study using intravascular ultrasound. *Circulation* 90:I-7, 1994.
49. Wiedermann JG, Wasserman HS, Weinberger JZ, Schwartz A, Apfelbaum M: Severe intimal thickening by intracoronary ultrasound predicts early death in cardiac transplant recipients. *Circulation* 90:I-93, 1994.
50. Rickenbacher PR, Pinto FJ, Lewis NP, et al: Prognostic importance of intracoronary ultrasound after cardiac transplantation. *Circulation* 90:I-639, 1994.
51. Heroux AL, Silverman P, Costanzo MR, O'Sullivan E, et al: Intracoronary ultrasound assessment of morphological and functional abnormalities associated with cardiac allograft vasculopathy. *Circulation* 89:272–277, 1994.

52. Sugimura T, Kato H, Inoue O, et al: Intravascular ultrasound of coronary arteries in children: assessment of the wall morphology and the lumen after Kawasaki Disease. *Circulation* 89:258–265, 1994.
53. Tuzcu EM, Hobbs RE, Rincon G, et al: Occult and frequent transmission of atherosclerotic coronary disease with cardiac transplantation. *Circulation* 91:1706–1713, 1995.
54. Collings CA: Exercise echocardiography in heart transplant recipients: a comparison with angiography and intracoronary ultrasonography. *J Heart Lung Transplant* 13:604–613, 1994.
55. Derumeaux G: Dobutamine stress echocardiography in orthotopic heart transplant recipients. *J Am Coll Cardiol* 25:1665–1672, 1995.
56. Schroeder JS, Gao S-Z, Alderman EL, Hunt S, Hill I, Stinson EB: Prevention of transplant accelerated coronary vascular disease with Diltiazem (abstr). *JACC* 23(3): 231A, 1994.
57. Nair R, Cao W, Morris R: Molecular mechanism of suppression of arterial intimal thickening by Leflunomide: demonstration of direct antiproliferative effect on murine smooth muscle cells in vitro and antagonism of action by Uridine. *J Heart Lung Transplant* 14(suppl): S54, 1995.
58. Nagamine S, Ohmi M, Tabayashi K, Iguchi A, Mohri H: Effects of cyclosporine and 15-deoxyspergualin on coronary arteriosclerosis after heart transplantation in the rat. *J Heart Lung Transplant* 13:895–898, 1994.
59. Halle A, Wilson RF, Massin EK, et al: Coronary angioplasty in cardiac transplant patients: results of a multicenter study. *J Am Coll Cardiol* 86:458–462, 1992.
60. Michler RE, Edwards NM, Hsu DT, et al: Pediatric retransplantation. *J Heart Lung Transplant* 12(suppl):S319–S327, 1993.

Chapter 9

Heart-Lung Transplantation

Pankaj S. Mankad, MD, FRCS
Marc R. de Leval, MD, FRCS

Introduction

The first clinically successful heart-lung transplant was performed in 1981 at Stanford University in a 45-year-old patient suffering from primary pulmonary hypertension.[1] This success was based on an extensive experimental work which began in the 1940s,[2,3] and was preceded by three unsuccessful clinical attempts in the late 1960s.[4-6] After extensive experiences with kidney, liver, and heart transplantation in children, pediatric heart-lung transplantation developed relatively rapidly with the adaptation of successful immunosuppressive therapy in this age group.

The number of heart-lung transplantations in children has increased significantly in the last few years. Between 1984 and 1993, almost 2000 infants and children with thoracic organ transplantation have been reported to the International Society for Heart and Lung Transplantation (ISHLT). Of these, 202 had heart-lung transplantation and 112 had lung transplantation.[7] Overall, the 5-year survival rate in children following heart-lung transplantation is around 40%.[7]

Indications and Recipient Selection

Heart-lung transplantation is considered for patients with severe respiratory or cardiac failure secondary to irreversible lung parenchymal or pulmonary vascular disease.[8] Due to the appreciable risks and complications involved, heart-lung transplantation is offered only as a last resort when the patient is unresponsive to all other forms of therapy. The potential recipients are severely symptomatic with a very poor quality of life and usually have a limited life expectancy (less than 2 years). The indications for heart-lung transplantation can be divided into those for pulmonary vascular disease and those for parenchymal lung disease.

From: Franco KL (ed). *Pediatric Cardiopulmonary Transplantation*. Armonk, NY: Futura Publishing Company, Inc.; © 1997.

167

Pulmonary Vascular Disease

Severe pulmonary hypertension secondary to an intracardiac shunt (Eisenmenger's syndrome) is the most common indication for heart-lung transplantation in the pediatric age group. It may also be considered for infants and children with complex pulmonary atresia who are unsuitable for conventional surgery.[9] These children pose a particular surgical problem, because of the presence of large bronchial collaterals in the mediastinum. In addition, a majority of them have previously undergone palliative surgery resulting in dense vascular adhesions in the mediastinum. These factors significantly increase the risk of peri- and postoperative hemorrhage.

Primary pulmonary hypertension and thromboembolic pulmonary hypertension are other anomalies requiring heart-lung transplantation. However, these patients are usually older. In patients with primary pulmonary hypertension, associated autoimmune disorders are occasionally encountered which may contraindicate the transplant. Patients with suspected thromboembolic pulmonary hypertension should undergo a thorough investigation of coagulation state prior to transplantation.

Patients with an elevated pulmonary vascular resistance secondary to long-standing left heart failure and pulmonary venous hypertension were, until recently, considered for heart-lung transplantation. However, some of these patients can now be managed by orthotopic cardiac transplantation by using donor hearts with hypertrophied right ventricles which are obtained from heart-lung transplant recipients with irreversible parenchymal lung disease. The donor right ventricle in this situation is better able to cope with the recipient's increased pulmonary vascular resistance. Furthermore, the intravenous administration of prostacyclin and the use of inhaled nitric oxide are additional useful adjuncts in this situation.

Parenchymal Lung Disease

Cystic fibrosis is the most common indication at our center for heart-lung transplantation. Other lung diseases that have been reported as successfully treated by heart-lung transplantation include emphysema (often due to alpha 1-antitrypsin deficiency or a familial emphysema of unknown origin), fibrosing alveolitis, primary pulmonary fibrosis, eosinophilic granuloma, pulmonary lymphangio-leiomyomatosis, and pulmonary sarcoidosis. A number of these patients with noninfective primary parenchymal lung disease may also be treated by either single or double lung transplantation.[10] Currently, there is a significant overlap in the indications for these procedures, and further experience will probably more clearly define the ideal procedure for a given patient. Optimal use of donor resources can be accomplished by heart-lung or double lung transplantation, as the normal heart from the heart-lung transplant recipient can be used as a donor heart. However, single lung transplantation offers potential benefit in terms of optimization of donor resources, as lungs can be used for two recipients. This may become an important consideration, due to the marked shortage of heart-lung donors.

Other Considerations for Recipient Selection

Recipients often have significant renal and/or hepatic dysfunction. If this is secondary to cardiorespiratory failure, it is usually reversible and is not an absolute contraindication to transplantation. If renal or hepatic failure is due to intrinsic disease, then a combined heart-lung plus liver or kidney transplantation could be considered. In patients with insulin-dependent diabetes mellitus, end-organ function should be thoroughly evaluated. In the absence of end-organ damage, insulin-dependent diabetes mellitus is not regarded as a contraindication to transplantation. A previous history of peptic ulceration is also not a contraindication, provided endoscopic healing has been achieved.

The majority of centers consider extensive previous cardiac or thoracic surgery as a relative contraindication to heart-lung transplantation. Previous thoracotomies are known to increase the morbidity and mortality of heart-lung transplantation, whereas previous median sternotomy does not appear to increase the risk of surgery. An alternative to the conventional method of transplantation has been suggested for patients with previous lateral thoracotomies. This is to perform a repeat lateral thoracotomy, free up all vascular adhesions, close the chest, and then to perform median sternotomy and transplantation. However, this also increases the morbidity and, therefore, each patient with a previous thoracotomy should be individually evaluated.

In patients with complex congenital heart disease, the presence of an abnormal atrial situs, left superior vena cava (SVC), or associated aortic arch anomalies requires technical modifications, and these conditions are not contraindications to transplantation.

A potential recipient often has to wait for a considerable period before a suitable donor organ becomes available. During this period, every effort should be made to optimize recipient medical management. Consideration should be given to the avoidance of malnutrition and multi-organ failure. Many children with parenchymal lung disease are on steroid therapy. High doses of steroid may impair healing of the tracheal anastomosis. It is advisable to reduce the dose of steroid to a minimum level prior to transplantation. However, it has been shown that the long-term use of low-dose prednisone before heart-lung transplantation does not preclude normal tracheal healing.[11]

It is important that patients be psychologically stable and have extremely strong family support. The way in which they have adapted to their end-stage heart and lung disease is often a good indication of the patient's and the family's ability to handle post-transplant complications and problems.

Donor Selection

In general, there are fewer suitable donors for lung transplantation than for heart and kidney transplantation. The criteria for donor selection vary between transplant centers. The broad principles of donor selection are outlined below. The assessment of a potential heart-lung donor includes general history, evaluation of cardiac and lung functions, chest x-ray, and screening for potential transmissible diseases.

The donor should be less than 40 years old, should not have a history of significant cardiopulmonary disease, and preferably should be a nonsmoker. Cardiac function should be satisfactory with either no or minimal inotropic support. If the donor is receiving large doses of inotropic support, then it is important to monitor central venous pressure and reevaluate the situation following adequate volume replacement. The donor sometimes has diabetes insipidus and is severely volume depleted.

Lung function is of vital importance in the evaluation. An arterial PO_2 of more than 14 kPa with an inspired oxygen of around 40% or an arterial oxygen of more than

35 kPa on 100% inspired oxygen is considered satisfactory. Airway pressure and minute ventilation should be within the normal range to maintain a normal arterial PCO_2. The length of mechanical ventilation is also an important consideration. There is an increased risk of pulmonary infection which is directly related to the length of mechanical ventilation. There should be no significant consolidation or contusion on chest x-ray, but radiologic evidence of neurogenic pulmonary edema in itself is not a contraindication. However, this must be differentiated from aspiration pneumonia which is frequently seen in potential donors with severe trauma and resuscitation.

The donor is screened for potential transmissible diseases especially hepatitis B surface antigen, and antibodies to the human immunodeficiency virus (HIV). Donors from groups at high risk of HIV infection should not be considered because of the danger of missing an early infection before an antibody risk has a chance to develop. There has been some debate about matching of donor-recipient pairs with respect to cytomegalovirus (CMV) status.[12,13] At this time, we consider it essential to match donor and recipient CMV status to reduce the risk of postoperative CMV infections which carry relatively high morbidity and mortality, especially in heart-lung transplant recipients.[14]

Once the donor is considered suitable, cultures are taken from the endotracheal tube and a cocktail of intravenous antibiotics is given prior to organ harvesting (flucloxacillin, gentamicin, metronidazole, and sodium fusidate). A stable hemodynamic state is maintained and the concentration of inspired oxygen is reduced to a minimum level that will achieve adequate arterial oxygen saturation.

Donor-Recipient Matching

Approximate matching of the donor and recipient chest sizes is required to prevent problems of cardiac compression, lung collapse, or persistent pneumothoraces and pleural effusions postoperatively. Matching of donor and recipient's chest x-ray is performed by measuring vertical and transverse diameters and cardiothoracic ratio, and by superimposition of the two x-rays. Some centers also use various external chest wall measurements of donor and recipient for size matching. We prefer comparing the estimated lung capacity of the donor, derived from normograms of height and sex, with the measured total lung capacity of the recipient.[15]

ABO blood group compatibility between donor and recipient is essential. If an Rh negative recipient is given an Rh positive organ, then a sufficient amount of anti-D is given intravenously to the recipient to prevent the formation of Rh antibodies. Human leukocyte antigen (HLA) typing of the donor and recipient is not used in assessing donor-recipient compatibility. However, from a retrospective analysis of data, Festenstein and colleagues have suggested that matching of class II (DR) antigens possibly influences patient survival.[16] If the recipient has preformed cytotoxic antibodies, then a specific negative cross-match between donor lymphocytes and recipient serum is also performed. However, it is likely that a positive lymphocytotoxic cross-match between the donor and recipient may not have a significant impact on survival.

Organ Harvesting and Preservation

Two different techniques are currently in use for organ harvesting and preservation. Some centers use a portable cardiopulmonary bypass machine to cool the donor organs to a core temperature of below 10°C, followed by arrest of the circulation and organ harvesting.[17] We prefer the alternative method of organ preservation which consists of pulmonary flush preservation and cold crystalloid cardioplegia for myocardial protection.[18] The Pittsburgh group has used a functioning heart-lung preparation, but subsequently abandoned this in favor of pulmonary flush preservation, because of the technical complexity of the autoperfusion system.[19] The pulmonary artery flush preservation technique is carried out in the following manner.

On arrival at the donor hospital, the hypertonic crystalloid solution for lung preservation (lung perfusate) is prepared. The composition of lung perfusate is outlined in Table 1. Midline sternotomy is performed. Thymic tissue is removed. Both pleurae are opened wide and the lungs are mobilized completely, including pulmonary ligaments. The anterior pericardium is then opened and right lateral pericardium is excised. The aorta, SVC, and inferior vena cava (IVC) are mobilized. The azygos vein is doubly ligated and divided, and 300 units/kg of heparin are given. The right and left lateral pericardium is excised back to the pulmonary veins. Purse-string sutures are inserted onto the main pulmonary artery and the ascending aorta. A catheter is inserted into the pulmonary artery through the purse-string which is connected to the pulmonary perfusate line. Prostacyclin infusion is given via the side arm of this catheter in the dosage of 5 to 10 ngm/kg per minute as tolerated. A cardioplegia needle is inserted in the ascending aorta. The aorta is cross-clamped. The SVC and IVC are divided, 20 mL/kg of cold crystalloid cardioplegia at 4°C is infused into the aortic root, and lung perfusate is infused into the main pulmonary artery. The left side of the heart is decompressed by excising the tip of the left atrial appendage. Cold saline is used as a topical cooling agent. Once the cardioplegia and lung perfusate are completed, the aortic cross-clamp is released. The dissection of the heart-lung block then begins. The heart and lungs are excised by first dividing the posterior pericardium. Posterior mediastinal pleura is then divided on both sides, just in front of the esophagus. A plane of dissection is developed anterior to the esophagus, keeping as close as possible to its wall to preserve peribronchial tissue with the organ block. On the left side, the aortic arch is transected. The dissection is continued superiorly on both sides. The ascending aorta is transected just below the origin of the innominate artery. A horizontal incision is made across the midportion of the aortic arch, between the two previous incisions, to leave a cuff of aortic tissue attached to the pulmonary artery by the ligamentum arteriosum. The endotracheal tube is pulled back at the level of the proximal trachea. The lungs are inflated with air, and the trachea is doubly clamped and divided. The organs are placed in a large bowl containing cold saline (4°C). The trachea is stapled immediately distal to the clamp. The organs are placed in a sterile plastic bag with about two liters of cold saline. The plastic bag containing the

Table

Lung perfusate

Component	*Amount*
Ringer solution	10 mL/kg
20% salt poor albumin	3 mL/kg
20% mannitol	1.5 mL/kg
IU heparin	150 units/kg
Blood	7 mL/kg

organs is sealed with two additional plastic bags, taking care to remove as much air as possible. The bags are placed into an air-cushioned cool-box for transport. The time of aortic cross-clamping is noted.

In experimental preparations, various additives to the pulmonary artery flush solutions, such as oxygen-free radical scavengers,[20] and platelet-activating factor antagonist,[21,22] have been claimed to provide superior lung preservation. Furthermore, in a bovine model of heart-lung transplantation, donor core cooling, leukocyte depletion, and addition of liposomal superoxide dismutase (SOD) are shown to enhance lung preservation.[23] There is a need to perform controlled clinical trials of different preservation protocols.

Recipient Operation

The technical aspects of the recipient operation can be divided into three stages: removal of the recipient heart and lungs; preparation of the donor organs; and implantation of the donor heart and lungs.[24] Slight modification in the removal of recipient organs is required if the recipient heart is to be used for "domino" transplantation into another recipient.

Once the suitability of the donor organs is confirmed by the harvesting team, the recipient is anesthetized. Median sternotomy is performed and the pericardium opened. If the recipient heart is to be used for "domino" transplantation, then both SVC and IVC are cannulated directly; otherwise the right atrium is cannulated as for conventional orthotopic cardiac transplantation. In either instance, the ascending aorta is cannulated directly proximal to the innominate artery. Cardiopulmonary bypass is established and the circulation is cooled down to about 25°C.

Both pleural cavities are opened wide. Excision of the heart is performed by cutting the atria at midatrial level leaving a cuff of the right atrium and interatrial septum (Figure 1). The pulmonary veins and the pulmonary artery are then divided, and the ascending aorta transected below the aortic cross-clamp. If the recipient heart is to be used for "domino" operation, then the SVC is divided just above the right atrium, taking care to avoid injury to the sinoatrial node (SA), and the IVC is divided close to its junction with the right atrium. Enough SVC and IVC tissues remain in the recipient for anastomosis to the respective donor vessels.

In preparation for excision of the lungs, pericardium around each hilum is incised circumferentially. The posterior pericardium, however, is left intact to prevent chances of subsequent bleeding and to provide support for the donor organs. During resection of the lungs, great care is taken to identify and safeguard phrenic, vagus, and left recurrent laryngeal nerves. The phrenic nerves are seen easily lying anterior to the hilum on the lateral aspect of the pericardium, while the vagus nerves lie posteriorly and are safeguarded by keeping the plane of dissection as close to the main bronchus as possible. The pulmonary arteries and veins are divided within the pleural cavities on both sides, and subsequently the remnants of the pulmonary arteries and veins are removed, leaving a cuff of left pulmonary artery in situ in the region of the ligamentum arteriosum to protect the left recurrent laryngeal nerve (Figure 2). The bronchial arteries are doubly ligated and divided. If the lungs are infected, both bronchi are

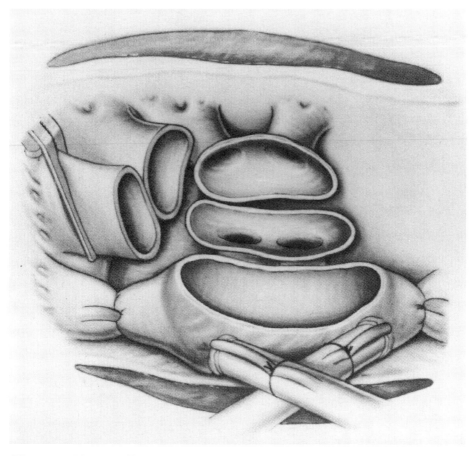

Figure 1. Diagram illustrating excision of the heart by a conventional technique.

clamped separately, the tracheobronchial tree sucked dry via the endotracheal tube, and the bronchi divided above the clamps. Suction can be applied to the trachea from below and the trachea divided approximately 1 cm above the carina (Figure 3). Alternatively, the trachea may be divided 1cm above the carina and both lungs removed en bloc through the incisions in the pericardium around the hilum. Stay sutures are applied to the cut end of the trachea. Little dissection is performed in the peritracheal tissue above the line of resection to prevent devascularization of the lower trachea. Once the heart and lungs are removed, complete hemostasis of the mediastinum is performed. This may be a tedious and time-consuming exercise, especially in children with Eisenmenger's syndrome.

Preparation of the donor organs then begins. The aorta is divided at a suitable level above the aortic valve. The right atrium is opened by an oblique incision from the IVC to the right atrial appendage, and the SVC closed with a continuous suture, safeguarding the SA. If the transplant procedure is part of a recipient "domino" operation, then the donor right atrium is kept intact and both SVC and IVC are anastomosed to the respective recipient vessels. The trachea is divided just above the bifurcation, and

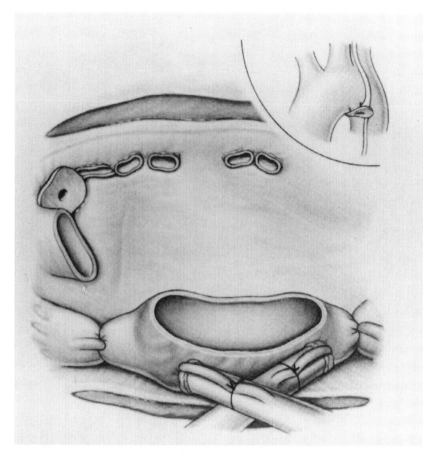

Figure 2. A small cuff of left pulmonary artery is left in situ at the site of ligamentum arteriosum to protect the left recurrent laryngeal nerve. The **inset** shows the course of the left vagus and recurrent laryngeal nerves.

the tracheobronchial tree cleared by suction. Cultures are sent both from the donor and recipient tracheobronchial tree for microbiology and antibiotic sensitivity. Minimal dissection of peritracheal tissue is performed, thus preserving the coronary bronchial collateral circulation in the heart-lung block.

The heart-lung block is then lowered into the recipient chest, and each lung is passed through the pericardial incision into the respective chest cavity (Figure 4). The recipient aorta is retracted and end-to-end anastomosis of the donor and recipient trachea is performed, using either polypropylene or a monofilament absorbable suture material. Previously inserted stay sutures on the recipient trachea aid in pulling it down in the operative field (Figure 5). The aortic anastomosis is then performed using the same suture material. The aortic cross-clamp is released, the heart de-aired, and the circulation rewarmed. The atrial anastomosis is then performed as for conventional orthotopic heart transplantation (Figure 6), or the SVC and IVC are anastomosed directly end-to-end in the "domino" technique. At normothermia, cardiopulmonary bypass is slowly weaned off. Inspired oxygen concentration is kept to the lowest possible

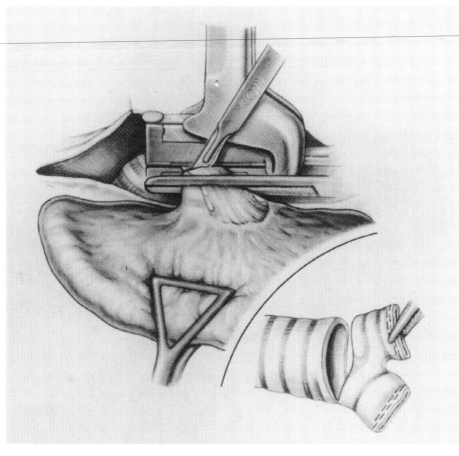

Figure 3. Excision of the lungs. The **inset** shows division of the trachea.

level in order to prevent the possibility of pulmonary injury. A renal dose of dopamine and a low dose of isoprenaline are usually given in the early postoperative period. An appropriate dose of methylprednisolone is also administered on releasing the aortic cross-clamp. Heparin is reversed using protamine, and hemostasis is secured. Three chest drains are inserted, atrial and ventricular pacing wires are left in situ, and the chest is closed in layers.

In case of a major mismatch between donor and recipient organs, successful transplant operation (by using bronchoplasty or pneumoreduction with a surgical stapler) has been reported.[25] However, with appropriate preoperative matching, we have not encountered a significant mismatch problem.

Technical modifications in the recipient operation are required in case of transplantations in the presence of left SVC, situs inversus, or other associated complex cardiac defects. If there is a left SVC without a communicating vein, it is dissected proximally toward the heart and a long length is obtained, including a part of coronary sinus. This facilitates insertion of donor organs. The left SVC is then brought either in front of the aorta, or is passed behind through the transverse sinus and anastomosed

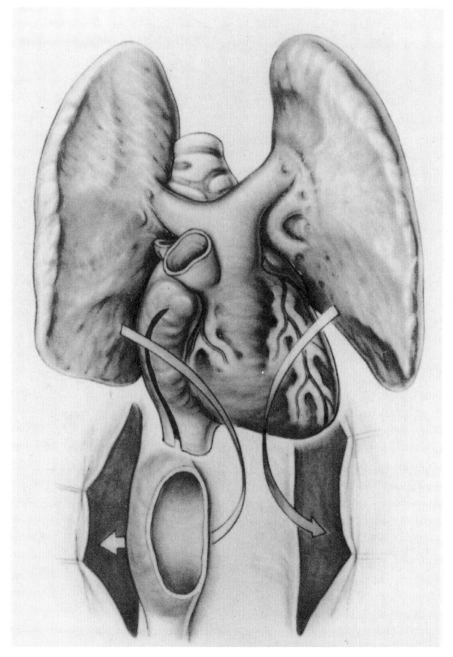

Figure 4. The donor organs are replaced into the recipient chest cavity as illustrated.

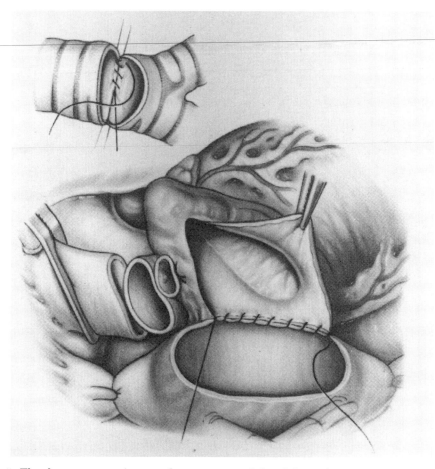

Figure 5. The donor organs, i.e., trachea, aorta, and the right atrium, are anastomosed to the respective recipient organs.

to the right atrial appendage.[26] In case of situs inversus, a large single atrium is created from the recipient right and left atria and is anastomosed to the donor right atrium.[27] Available donor tissues can be utilized to correct defects in the recipient, such as interrupted aortic arch.[28]

Postoperative Care

The general principles of postoperative management are similar to those applied to patients undergoing open-heart surgery.[29] In addition, extra precaution is taken to avoid fluid overload, as ischemic lungs are prone to noncardiogenic pulmonary edema. Colloid transfusions are given to maintain adequate filling pressures and inotropic support is continued for as long as necessary. A renal dose of dopamine is usually administered until the time of extubation.

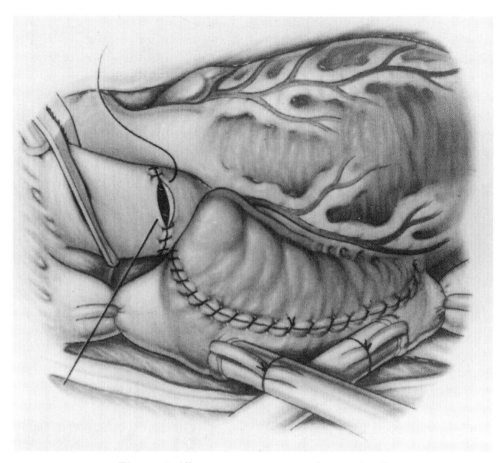

Figure 6. All anastomoses are nearly completed.

Bleeding is a serious complication following heart-lung transplantation. Due attention is, therefore, given to clotting parameters, and any abnormality of coagulation is immediately and completely corrected. Aprotinin is continued for a few hours after surgery. If, despite these measures, blood loss is still excessive, then reopening the chest is indicated without undue delay, as a large volume of blood transfusion is poorly tolerated by the transplanted lungs.

Prophylactic antibiotics are continued for the first few days. The type of antibiotic regimen is often dictated by the sensitivity report of the donor and recipient endotracheal secretions. In addition, nystatin, acyclovir, and low-dose cotrimoxazole are administered as a prophylaxis against candida, herpes, and pneumocystis infection, respectively.

Patients are weaned off mechanical ventilation as soon as possible. Patients who had chronic CO_2 retention prior to surgery may pose specific problems in weaning, if normal arterial PCO_2 levels are maintained after surgery. Instead, these patients are maintained on high arterial PCO_2 levels, but maintain a normal arterial pH. They are weaned off slowly on synchronized intermittent mandatory ventilation (SIMV) mode of ventilation.

Immunosuppression

Immunosuppression protocols vary from center to center. Our regimen for heart-lung transplant recipients is based primarily on cyclosporine (CsA) and azathioprine therapy.[30] Preoperatively, at the time of the patient's admission, azathioprine is given orally at a dose of 2 mg/kg with the premedication. CsA is also given orally at a dose of 5 to 10 mg/kg with the premedication according to renal function. If the patient is critically ill, we do not give CsA. A skin test for antilymphocyte globulin (ALG) is also performed at this stage.

Intraoperatively, once the aortic cross-clamp is released, 10 mg/kg of methylprednisolone is given intravenously (IV), followed by an IV administration of chlorpheniramine (5 to 10 mg). ALG or ATG is also given. We use an equine preparation (marketed by Merieux) in a dose of 0.5 mg/kg given over 6 hours.

Postoperatively, azathioprine is continued in the dose range of 1 to 2 mg/kg once daily, given either intravenously or orally. The dose of azathioprine is adjusted depending upon total white cell count which should be kept above 5000. CsA is given at a dosage of 5 to 20 mg/kg per day in three divided doses according to renal function. On the first postoperative day, we normally commence at a dose of 3 mg/kg three times a day, and if renal function remains satisfactory, gradually increase the dosage to obtain a trough cyclosporine level of 450 to 550 ngm/mL during the first 2 months after surgery. Our experience suggests that it is advisable to reduce the dosage of CsA if there is impending renal dysfunction. Two additional doses of ALG are given on days 2 and 3. The actual dosage depends on absolute T cell count, the aim being to lower the total number to between 100 to 200 T cells. If the total number of T cells has not been adequately depressed, then the dose of ALG is increased to about 0.7 to 0.8 mg/kg, and if the absolute number is between 50 and 100, then the dose of ALG may be reduced. Should the total count fall below 50, then the ALG may be withheld. The T cells should be measured for at least the first 5 postoperative days or until the total count goes below 500.

Our maintenance of long-term immunosuppression for heart-lung recipients consists of azathioprine and CsA. In case of acute rejection occurring in the first 3 months after surgery, augmented immunosuppression is given in the form of intravenous methylprednisolone 10 mg/kg per day for 3 days, followed by a reducing oral prednisolone starting at 1 mg/kg per day. If rejection is recurrent or difficult to control, then long-term oral steroids may be considered. The precise role of a new immunosuppressive agent FK 506 is as yet not established; however, early results are promising.[31]

Complications

Complications in a heart-lung transplant recipient may be related to surgery, to the donor organs, and to immunosuppression. Surgical complications include: bleeding, injury to the phrenic, left recurrent laryngeal, and vagus nerves; and those related to healing of the airways.[32] We have already discussed the postoperative bleeding problem. The risk of trauma to the nerves is minimized by careful surgical techniques. In an occasional patient who has had previous surgery, damage to the recurrent laryngeal nerve is seen postoperatively. Usually this is transient and improves with time. However, careful airway management and vigorous physiotherapy are required in the initial postoperative period, as the patient may have difficulty in generating an adequate cough reflex to clear pulmonary secretions. Successful augmentation of vocal cords in the acute phase using Teflon injection has been reported.[33] Damage to the phrenic nerves is uncommon and is usually well tolerated in an older child. Trauma to the vagal trunks can result in functional gastric outlet obstruction. This is also a transient paresis and resolves within a few weeks. Since the transplant operation interrupts the systemic arterial blood supply to the major airways, complications related to healing of the airways are at times a concern. In recent years, with careful operative technique, avoidance of pre- and postoperative steroids, and improvement in pulmonary preservation, this risk has been minimized. Occasionally, ischemia of the major airways below the anastomosis can result in bronchial stenosis as a result of healing with exuberant granulation tissue. This usually occurs between 2 to 3 weeks after the operation, and may respond to bronchial dilatation or cryotherapy. In our experience, the insertion of bronchial stents is rarely required.[34]

Donor organ-related complications are allograft rejection, obliterative bronchiolitis, and development of coronary artery disease (CAD). Acute pulmonary rejection is more common in heart-lung transplant recipients than cardiac allograft rejection.[35,36] This usually occurs in the first 3 months after surgery. Clinically, pulmonary rejection is associated with general symptoms of fever, malaise, and sometimes myalgia, with respiratory symptoms in the form of shortness of breath, dry cough, and falling oxygen saturations. The respiratory signs are not specific and include pulmonary crepitations. Chest x-ray shows interstitial infiltrate, which is often difficult to differentiate from conventional or opportunistic respiratory infection. Respiratory function tests reveal reduction in forced expiratory volume in one second (FEV_1). Serial parametric measurements of respiratory function are useful in detecting the onset of rejection. The diagnosis of rejection can be confirmed by fiberoptic bronchoscopy coupled with bronchoalveolar lavage and transbronchial biopsy. The lavage fluid should be cultured for various infective organisms. In addition, monoclonal antibody stains are performed for pneumocystis and CMV infection. Transbronchial biopsy shows characteristic features not only in pulmonary rejection, but also in certain pulmonary infections such as CMV and pneumocystis. Early diagnosis and treatment of allograft rejection is important to prevent permanent graft damage. The principles of treatment of rejection have already been outlined. Acute cardiac allograft rejection is relatively uncommon without pulmonary rejection. Obliterative bronchiolitis has emerged as the most serious late complication of heart-lung transplantation. This was first reported by Burke et al,[37] and consists of an inflammatory disorder of the pulmonary bronchioles that results in distortion, narrowing, and plugging with granulation tissue of the small airways.[38] It may represent a form of chronic rejection, although episodes of infection may also contribute to this condition. Histologically, there is destruction of the small airways and surrounding lung parenchyma with associated fibrosis. It usually occurs within 6 months to 2 years after operation. Initial clinical manifestations consist of a nonproductive or minimally productive cough followed by dyspnea. The chest x-ray in the early stages shows minimal changes which progress to small pulmonary infiltrates. Eventually, the characteristic changes of hyperinflation of the lung fields appear, associated with patchy shadowing and bronchial thickening. The lung function tests usually show an obstructive pattern with reduction in FEV_1/FVC ratio. Transbronchial biopsy is not always diagnostic of the condition, unless suitably sized airways are included in the sample. Open lung biopsy can be diagnostic, but this is associated with significant scarring and will add to the risk of any subsequent transplant procedure.

In the early days of heart-lung transplantation, a number of patients with obliterative bronchiolitis died due to the development of severe pulmonary failure. In recent years, early detection and expeditious treatment of rejection and viral pneumonitis has resulted in a real decrease in the incidence of this complication. The condition may respond to a prolonged course of augmented immunosuppression, which can be achieved by intravenous methylprednisolone followed by oral steroids.[39] Some patients, however, do not respond to augmented immunosuppression and may be considered for retransplantation. This should not be taken lightly, as extensive adhesions from the previous surgery carries significant risk for retransplantation. If there is no bronchial stenosis and the lung is free of infection, then single lung transplantation may be considered for this subset of patients. Early results of single lung transplantation in this condition have been encouraging.

Accelerated CAD is relatively uncommon in recipients of heart-lung transplantation. It occurs in perhaps 5% to 10% of those with long-term follow-up, and many of these patients also have manifestations of obliterative bronchiolitis.[40] This is also believed to be a manifestation of chronic allograft rejection.

Infection is a relatively common complication as a result of chronic immunosuppression.[41] The transplanted lung is continuously exposed to the external environment and is, therefore, vulnerable to infection. Furthermore, the donor organs have impaired normal ciliary defense mechanisms, and disrupted lymphatic drainage resulting in increased vulnerability to infection. Bacterial infections are especially a problem in patients with cystic fibrosis in whom the transplanted lungs may become colonized by bacteria. The management of acute bacterial infection consists of the use of appropriate antibiotics and supportive treatment in the form of physiotherapy and bronchoscopy. Opportunistic respiratory infection is also common, especially with CMV. This is treated with intravenous ganciclovir combined in severe cases with intravenous hyperimmune globulin. Despite aggressive treatment, mortality secondary to CMV pneumonitis in heart transplant recipients remains around 50% to 70%. Polymerase chain reaction amplification can detect increasing titers of CMV DNA in bronchoalveolar lavage specimens, prior to the onset of clinical symptoms or detection of infection by conventional techniques.[42] The technique, if available, may be used in patients at high risk of developing CMV to detect and treat the infection in its latent period. Routine prophylaxis with low-dose cotrimoxazole has significantly reduced the incidence of infection with pneumocystis. If there is a mismatch for toxoplasma gondii between donor and recipient, pyrimethamine may be given prophylactically.[43] Pulmonary allografts in heart-lung transplant patients are particularly vulnerable to the development of Epstein-Barr virus (EBV)-associated B cell lymphoma. Inhibition or destruction of preformed circulating T cells, specifically cytotoxic to EBV-infected B lymphocytes, allows outgrowth of virally transformed cells resulting in B-cell lymphomas. Treatment involves reduction of immunosuppression and intravenous acyclovir. The Pittsburgh group has reported two distinct forms of lymphoproliferative disease after heart-lung transplantation. Early onset disease (less than 1 year post-transplant) has a low mortality and usually responds to reduction in immune therapy; in contrast, the late onset disease (more than 1 year post-transplant) is often disseminated, has a high mortality, and usually does not respond to reduction in immunotherapy.[44]

Other complications of long-term immunosuppression include hypertension and nephrotoxicity, neurologic complications in the form of universal hand tremor, seizures, weight gain, Cushingoid changes secondary to steroid, and hirsutism. Major abdominal complications occur in 5% to 10% of transplant recipients. These include acute pancreatitis, peptic ulceration with bleeding, pseudo-obstruction, and bowel perforation. These often have atypical presentations. Successful management of these complications requires prompt diagnosis and treatment.[45,46]

Results

Pediatric heart-lung transplantation has been performed with increasing frequency and success. Successful transplantation can result in a marked improvement in both symptoms and quality of life. A 2-year actuarial survival rate of just over 40% has been reported for pediatric heart-lung recipients from Stanford University. This is less than the survival of 67% reported in adult patients.[47] Although the immediate postoperative survival rate for children with heart-lung transplantation is not substantially different from the adult population, pediatric patients have substantially increased morbidity and mortality after 3 months. Late deaths are commonly due to sepsis, airway problems, obliterative bronchiolitis, or diffuse CAD.

Despite the limitation of suitable donors, pediatric heart-lung transplantation is on the increase. Reducing postoperative mortality, especially in the post 3-month period, is the major task for the future. Continuing improvement in immunosuppression, and perhaps the development of selective immune tolerance, may pave the way for a better future. Perhaps, ultimately, xeno-transplantation will be the alternative that may overcome the donor organ limitation. Heart-lung transplantation will certainly be offered to patients with end-stage heart and lung disease, due to significant complexities of the procedure. However, current results support the continued efforts to perform transplantations in children with end-stage conditions.

References

1. Reitz BA, Wallwork JL, Hunt SA, et al: Heart-lung transplantation: successful therapy for patients with pulmonary vascular disease. *N Engl J Med* 306:557–564, 1982.
2. Neptune WB, Cookson BA, Bailey CP, et al: Complete homologous heart transplantation. *Arch Surg* 66:174–178, 1953.
3. Marcus E, Wong SNT, Luisada AA: Homologous heart grafts. *Arch Surg* 66:179, 1953.
4. Cooley DA, Bloodwell RD, Hallman GL, et al: Organ transplantation for advanced cardiopulmonary disease. *Ann Thorac Surg* 8:30–46, 1969.
5. Wildevuur CRH, Benfield JR: A review of 23 human lung transplantations by 20 surgeons. *Ann Thorac Surg* 9:489–515, 1970.
6. Losman JG, Campbell CD, Replogle RL, Bernard CN: Joint transplantation of the heart and lungs: past experience and present potentials. *J Cardiovasc Surg* 23:440, 1982.
7. Miller WW, Kaye MP, Baum D: Pediatric heart, heart-lung and lung transplantation: the world experience from 1984–1993. *Prog Pediatr Cardiol* 11:4–8, 1993.

8. Smyth RL, Scott JP, Whitehead B, et al: Heart-lung transplantation in children. *Transplant Proc* 22:1470–1471, 1990.
9. Starnes VA, Oyer PE, Bernstein D, et al: Heart, heart-lung, and lung transplantation in the first year of life. *Ann Thorac Surg* 53:306–310, 1992.
10. Bolman RM, Shumway SJ, Estrin JA, Hertz MI: Lung and heart transplantation: evolution and new applications. *Ann Surg* 214:456–470, 1991.
11. Novick RJ, Menkis AH, McKenzie FN, et al: The safety of low-dose prednisone before and immediately after heart-lung transplantation. *Ann Thorac Surg* 51:642–645, 1991.
12. Novick RJ, Menkis AH, McKenzie FH, Reid KR, Ahmad D: Should heart-lung transplant donors and recipients be matched according to cytomegalovirus serologic status? *J Heart Transplant* 9:699–706, 1990.
13. Hutter JA, Scott J, Wreghitt T, Higenbottam T, Wallwork J: The importance of cytomegalovirus in heart-lung transplant recipients. *Chest* 95:627–631, 1989.
14. Smyth RL, Scott JP, Borysiewicz LK, et al: Cytomegalovirus infection in heart-lung transplant recipients: risk factors, clinical associations, and response to treatment. *J Infect Dis* 164:1045–1050, 1991.
15. de Leval MR, Smyth R, Whitehead B, et al: Heart and lung transplantation for terminal cystic fibrosis. *J Thorac Cardiovasc Surg* 101:633–642, 1991.
16. Festenstein H, Banner N, Smith J, et al: The influence of matching and lymphocytotoxic antibody status on surviving heart-lung allograft recipients receiving cyclosporine and azathioprine. *Transplant Proc* 21:797–798, 1989.
17. Yacoub M, Khaghani A, Banner N, et al: Distant organ procurement for heart-lung transplantation. *Transplant Proc* 21:2548–2550, 1989.
18. Wallwork J, Jones DK, Cavorocchin N, et al: Distant procurement of organs for clinical heart-lung transplantation using a single flush technique. *Transplantation* 44:654–658, 1987.
19. Hardesty RI, Griffith BP: Autoperfusion of the heart and lungs for preservation during distant procurement. *J Thorac Cardiovasc Surg* 93:11–18, 1987.
20. Cremer J, Jurmann M, Dammenhayn L, Wahlers T, Haverich A, Borst HG: Oxygen free radical scavengers to prevent pulmonary reperfusion injury after heart-lung transplantation. *J Heart Transplant* 8:330–336, 1989.
21. Qayumi AK, Jamieson WRE, Poostizadeh A: Effects of platelet-activating factor antagonist CV-3988 in preservation of heart and lung for transplantation. *Ann Thorac Surg* 52:1026–1032, 1991.
22. Wahlers T, Hirt SW, Haverich A, Fieguth HG, Jurmann M, Borst HG: Future horizons of lung preservation by application of a platelet-activating factor antagonist compared with current clinical standards: Euro-Collins flush perfusion versus donor core cooling. *J Thorac Cardiovasc Surg* 103:200–205, 1992.
23. Bando K, Schueler S, Cameron DE, et al: Twelve-hour cardiopulmonary preservation using donor core cooling, leukocyte depletion, and liposomal superoxide dismutase. *J Heart Lung Transplant* 10:304–309, 1991.
24. Vouhe PR, Dartevelle PG: Heart-lung transplantation: technical modifications that may improve the early outcome. *J Thorac Cardiovasc Surg* 97:906–910, 1989.
25. Noirclerc M, Shennib H, Giudicelli R, et al: Size matching in lung transplantation. *J Heart-Lung Transplant* 11:S203–S208, 1992.
26. Yacoub M, Mankad P, Ledingham S: Donor procurement and surgical techniques for cardiac transplantation. *Semin Thorac Cardiovasc Surg* 3:47–56, 1990.
27. Miralles A, Muneretto C, Gandjbakhch I, et al: Heart-lung transplantation in situs inversus: a case report in a patient with Kartagener's syndrome. *J Thorac Cardiovasc Surg* 103:307–313, 1992.
28. Aranki S, Musumeci F, Khaghani A, Radley-Smith R, Yacoub M: One-stage correction of interrupted aortic arch combined with heart-lung transplantation. *J Thorac Cardiovasc Surg* 98:285–288, 1989.
29. Scott JP, Fradet G, Smyth RL, Solis E, Higenbottam TW, Wallwork J: Management following heart and lung transplantation: five years experience. *Eur J Cardiothorac Surg* 4:197–201, 1990.

30. Whitehead B, James I, Helms P, et al: Intensive care management of children following heart and heart-lung transplantation. *Intensive Care Med* 6:426–430, 1990.
31. Griffith BP, Hardesty RL, Armitage JM, et al: Acute rejection of lung allografts with various immunosuppressive protocols. *Ann Thorac Surg* 54:846–851, 1992.
32. Starnes VA, Marshall SE, Lewiston NJ, Theodore I, Stinson EB, Shumway NE: Heart-lung transplantation in infants, children and adolescents. *J Pediatr Surg* 26:434–438, 1991.
33. Murty GE, Smith MC: Recurrent laryngeal nerve palsy following heart-lung transplantation: three cases of vocal cord augmentation in the acute phase. *J Laryngol Otol* 103:968–969, 1989.
34. Spatenka J, Khaghani A, Irving JD, Theodoropoulos S, Slavik Z, Yacoub MH: Gianturco self-expanding metallic stents in treatment of tracheobronchial stenosis after single lung and heart and lung transplantation. *Eur J Cardiothorac Surg* 5:648–652, 1991.
35. Baldwin JC, Oyer PE, Stinson EB, Starnes VA, Billingham ME, Shumway NE: Comparison of cardiac rejection in heart and heart-lung transplantation. *J Heart Transplant* 6:352–356, 1987.
36. Griffith BP, Hardesty RL, Trento A, Bahnson HT: Asynchronous rejection of the heart and lungs following cardiopulmonary transplantation. *Ann Thorac Surg* 40:488–493, 1985.
37. Burke C, Theodore J, Dawkin K, et al: Post-transplant obliterative bronchiolitis and other late lung sequalae in human heart-lung transplantation. *Chest* 86:824–829, 1984.
38. Theodore J, Starnes VA, Lewiston NJ: Obliterative bronchiolitis. *Clin Chest Med* 11:309–321, 1990.
39. Glanville AR, Baldwin JC, Burke CM, Theodore J, Robin ED: Obliterative bronchiolitis after heart-lung transplantation: apparent arrest by augmented immunosuppression. *Ann Intern Med* 107:300–304, 1987.
40. Miller LW: Transplant coronary artery disease: editorial. *J Heart Lung Transplant* 11:S1–S4, 1992.
41. Dauber JH, Paradis IL, Dummer JS: Infectious complications in pulmonary allograft recipients. *Clin Chest Med* 11:291–308, 1990.
42. Cagle PT, Buffone G, Holland VA, et al: Semiquantitative measurement of cytomegalovirus DNA in lung and heart-lung transplant patients by in vitro DNA amplification. *Chest* 101:93–96, 1992.
43. Wreghitt TG, Gray JJ, Pavel P, et al: Efficacy of pyrimethamine for the prevention of donor acquired Toxoplasma gondii infection on heart and heart-lung transplant patients. *Transplant Int* 5:197–200, 1992.
44. Armitage JM, Kormos RL, Stuart RS, et al: Post-transplant lymphoproliferative disease in thoracic organ transplant patients: ten years of cyclosporine-based immunosuppression. *J Heart Lung Transplant* 10:877–887, 1991.
45. Augustine SM, Yeo CJ, Buchman TG, Achuff SC, Baumgartner WA: Gastrointestinal complications in heart and in heart-lung transplant patients. *J Heart Lung Transplant* 10:547–556, 1991.
46. Watson CJ, Jamieson NV, Johnston PS, et al: Early abdominal complications following heart and heart-lung transplantation. *Br J Surg* 78:699–704, 1991.
47. Nisco SJ, Reitz BA: Pediatric heart-lung and lung transplantation. *Prog Pediatr Cardiol* 2:47–58, 1993.

Chapter 10

Heart and Heart-Lung Transplantation in Children:

A Review of the International Society of Heart and Lung Transplantation/United Network for Organ Sharing Registry Data

Stuart Berger, MD; Jeffrey D. Hosenpud, MD

Introduction

Cardiac transplantation and heart-lung transplantation in neonates, infants, children, and adolescents have grown immensely over the last decade, and are now an accepted modality of treatment for end-stage myocardial dysfunction, as well as for treatment of palliated congenital heart disease with severe myocardial dysfunction. In some cases, and at some centers, it is the preferred therapy for some forms of congenital heart disease even prior to palliation. The utility of this therapy is limited primarily by the availability of acceptable organ donors. This chapter reviews the current experience in heart and heart-lung transplantation in neonates, infants, children, and adolescents based upon the current International Society of Heart and Lung Transplantation (ISHLT) data.

Cardiac Transplantation

Heart Transplantation in Neonates and Infants Under 1 Year of Age

The major indication for cardiac transplantation in this age group is congenital heart disease (Figure 1). The largest subset within this category includes those infants

From: Franco KL (ed). *Pediatric Cardiopulmonary Transplantation.* Armonk, NY: Futura Publishing Company, Inc.; © 1997.

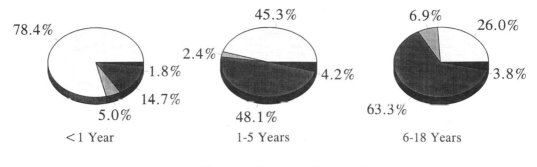

Heart Transplantation

☐Congenital ▨Other ▧Myopathy ■ReTx

Figure 1. Indications for heart transplantation by age group. (Reproduced with permission from Hosenpud JD, Novick RJ, Breen TJ, et al: The Registry of the International Society for Heart and Lung Transplantation—1995. *J Heart Lung Transplant* 14:805–815, 1995.)

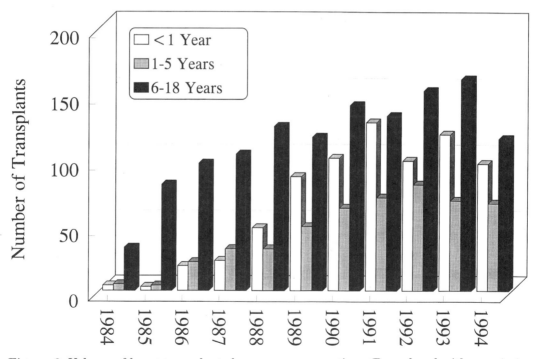

Figure 2. Volume of heart transplants by age group over time. (Reproduced with permission from Hosenpud JD, Novick RJ, Breen TJ, et al: The Registry of the International Society for Heart and Lung Transplantation—1995. *J Heart Lung Transplant* 14:805–815, 1995.)

with hypoplastic left heart syndrome (HLHS) and its variants. This comprised 78.4% of the heart transplants performed in infants under 1 year of age. A relatively smaller group in this age was that of dilated cardiomyopathy (14.7%), while 1.8% of the transplants performed were in fact retransplants.

The number of transplants performed in infants less than 1 year of age has grown progressively over the years (Figure 2). In 1984, this therapy was performed in very few infants, while in 1993 and 1994 over 100 transplants in this age group were performed in each year. The slight decrease from 1993 to 1994 may be a result of donor availability.

The actuarial survival curves for pediatric heart transplantation are represented in Figure 3. A total of 645 transplants in infants less than 1 year of age, since 1984, has resulted in an overall 1-year survival of 66% and a 2-year survival of 65%. The 30-day mortality figures (Figure 4) depict a 25% mortality. It should be pointed out that this data includes all transplants in this age group since 1984. Comparing the more current transplant era (1988 to 1994) to the earlier experience suggests a substantial improvement in outcome (Figure 5). Some single center studies currently report as high as a 90% "immediate" and 84% 5-year survival.[1]

Heart Transplantation in Patients 1 to 18 Years of Age

The majority of patients receiving heart transplantation in this age group are for the indication of cardiomyopathy. An indication with increasing frequency, however,

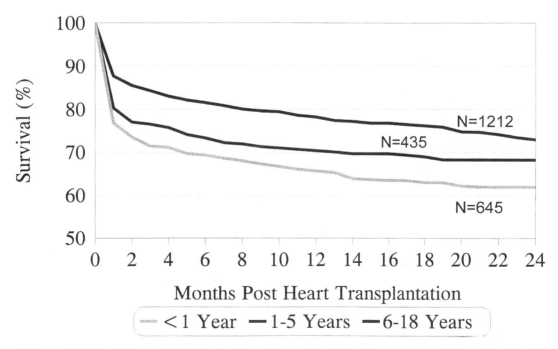

Figure 3. Actuarial survival following heart transplantation by age group. (Reproduced with permission from Hosenpud JD, Novick RJ, Breen TJ, et al: The Registry of the International Society for Heart and Lung Transplantation—1995. *J Heart Lung Transplant* 14:805–815, 1995.)

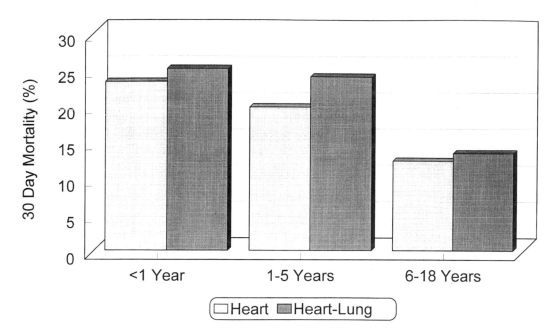

Figure 4. Thirty-day morality for heart and heart-lung transplantation by age group. (Reproduced with permission from Hosenpud JD, Novick RJ, Breen TJ, et al: The Registry of the International Society for Heart and Lung Transplantation—1995. *J Heart Lung Transplant* 14:805–815, 1995.)

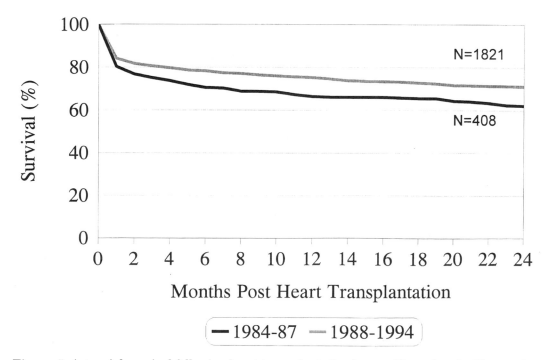

Figure 5. Actuarial survival following heart transplantation by era. (Reproduced with permission from Hosenpud JD, Novick RJ, Breen TJ, et al: The Registry of the International Society for Heart and Lung Transplantation—1995. *J Heart Lung Transplant* 14:805–815, 1995.)

is that of palliated congenital heart disease. If one further subdivides this age range (Figure 1), one notes that in the group of children 1 to 5 years of age, 48.1% of transplants were for cardiomyopathy, while 45.3% were for children with congenital heart disease, 4.2% of the transplants were retransplants. In the 6- to 18-year old group, 63.3% of the transplants were for cardiomyopathy, 26.0% for congenital heart disease, and 3.8% for retransplantation.

In 1993 and 1994, 80 transplants were performed in the 1- to 5-year age group (Figure 2). The number has grown since the 1980s, but has been relatively constant over the last 4 years. In the 6- to 18-year age group, in 1993 and 1994, 175 and 130 transplants were performed in this age group, respectively (Figure 2). Once again, the decrease in number may be due to donor availability, as well as the fact that older adolescents must compete with adults for this limited resource.

In the 1- to 5-year age group, of the 435 transplants performed, the actuarial 1-year survival was 70% with a 5-year survival of 68% (Figure 3). This data is cumulative since 1984, and more recent statistics suggest an improvement in both 1-year as well as 5-year survival. Thirty-day mortality figures suggest an approximate mortality of 23% (Figure 4). In the 6- to 18-year age group, of the 1212 transplants performed, the actuarial 1-year survival was 78% with a 5-year survival of 75% (Figure 3). This is comparable to survival in adult patients.[2] Thirty-day mortality in this group is 13%, once again suggesting, as in the other age groups, that the highest mortality occurs in the first 1 to 2 months after transplantation (Figure 4).

Heart-Lung Transplantation

Heart-Lung Transplantation in Neonates and Infants Under 1 Year of Age

There are relatively few indications for this therapy in neonates and infants. Such therapy has, therefore, not been performed with any degree of regularity. Indications would include pulmonary vascular disease, either secondary to congenital heart disease, or primary pulmonary hypertension. Either of these diagnoses are rare in the infant less than 1 year of age, especially the former. Primary pulmonary hypertension is likely to be palliated medically, especially within the first year of life. In addition, current practice has resulted in lung transplantation, rather than heart-lung transplantation as the preferred method of surgical therapy. Fewer than five heart-lung transplants per year have been performed in this age group. This has not changed appreciably over the years (Figure 6).

Thirty-day mortality for heart-lung transplantation in infants less than 1 year of age is 27% (Figure 4). This is comparable to the 30-day mortality for heart transplantation in this age group.

Heart-Lung Transplantation in Children 1 to 18 Years of Age

The indications for heart-lung transplantation include intractable and terminal pulmonary and/or cardiopulmonary diseases, for which conventional medical or surgical treatment, including heart transplantation, would be ineffective. Major indications

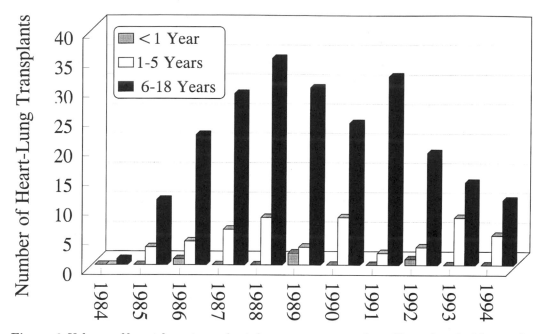

Figure 6. Volume of heart-lung transplants by age group over time. (Reproduced with permission from Hosenpud JD, Novick RJ, Breen TJ, et al: The Registry of the International Society for Heart and Lung Transplantation—1995. *J Heart Lung Transplant* 14:805–815, 1995.)

have included primary pulmonary hypertension and irreversible pulmonary vascular obstructive disease (Eisenmenger's syndrome) secondary to congenital heart disease (Figure 7). Other indications have included end-stage chronic obstructive lung disease, interstitial pulmonary fibrosis, cystic fibrosis, and irreversible physical or chemical damage to the airways. Finally, certain rare forms of congenital heart disease that involve severe pulmonary artery or pulmonary vein stenosis, hypoplasia or atresia, with or without pulmonary hypertension, may be candidates for heart-lung transplantation. It should be pointed out that the current trend suggests that it is preferable, in situations where it is appropriate, to transplant one or two lungs rather than the heart-lung block itself. If the heart is structurally normal or can be easily repaired at the time of transplant, and the left ventricle is functionally normal, unilateral or bilateral lung transplantation, as opposed to heart-lung transplantation, may be preferable.

In the 1- to 5-year age group, the number of heart-lung transplants performed is still relatively small (Figure 6). Over the last 2 years, this therapy has been instituted in 7 to 10 children per year. In the 6- to 18-year age group, the numbers are a bit larger, but still significantly less than patients of this age who receive heart transplantation. The peak numbers for this therapy were in 1987 to 1991, where 30 to 35 heart-lung transplants per year were performed. The last 3 years have represented a progressive decrease in the total number of heart-lung transplants per year across all age groups. In 1993 and 1994, only 15 and 13 heart-lung transplants, respectively, were performed in this age group. The reason for this, as mentioned earlier, is that many of the patients who would have been appropriate candidates for heart-lung transplantation are

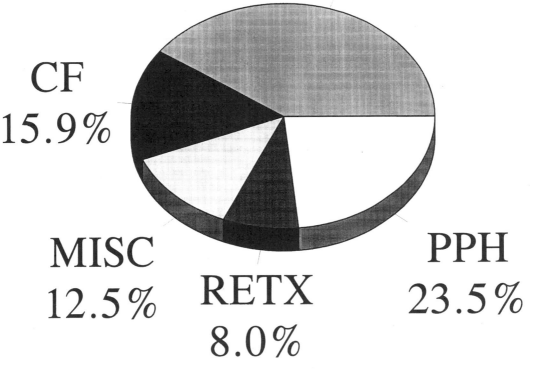

Figure 7. Indications for heart-lung transplantation. (Reproduced with permission from Hosenpud JD, Novick RJ, Breen TJ, et al: The Registry of the International Society for Heart and Lung Transplantation—1995. *J Heart Lung Transplant* 14:805–815, 1995.)

also very appropriate candidates for either unilateral or bilateral lung transplantation. The additional advantage of this approach allows for the use of the donor heart in another patient waiting for heart transplantation. This seems to be a much better use of resources that are significantly limited.

In the 1- to 5-year age group, the 30-day mortality for heart-lung transplantation was 25% (Figure 4). This is slightly higher, but not significantly different from patients in this age group who receive heart transplantation. In the 6- to 18-year age group, the 30-day mortality for heart-lung transplantation was 13%. This also was comparable to patients in this age group who have received cardiac transplantation. The 3-year actuarial survival for the two latter age groups are presented in Figure 8. As with heart transplantation, the 1- to 5-year age group had poorer survival than the 6- to 18-year age group. This difference was as high as 25% by 1 year, but narrowed to approximately 15% by 3 years post-transplantation.

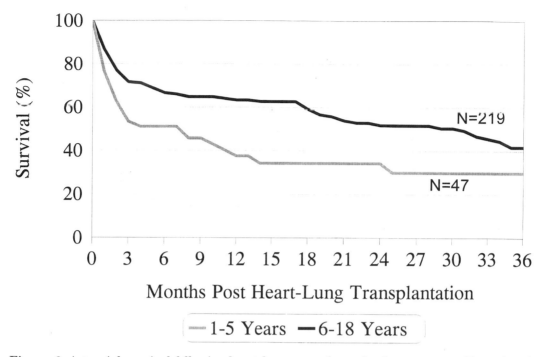

Figure 8. Actuarial survival following heart-lung transplantation by age group. (Reproduced with permission from Hosenpud JD, Novick RJ, Breen TJ, et al: The Registry of the International Society for Heart and Lung Transplantation—1995. *J Heart Lung Transplant* 14:805–815, 1995.)

Retransplantation

Although uncommon, retransplantation carries a very high mortality for both heart and heart-lung transplantation (Figure 9). The 2-year survival for heart retransplantation is approximately 40% (compared to approximately 70% for first time heart transplantation), and for heart-lung retransplantation is approximately 22% (compared to between 40% and 50% for first time heart-lung transplantation). This is comparable to the magnitude of the reduction in outcome seen in the adult population,[2] but is even more discouraging in absolute survival.

Summary and Conclusions

This ISHLT/UNOS (United Network for Organ Sharing) data suggests that cardiac transplantation continues to be an acceptable and viable therapy for select clinical problems in pediatric cardiology. It continues to be an important therapy for children with end-stage cardiomyopathy. The actuarial data suggests that cardiac transplantation will result in improved morbidity and mortality, and should be a therapy for children with cardiomyopathy, whose predicted 1-year survival is less than that

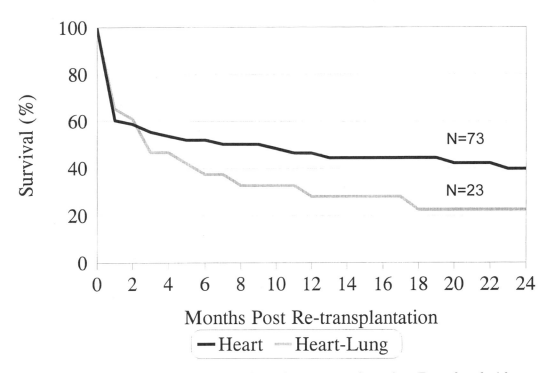

Figure 9. Actuarial survival for heart and heart-lung retransplantation. (Reproduced with permission from Hosenpud JD, Novick RJ, Breen TJ, et al: The Registry of the International Society for Heart and Lung Transplantation—1995. *J Heart Lung Transplant* 14:805–815, 1995.)

of cardiac transplantation. Though this of course is extremely difficult to predict, recent data does suggest an overall improved survival with cardiac transplantation performed more recently.

An additional group of infants and children who might be considered for cardiac transplantation include those infants or children with congenital heart disease, with either a poorly functioning or inadequate-sized systemic ventricle, who may or may not have had a prior cardiac operation. This indication comprises a relatively larger number of cardiac transplants in the under 1-year age group and the 1- to 5-year age group. The decision to offer cardiac transplantation, and the results, are similar to the criteria as discussed for dilated cardiomyopathy. However, unoperated neonates with serious congenital heart disease represent a special group. The prototypic example of this group is represented by the neonate with hypoplastic left heart syndrome (HLHS). In this group of infants, an alternate approach to heart transplantation does exist. The Norwood approach requires three operations and the ultimate result is a Fontan-like repair with single ventricle anatomy and physiology. The morbidity and mortality is variable, but at some centers is quite low. The decision to recommend cardiac transplantation as opposed to Norwood palliation for this group of patients is philosophical, and varies from one institution to another.

The ISHLT/UNOS data suggests that heart-lung transplantation is occurring much less frequently. This can be explained by the fact that lung transplantation seems to be a very acceptable therapy for many of the indications that previously required heart-lung transplantation. The additional usefulness of this approach will allow for the use of the donor heart in a different, separate, appropriate patient. This clearly is a more efficient use of an extremely limited resource. Heart-lung transplantation will still be necessary and indicated for children with complex congenital heart disease, and pulmonary artery hypertension, or for children with pulmonary artery hypoplasia/atresia or pulmonary vein hypoplasia/atresia, with complex congenital heart disease and/or a poorly functioning or inadequate-sized systemic ventricle. These would be situations where lung replacement alone might not be sufficient.

Finally, repeat thoracic organ transplantation results in extremely poor outcomes. Given the serious shortage of donor organs, one must question the use of this extremely limited resource for retransplantation.

References

1. Bailey LL, Gundry SR, et al: Bless the babies: one hundred fifteen late survivors of heart transplantation during the first year of life. *J Thorac Cardiovasc Surg* 105:805–815, 1993.
2. Hosenpud JD, Novick RJ, Breen TJ, Daily OP: The Registry of the International Society for Heart and Lung Transplantation: eleventh official report—1994. *J Heart Lung Transplant* 13:561–570, 1994.

Chapter 11

Lung Preservation

David P. Kapelanski, MD, FACS
Stuart W. Jamieson, MB, FRCS

Introduction

During the past 30 years, transplantation of the lung has evolved from a laboratory curiosity with limited therapeutic potential to an essential option in the management of patients with terminal pulmonary disease. Unequivocally, the contingent factor in this transition was the introduction of cyclosporine-based immunosuppresion. While the current success rates are predicated on a collaborative endeavor encompassing recipient and donor selection, implantation, and peri- and postperative care, the defining process is the replacement of a dysfunctional lung with a physiologically competent one. This chapter provides a comprehensive analysis of those factors critical to the immediate function of the grafted organ. Drawing from an extensive literature not solely confined to the lung, a formal examination of the general pathophysiology of reperfusion injury is, thus, an obiigatory preface, and defines a common context from which to understand the art as currently practiced. We proceed with an analysis of the causes of abnormal oxygenation following lung reperfusion, and follow with a brief discourse on the strategies we employ to assure the immediate function of the pulmonary graft. We conclude with our thoughts on the future of experimental work.

Our intent in this chapter is to provide a global perspective on the phenomenon and mechanisms that are believed to contribute to dysfunction of the lung following hypothermic preservation and reperfusion. The subject of pulmonary preservation has been amply reviewed in the past, and at each iteration, new data is added from a rich and evolving body of work.[1–7] In deference to others who have covered many of the individual topics embraced in this section in greater detail, our goal is to emphasize newer information at the relative expense of well-accepted doctrine. While we propose to catalog each of the major features pertinent to a discussion of lung preservation, no attempt is made to be encyclopedic.

We have gleaned our interpretation of the pathogenesis of reperfusion injury from work accomplished in systems spanning the spectrum from cultured cells to whole or-

From: Franco KL (ed). *Pediatric Cardiopulmonary Transplantation.* Armonk, NY: Futura Publishing Company, Inc.; © 1997.

ganisms, studying diverse mammalian and (rarely) avian species. Unless otherwise specified, citations describing the outcome of whole organ ischemic challenges were conducted at physiologic temperature, and in the absence of attempts to alter the subsequent development of injury. We have been more circumspect in our analysis of preservation work, although, unlike others, we do not believe the fundamental repertoire of interactions available to host and graft is determined by any extent of ischemia short of cell death.[5]

The Pathogenesis of Reperfusion Injury

In part attributable to an approach that was focused on sustaining or restoring oxidative metabolism in the parenchymal cells of those organs with intrinsically high metabolism, the endothelium's role in transducing, interpreting, and modulating the discourse between the circulation and the parenchymal cells was largely ignored in early discussions of organ preservation. The vascular endothelium is no longer viewed as the innermost layer of a passive and metabolically inert conduit, but rather as the most active paracrine organ in the body.[8,9] From this vantage, many of the pathophysiologic manifestations of postischemic injury can be viewed as the consequence of deranged signal processing by the endothelium. As will be seen, many of the messages emitted during reperfusion were difficult to perceive because they are ephemeral. Other signals were difficult to recognize because they are not released into the general circulation, but are rather restricted within the cell of origin, or displayed only on the surface membrane, with their intended audience a restricted subset of the itinerant leukocytes. Apart from the initial difficulties encountered in detecting these signals, their limited expression made it difficult to determine the nature of the stimulus that incited transmission. In many instances, these problems have been overcome using monoclonal antibodies (mAb) as specific probes for detecting and interfering with the function of cell surface molecules, and by the refinement of techniques which indirectly allow the expression of specific genes to be monitored within individual cells.

Although leukocyte infiltration occurs late in reperfusion, we begin our discussion of the pathogenesis of reperfusion injury at this terminal phase for four reasons. First, as will be demonstrated, the process is well defined, and the nature of the signals, the content of the message, and the response of the recipient have been described in considerable depth. The terminal phase of leukocyte infiltration, thus, constitutes a prototype, and provides a framework within which to interpret other phenomena not yet as well characterized. Second, because it occurs at a relatively late stage, the process of leukocyte recruitment and activation represents a response that both integrates and amplifies a composite of antecedent messages and, thus, demarcates a point beyond which time strategies intent on precluding injury can by definition no longer be effective. Third, because leukocyte activation during reperfusion occurs in an environment rich in messages, a top down approach provides an opportunity to initiate our discussion of these signals from the perspective of an integrated context and, thus, discern the coordinate behavior, rather than the piecemeal response. The final, and, from our clinical perspective, most important reason we initiate our discussion with this topic is that the signals which promote leukocyte trafficking and activation can be interfered with, and in a manner that ameliorates reperfusion injury.

Leukocytes and Leukocyte Adhesion

Within the past decade, extraordinary progress has been made in deciphering the nature and sequence of interactions governing the attraction, activation, and extravascular migration of circulating leukocytes during inflammation. While the broader topic of leukocyte trafficking encompasses several shared and parallel processes central to specific immune recognition and graft rejection, the following discussion focuses primarily on the details of leukocyte recruitment in postischemic tissue.[10,11]

When time-lapse video techniques are used to examine the microcirculation after an ischemic insult, dilation of the postcapillary venules is evident within moments of the onset of reperfusion.[12–14] As the vessel caliber increases, the velocity of individual cells within the bloodstream is reduced, particularly adjacent to the endothelium. Within this marginal layer of reduced flow, the proportion of neutrophils becomes progressively greater. Individual neutrophils can be seen tumbling or "rolling" along the vessel wall for variable intervals; some recoil and reenter the central flowing stream, while others slow, then halt. These immobilized cells then deform, first flattening against the endothelium, then progressively insinuating, in ameboid fashion, through the vessel wall and into the extravascular space. It is now recognized that each of these distinct phases of leukocyte emigration is mediated by the specific interaction of endothelial and leukocyte cell surface molecules belonging to one of three gene families: the selectins, the integrins, and the immunoglobulin superfamily.[15] An abridged review of the essential functions and regulation of the individual proteins encoded by these genes, followed by a description of their coordinate interactions provides a useful perspective from which the mechanisms of neutrophil amplification of reperfusion injury can be viewed (Figures 1, 2, and 3).

The selectins are a group of three endothelial and leukocyte surface monomers individually characterized by their binding affinity for glycoproteins and, in particular, those displaying the tetrasaccharide sialyl Lewis X.[16,17] Only after each molecule was cloned and sequenced was the structural homology of the group evident. Each member of the selectin family contains an amino-terminal calcium-dependent lectin-binding domain, an epidermal growth factor-like region, a variable number of short consensus repeat sequences analogous to those found in the complement regulatory proteins, a transmembrane region, and a short cytoplasmic tail.[18–20] Notwithstanding their comparable structure, the cellular distribution and regulation of the selectins are quite disparate.

L-selectin (CD62L, LECAM-1, LAM-1, gp90MEL-14) is constitutively expressed by essentially all circulating leukocytes. On unstimulated neutrophils, L-selectin is preferentially distributed to the microvilli, the site of initial cell to cell contact.[21] Within minutes of activation in vitro by exposure to C5a, tumor necrosis factor (TNF), leukotriene B4, or the chemotactic peptide n-formyl-methionly-leucyl-phenylalanine (fMLP), L-selectin expression is virtually abolished by a process in which the molecule is shed from the surface of the neutrophil.[22–26] Even in the absence of inflammatory stimuli, high levels of the soluble shed form are detected in the peripheral blood, presumably reflecting leukocyte emigration during ongoing surveillance.[27] Since the soluble molecule inhibits L-selectin-dependent leukocyte attachment at physiologic concentrations in vitro, rapid shedding provides a dual mechanism for tempering what has proved to be a very early event in the leukocyte emigration sequence.[28]

Despite considerable effort, the endothelial ligand for neutrophil L-selectin has,

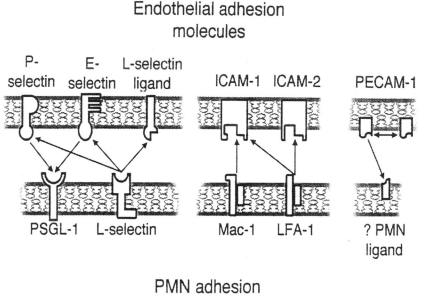

Figure 1. The binding interaction of endothelial and PMN leukocyte adhesion molecules in acute inflammation are depicted by **arrows.** In unstimulated endothelium, PECAM-1 homophilically binds to PECAM-1 on adjacent endothelial cells; during acute inflammation, it heterophilically binds an unknown PMN ligand. The endothelial L-selectin ligand has not been identified.

thus far, defied attempts at identification. Several sialomucin-like glycoproteins have been isolated from the high endothelial venules of peripheral lymph nodes, and have been demonstrated to function as important homing receptors for L-selectin mediated lymphocyte emigration.[29–31] With the exception of CD34, none of these ligands is widely enough distributed to warrant consideration as mediators of neutrophil trafficking in nonlymphoid tissue.[32] In an unusual example of a bidirectional interaction, however, neutrophil L-selectin also serves as a ligand for both of the inducible endothelial selectins (see below) by presentation of sialyl Lewis X.[21,33,34]

Both endothelial cells and platelets constitutively express P-selectin (CD62P, GMP-140, PAD-GEM).[35,36] In the absence of stimulation, P-selectin surface expression by either lineage is limited, with the vast majority of detectable molecule stored in the alpha granules of platelets and the Weibel-Palade bodies of the endothelial cells. Within minutes of exposure to hydrogen peroxide, histamine, thrombin, platelet-activating factor (PAF), or the complement membrane attack complex, C5b-9, P-selectin surface expression is upregulated by exocytosis utilizing a calcium-calmodulin and protein kinase C dependent mechanism, and PAF is simultaneously coexpressed by the endothelial cell.[37–43] Endothelial P-selectin surface expression is then rapidly downregulated by internalization and subsequent degradation.[44] PSGL-1, the high-affinity ligand for P-selectin, is a glycoprotein constitutively expressed by all leukocytes.[45,46] PSGL-1 is uniformly dispersed on the surface microvilli of unstimulated neutrophils, but is preferentially redistributed to the uropod of the polarized neutrophil following activation.[47,48]

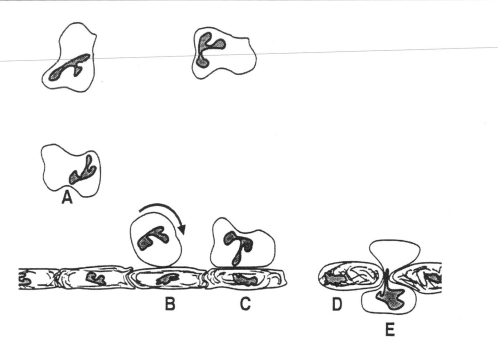

Figure 2. The multistep model of leukocyte emigration. In the absence of inflammation, neutrophils are dispersed in the vascular lumen; the endothelial cytoskeleton is organized at the periphery (**A**). During acute inflammation, neutrophils marginate and roll along the activated endothelium (**B**), are then tethered and become firmly adherent to the endothelium (**C**). The endothelial cytoskeleton condenses, causing centripetal retraction of individual endothelial cells, allowing gaps to develop between formerly adjoining cells (**D**). Leukocyte are activated during firm adhesion (C), and emigrate from the vessel through the gaps between endothelial cells.

E-selectin (CD62E, ELAM-1) is expressed only by cytokine (interleukin-1 [IL-1], TNF) stimulated endothelial cells.[18,49–51] Upregulation of E-selectin is by transcriptional activation and, thus, peak surface expression is delayed until several hours after exposure to the inciting stimulus, after which time expression progressively diminishes.[18,52,53] Like P-selectin, E-selectin binds to sialylated glycoproteins, including L-selectin and PSGL-1, although the binding affinity for the latter is much lower than between P-selectin and PSGL-1.[54,55]

The integrins are a family of cell surface glycoproteins functionally characterized by their capacity to mediate adhesion between leukocytes and other leukocytes; between leukocytes and other cells of nonmyeloid lineage, including endothelium; and between leukocytes and components of the extracellular matrix, including fibrinogen, fibronectin, laminin, collagen, iC3b, and factor X.[10,56,57] Five known members of the integrin family mediate leukocyte adhesion to endothelium: the β-1 integrin VLA-4 (very late antigen, α-4/β-1, CD49d/CD29); the β-7 integrin LPAM-1 (murine mucosal homing receptor, α-4/β-7, CD49d/CDxx), and the three β-2 integrins. Neither the timing of expression nor the lineage of cells expressing VLA-4 and LPAM-1 suggest either is likely to influence events within the initial hours of organ reperfusion. In contrast, a growing body of data has delineated a critical role for the β-2 integrins in the pathophysiology of ischemia-reperfusion injury.

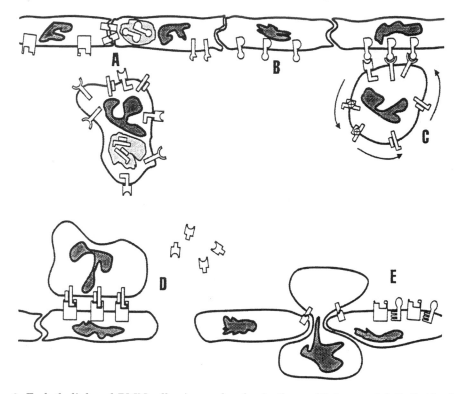

Figure 3. Endothelial and PMN adhesion molecules in the multistep model. Individual receptors are as shown in Figure 1. Unstimulated PMNs express L-selectin, PSGL-1, and LFA-1 on the surface membrane, while inactive Mac-1 is dispersed in cytoplasmic granules (**A**). Unstimulated endothelial cells express low levels of ICAM-1, ICAM-2, and the L-selectin ligand on the lumenal membrane, with P-selectin sequestered in the Weibel-Palade bodies (**A**). In acute inflammation, P-selectin is rapidly expressed at the surface membrane (**B**), and mediates the low affinity binding to L-selectin and PSGL-1 on PMNs that allow the development of rolling and tethering (**C**). The coexpression of PAF and P-selectin by the endothelial cells stimulates the rolling PMN to translocate Mac-1 to the surface membrane and increases the binding affinity of both LFA-1 and Mac-1 for their ligands. Firm adherence and leukocyte activation is mediated by LFA-1 and Mac-1 binding to ICAM-1 and ICAM-2 (**D**); L-selectin is shed from the PMN coincident with activation. Emigration at intercellular gaps is mediated by the coordinate interaction of the β-2 integrins and the ICAMs, as well as by the binding of PECAM-1 with its PMN ligand (**E**). Transcriptional activation during acute inflammation promotes the delayed expression of E-selectin and increases the expression of ICAM-1 (E).

Structurally, the β-2 integrins are distinguished by a common beta subunit (CD18) noncovalently associated with one of three homologous alpha subunits (CD11a, CD11b, and CD11c), thus forming three functionally discrete heterodimers: LFA-1 (lymphocyte function associated antigen-1, CD11a/CD18); Mac-1 (Macrophage-1 antigen, CD11b/CD18, complement receptor 3 [CR3]), and p 150,95 (CD11 c/CD18, complement receptor 4 [CR4]). The β-2 integrins are transmembrane molecules that display an extracellular ligand binding domain in close proximity to a divalent cation (calcium, magnesium) binding region, a transmembrane domain, and a cytoplasmic tail.[58,59] While LFA-1 is constitutively expressed by essentially all myeloid derivatives, surface expression of Mac-1 and p150,95 is limited to phagocytic cells, including alveolar macrophages, as well as a restricted population of lymphocytes.[10,56,60,61]

The cell surface counterreceptors for the β-2 integrins are three monomeric members of the immunoglobulin superfamily: ICAM-1 (intercellular adhesion molecule-1, CD54); ICAM-2; (CD102) and ICAM-3 (CD50).[59,62–65] Each of the ICAMs is an integral plasma membrane glycoprotein with an extracellular domain consisting of a variable number of immunoglobulin-like motifs, a single transmembrane region, and short cytoplasmic tail. ICAM-1 is widely distributed, and is displayed on diverse cellular elements within the lung, including capillary endothelium, alveolar lining cells, type I and type II pneumocytes, and alveolar macrophages.[59,66] ICAM-2 is expressed by monocytes, interstitial lymphoid cells, platelets, and endothelium, including pulmonary capillary endothelium, while ICAM-3 is expressed only by leukocytes.[64,67,68] ICAM-1 exhibits high-affinity binding to LFA-1 and lower affinity binding to Mac-1, while ICAM-2 and ICAM-3 bind exclusively to LFA-1.[62–64,69–72]

As with the selectins, there are two fundamental mechanisms by which control of the adhesive interaction between the β-2 integrins and their ligands is asserted: alteration of surface expression, and control of receptor affinity. Thus, ICAM-1 expression by unstimulated endothelial cells is low, but is slowly upregulated in response to TNF, IL-1, interferon-γ (IFNγ) and hydrogen peroxide.[64,66,73–79] Enhanced expression requires de-novo messenger RNA and protein synthesis, is initially detectable within 4 hours of stimulation, and peaks at about 24 hours. In contrast, surface expression of endothelial ICAM-2 appears invariant in response to acute inflammatory stimuli, while ICAM-3 undergoes rapid (less than 1 minute), but transient phosphorylation after neutrophil chemotactic stimulation (fMLP, PAF), and surface expression quickly declines by proteolytic degradation after neutrophil exposure to the protein kinase C activator phorbol myristate acetate (PMA) or calcium ionophores.[80,81] In spite of regulation by initiators of nonspecific inflammation, the functional role of ICAM-3, thus far, appears to be restricted to the induction of specific immunity.[68,71] Finally, while the extent of ICAM-1 glycosylation influences the binding affinity of Mac-1, it is not firmly established that this represents an important control mechanism in vivo.[82]

While LFA-1 is constitutively expressed by leukocytes, it is not constitutively avid for the ICAMs, and control of the adhesive interaction mediated by LFA-1 is asserted by modulating its affinity for ligands. Thus, ligation of the T-cell receptor induces a rapid, but ephemeral increase in LFA-1 avidity for ICAM-1.[59,83] The increase in affinity can be reinvoked by repetitive stimulation, suggesting a conformational rather than structural alteration in LFA-1, and this cycling capability has subsequently been demonstrated to be dependent in part on phosphorylation of a serine residue within the cytoplasmic domain of the beta chain CD18.[84,85] A functionally comparable mechanism has been demonstrated to alter LFA-1 affinity in neutrophils and monocytes.[86]

In contrast to LFA-1 , Mac-1 surface expression is relatively low on unstimulated neutrophils, accounting for less than 5% of the available cellular pool.[87] Within minutes of activation by diverse stimuli (fMLP, GM-CSF, IL-8, leukotriene B4, PAF, TNF, C5a) surface expression dramatically increases by translocation from secretory vesicles to the plasma membrane, and the magnitude of this enhanced expression is tightly coupled to the intensity of the stimulus.[87–90] L-selectin expression reciprocally declines coordinate with the upregulation of Mac-1, which becomes uniformly distributed over the surface of the neutrophil as it is expressed.[91] Only a limited subset of the newly expressed Mac-1 displays an activation specific epitope which is essential for adhesion to ICAM-1 and fibrinogen.[92] Since this marker is not detectable in quiescent neutrophils, the affinity of Mac-1 for its ligands appears subject to conformational regulation, as previously noted for LFA-1.

By comparison to LFA-1 and Mac-1, relatively limited information exists regarding the function of p150,95. Monocyte p150,95 and Mac-1 are both upregulated by stimulation with the chemokines monocyte chemoattractant protein-1 (MCP-1), macrophage inflammatory protein 1 (MlP-1a), and RANTES (regulated on activation, normal T expressed and secreted); no comparable data exists concerning the regulation of neutrophil p150,95.[93] Purified p150,95 adheres to an unknown inducible ligand on IL-1 and lipopolysaccharide (LPS) stimulated endothelial cells.[94] p150,95 transfected cells bind iC3b-coated erythrocytes, fibrinogen, and LPS, and LPS binding has been shown to initiate macrophage-like behavior in transfected fibroblasts through translocation of the transcription promoter nuclear factor kappa B.[61,95–97] Since p150,95 does not bind any of the ICAMs, its primary function may be to promote phagocytosis in the extravascular space through recognition of iC3b.[61,98] Paradoxically, even though it does not recognize native ICAM-2, an ICAM-2-derived synthetic peptide triggers high affinity binding of p150,95 for immobilized fibrinogen and iC3b.[97]

One more recently characterized member of the immunoglobulin family merits consideration in this discussion of leukocyte emigration mechanisms relevant to reperfusion injury. PECAM-1 (platelet-endothelial cell adhesion molecule-1, CD31) is an integral membrane glycoprotein constitutively expressed by endothelial cells, platelets, and leukocytes.[99,100] In unstimulated endothelial cells, PECAM-1 is localized at intercellular junctions, where it binds with PECAM-1 on adjacent cells.[101] TNF or IFNγ induce a dose-dependent redistribution of PECAM-1 away from the intercellular junctions, and facilitate calcium dependent neutrophil binding which is mediated by a distinct and as yet unidentified neutrophil ligand.[100,102,103] This heterophilic aggregation is inhibited by heparin or recombinant soluble PECAM-1, suggesting a regulatory mechanism analogous to that of soluble L-selectin.[104] Inhibition of PECAM-1 by either specific mAb or recombinant soluble PECAM-1 almost completely inhibits transmigration of monocytes and neutrophils across cytokine activated endothelium, and microscopic examination demonstrates that the blocked cells are tightly bound to the endothelial cells at the intercellular junction.[105] In a now familiar fashion, engagement of PECAM-1 transiently increments the avidity of Mac-1 and LFA-1, while coligation with monocyte FcgRll induces the release of TNF, IL-1, and IL-8 by the leukocytes.[106–108]

The individual functions and coordinate regulation of the selectins, the β-2 integrins, the ICAMs, and PECAM-1 in the sequence of rolling, tethering, firm adhesion, and transendothelial migration have been dissected in a series of creative and elegant in vitro and in vivo studies. Thus, rolling of unstimulated leukocytes occurs on artificial lipid bilayers containing purified P-selectin and E-selectin under shear flow conditions that replicate those in the postcapillary venule.[109,110] With increasing shear stress, the maximum rolling velocity attained correlates with the density of selectin embedded in the artificial surface.[110] During equivalent flow, neutrophils fail to adhere to lipid bilayers displaying only ICAM-1, while under static conditions activated neutrophils develop an attachment that is one hundredfold more resistant to shear than the adhesion formed with P-selectin.[31,109] Both rolling and subsequent firm attachment in shear flow by cytokine-activated neutrophils occur on bilayers displaying

P-selectin and ICAM-1. Analogous results have been demonstrated during shear flow with cell lines stably transfected with either E-selectin or P-selectin, and with endothelial monolayers stimulated to express the vascular selectins.[53,111] Similarly, rolling capability can also be conferred by stable transfection with L-selectin.[34,112]

The fine details of the general multistep model of leukocyte emigration emerge with increasing clarity when further dissected using specific mAb and signal transduction inhibitors, and can be summarized as follows. Endothelial activation by diverse stimuli induces rapid translocational expression of of P-selectin, rapid synthesis of PAF, and delayed transcriptional expression of E-selectin and ICAM-1.[113] Under conditions of shear flow in the postcapillary venule of most tissues, but in the alveolar capillaries of the lung a series of low-affinity, reversible binding interactions occur with neutrophils constitutively displaying L-selectin and PSGL-1, resulting in the characteristic rolling behavior and the formation of circulating platelet-leukocyte aggregates.[53,111,114–121] Transmembrane signaling in the neutrophil, mediated by selectin engagement and pertussis toxin sensitive and insensitive guanine nucleotide binding proteins, induces intracellular calcium release, superoxide anion production, and induction of messenger RNA for the production of interleukin-8 (IL-8) and TNF, either of which may further modulate the adherence and activation response.[122–127] If the transiently tethered neutrophils are exposed to any of a variety of coactivation signals in this microenvironment, including PAF, L-selectin is shed, and high-affinity Mac-1 is simultaneously expressed by the neutrophils.[15,25,39,127–131] With activation, the cytoskeleton undergoes a conformational change, leading to leukocyte polarization, redistribution of cellular adhesion receptors, and disengagement from the selectin mediated bonds.[48,117,128,132] Firm endothelial attachment and subsequent transendothelial migration are selectin independent, but require LFA-1, Mac-1, ICAM-1, ICAM-2, and PECAM-1, and engagement of these receptors may signal additional alterations in their affinity for ligands.[25,75,98,108,114,133–138]

Although ischemia and other forms of oxidant stress induce injury by processes not initially dependent on leukocytes, the evidence that leukocytes are essential for the full expression of reperfusion injury is extensive. In virtually all models of ischemia and in particular following pulmonary ischemia, histologic examination in the late hours of reperfusion demonstrates neutrophil extravasation and increased tissue myeloperoxidase activity, the latter being an enzyme uniquely expressed by leukocytes that catalyzes the production of hypochlorous acid from hydrogen peroxide and chloride ion.[139–157] Immunoreactive E- and P-selectin and ICAM-1 are upregulated in heart, lung, and kidney during reperfusion, and the timing of their coordinate expression corresponds with other indices of activation.[144,151,152,158–161] In the heart, the upregulation of ICAM-1 mRNA has further been shown to occur exclusively in the previously ischemic region, but not in cells with contraction band necrosis, and the intensity of upregulation is greatest in the border zone of viable muscle immediately adjacent to the necrotic zone.[152,155,156] When the efficacy of cardiac protection following warm ischemia is judged by criteria including the extent of reduction in infarct size, leukocyte infiltration, tissue myeloperoxidase actity, and preservation of endothelium dependent vasodilation, mAb individually directed against ICAM-1, Mac-1, LFA-1, P-selectin, and L-selectin have each been shown to be effective, and comparable improvements have been demonstrated with administration of sialyl Lewis X containing oligosaccharides that inhibit P- and E-selectin mediated adherence.[140,148,151,158,162–166] Even following hypothermic, cardioplegic preservation, interference with β-2 integrin mediated adhesion can lead to improvements in myocardial contractility, coronary flow reserve, and myocardial oxygen consumption.[167] Somewhat surprisingly, in at least one study of myocardial reperfusion, the efficacy of an mAb directed against CD18 was reduced unless it was administered well in advance of reperfusion, although some treatment effect was still retained when administration was delayed until 5 minutes after the onset of reperfusion. It is not certain if this reduction of efficacy reflects different binding kinetics of the mAb in the animal model studied, or indicates that species dependent variability may exist in the regulation of β-2 integrin expression.[168]

The precept that leukocytes contribute to reperfusion injury has also been validated in the lung, although the body of evidence is less extensive than in many other organs. Using in-line filters that on average reduce circulating leukocyte counts by more than 95%, tissue malondialdehyde accumulation, an index of lipid peroxidation, was reduced following 2-hour warm ischemia and reperfusion, although there was no change in the levels of the lipoxygenase products, leukotriene B4 and leukotriene C4.[169] When rabbit lungs were hypothermically preserved for up to 24 hours with modified Collins solution, then reperfused in vitro, leukapheresed blood prevented the development of increased microvascular permeability and lung edema.[170] In that same study, the salutary benefit of leukocyte depletion was sustained if leukocytes were added after the initial hour of reperfusion, but was abrogated by leukocyte repletion at the onset of reperfusion. This technique was then examined in a model employing donor core cooling with cardiopulmonary bypass for heart-lung procurement, followed by 12-hour, hypothermic storage, and subsequent reimplantation.[171] When contrasted with controls not undergoing leukapheresis during reimplantation, early mortality (within 6 hours) was eliminated by leukocyte depletion, and significant advantages were demonstrated in both respiratory gas exchange and lung edema accumulation. These workers affirmed these initial results and expanded their observations in a companion work in which leukocyte filters were employed both during procurement and reimplantation, and further tested for an additive benefit of liposomal superoxide dismutase (SOD).[172] In that protocol, leukapheresis was associated with less reperfusion injury than SOD alone, and a modest synergistic effect was demonstrated by the combined intervention. The beneficial effects of leukocyte filtration were subsequently verified even with preservation intervals as long as 24 hours in a double lung transplant model employing donor core cooling and hypothermic storage in donor blood.[173] Only one other group has contrasted the effects of leukapheresis with oxygen radical scavengers administered during reperfusion.[174] In that study, reperfusion of isolated lungs with leukocyte depleted blood significantly reduced lung edema and tissue malondialdehyde accumulation as anticipated, while combination therapy with the extracellular radical scavengers SOD and catalase reduced lung edema formation without influencing lipid peroxidation.

Relatively less work has been accomplished using mAb against leukocyte adhesion receptors to modify lung reperfusion injury. Nevertheless, the treatment effect has been broadly equivalent to those achieved with the identical strategy in modifying experimental myocardial reperfusion injury, and with modification of lung reperfusion injury by leukapheresis. To date, none have attempted a strict comparison of leukapheresis versus leukocyte adhesion inhibition in studies of lung reperfusion injury. When examining the effect of an mAb directed against CD18 in a model of reperfusion following 24-hour normothermic ischemia, mAb recipients developed less lung edema and microvascular permeability, and accumulated less tissue myeloperoxidase than controls treated with an indifferent control mAb.[143] In a companion study employing a different anti-CD18 mAb, and contrasting the results of leukocyte adhesion inhibition with leukocyte depletion following hydroxyurea administration (89% reduction in leukocyte count), neither treatment limited the initial reductions in pulmonary flow that occur in that model during reperfusion, but both interventions promoted an essentially equivalent improvement in flow as reperfusion progressed.[175] In a similar model of prolonged normothermic ischemia, increases in gravimetric lung water and tissue myeloperoxidase activity were attenuated to approximately the same extent by administration of mAb directed against either ICAM-1 or CD18.[144] When pulmonary capillary permeability was examined in an isolated lung model following short-term (2 hour) normothermic ischemia and reperfusion, equivalent preservation of microvascular integrity was demonstrated by inhibiting xanthine oxidase activity, by scavenging hydroxyl radicals with catalase, or by interfering with β-2 integrin mediated adhesion.[176] When assessing the relative contribution of the selectin and β-2 integrin mediated adhesion pathways in the development of increased pulmonary permeability and lung leukocyte infiltration following 2-hour lung ischemia in rats, mAb directed against P-selectin, CD18, and ICAM-1 were individually demonstrated effective, yet interference with the function of L-selectin conferred no benefit.[177] Conversely, in a sheep model of 3-hour normothermic ischemia, provision of an mAb that binds both E- and L-selectin both improved short-term (6-hour) survival, and preserved respiratory gas exchange when compared to unmodified reperfusion or reperfusion with an isotype matched indifferent mAb.[178] Because transcriptional upregulation of E-selectin should have been negligible in the initial hours of this study, when mortality in controls was highest, the treatment effect with the study mAb implied interference with the constitutively expressed L-selectin and, with data from other models, suggests that the relative contribution of different adhesion pathways in inflammation may vary both between species and between injury models.[178]

Only two groups have explored the role of leukocyte adhesion inhibition as an adjunct to the management of reperfusion following hypothermic lung preservation. When a leucine analog (NPC 15669) that interferes with receptor coupled signal transduction and, thus, prevents neutrophil activation and Mac-1 upregulation was administered to isolated rabbit lungs reperfused with whole blood after hypothermic preservation with modified Euro-Collins solution, pulmonary flow and static lung compliance were well preserved even with 24-hour storage, and while lung edema formation was reduced in lungs stored for only 12 hours, this advantage was lost with 24-hour storage.[179,180] Disappointingly, oxygen transfer was not influenced by this agent. When 4-hour hypothermic preservation with modified Euro-Collins solution was examined in a canine model, an mAb that blocks CD18 improved respiratory gas exchange and gravimetric lung water, but failed to prevent reductions in compliance and pulmonary vascular resistance over the 6-hour reperfusion period.[181]

If, on the basis of the preceding we accept that the process of leukocyte adherence and activation is an obligatory prelude to neutrophil-mediated tissue injury during organ reperfusion, the stimuli that provoke this process merit equivalent consideration. Many of these stimuli are already familiar to most with an interest in organ transplantation, either because they are known to play a role in the induction of specific immunity, or because they configure the host response during other inflammatory disorders, including sepsis. None of the molecules discussed in this section are the primary signal; indeed, each has a characteristic panel of antecedent stimuli, but with their description, we move closer to the prime causes of reperfusion injury. Some are directly cytotoxic; others are important to the pathogenesis of reperfusion injury because they assert a regulatory function. Their individual contribution to the pathogenesis of reperfusion injury has only lately been subject to scrutiny.

Tumor Necrosis Factor

Among the best characterized of the cytokines, TNF is produced principally by myeloid derivatives and endothelial cells in response to numerous inflammatory stimuli including endotoxin; among those particularly relevant to this discussion are C5a, leukotriene B4, and superoxide radical.[182-184] Paradoxically, hydrogen peroxide, a product of activated neutrophils, reversibly inhibits the binding of TNF to its endothelial receptors and, thus, tempers TNF-induced gene expression.[77] A limited recapitulation of several recent studies will suffice to demonstrate the diverse functions of TNF during acute inflammation, and will further illustrate why TNF is generally held to play a pivotal role in the promotion of postischemic injury.

TNF, alone, and synergistically with IFNγ, promotes the synthesis and release of IL-1 by monocytes and the expression of ICAM-1 by endothelial cells and cardiac myocytes.[74,185,187] TNF simultaneously induces L-selectin shedding and upregulation of Mac-1 expression by neutrophils; in yet another instance of autocrine amplification, engagement of L-selectin induces TNF mRNA production.[86,91,127] Following binding of either one of its two discrete membrane receptors, subsequent endocytosis, and activation of nuclear factor kappa B, TNF promotes the expression of endothelial E-selectin. The capacity for restricted activation of distinct vascular beds may signal either a variable response to TNF by endothelium of different tissues, a specific and discrete response to a limited and highly localized elaboration of TNF, or the effect of costimulation by other locally released cytokines, including IFNγ.[18,186,188-193] TNF also promotes endothelial expression of VCAM-1 (CD106) which mediates the specific late recruitment of monocytes through its interaction with VLA-4; this process is further enhanced by the TNF mediated transcriptional activation of MCP-1 and monocyte colony-stimulating factor (CSF-1).[193-197] In endothelium, TNF promotes transcriptional activation of β-galactoside α-2,6-sialyltransferase, an enzyme which can participate in the sialylation of and, thus, alter the activation state of its substrates, among which are E-selectin, ICAM-1, and VCAM-1.[197] Paradoxically, TNF confers limited tolerance to subsequent cardiac ischemia. Within hours of TNF administration, neutrophils accumulate within the myocardium, locally increasing hydrogen peroxide production, and in consequence inducing both catalase and MnSOD.[198-200] Finally, while the mechanism is as yet poorly characterized, TNF blunts the vasodilator response to acetycholine customarily observed in intact, perfused carotid arteries; whether the pulmonary vascular bed responds in like fashion is not known.[201]

The kinetics of TNF release follow a fairly consistent pattern in the majority of studies examining either regional or global organ ischemia. The initial induction of TNF mRNA and release of TNF protein generally occurs within a few minutes of the onset of reperfusion, peaks shortly thereafter at levels as high as fifteen times control values, and then rapidly declines to baseline values, often within the initial hour of the onset of reperfusion.[202–216] The rapid release of TNF during the initial minutes of reperfusion suggests a washout phenomenon, but none have specifically probed for TNF mRNA during the ischemic interval.[213] While the preponderance of evidence suggests TNF is released as a consequence of ischemia, this finding has not been universal, and studies spanning the spectrum from canine gracilis muscle ischemia to human orthotopic liver transplantation have failed to demonstrate significant TNF induction during reperfusion, although it must be noted that in each of the confounding studies cited, TNF protein was assayed, rather than TNF mRNA, and it may well be that the more sensitive assay would resolve this apparent discrepancy.[217–219] As further affirmation of the role of TNF in the pathogenesis of reperfusion injury, polyclonal TNF neutralizing antibodies, soluble TNF receptor antagonists, and soluble TNF receptors have each been demonstrated to significantly attenuate both the local and remote injuries characteristic of the various ischemic models in which they were employed.[202–204,209,210,216,220] Disappointingly, only limited work has specifically addressed the potential role of TNF in lung reperfusion injury. Although serum TNF levels were unaltered, TNF was significantly increased in the alveolar space within 1 hour of reperfusion following 4-hour hypothermic preservation of canine pulmonary allografts, thereafter declining to control levels within 24 hours; an analogous pattern was not found when preserved pulmonary autografts were studied in identical fashion.[221,222]

Interleukin-1

In many ways similar to TNF, IL-1 is a proinflammatory cytokine with diverse biologic effects central to the pathophysiology of postischemic states. Although expressed primarily by monocytes and macrophages, multiple cell lines, including neutrophils and endothelium, produce IL-1. Leukotriene B4, C5a, and TNF are all potent stimuli for the production of IL-1 by monocytes and the response to TNF is significantly enhanced by costimulation with IFNγ.[182,185] Xanthine oxidase-derived radicals promote the expression of IL-1 mRNA by pulmonary mononuclear cells; whether other forms of oxidant stress induce IL-1 is unknown, while, as with TNF, subinjurious concentrations of hydrogen peroxide antagonize the effect of IL-1 on endothelium.[77,184] IL-1 stimulates serine/threonine kinase activity in cells withn minutes of binding to its receptor, stimulating the release of heat shock protein-27, and activation of the transcription promoter nuclear factor kappa B and the epidermal growth factor receptor.[223,224] Like TNF, IL-1 induces the endothelial expression of MCP-1, E-selectin, and ICAM-1, and, in keeping with the foregoing description of selectin function, the microvascular expression of E-selectin is preferentially enhanced in venules. [73,120,186,194,225] In contrast to the synergistic interaction of IFNγ and TNF, however, the IL-1 induced expression of E-selectin and ICAM-1 is not substantially influenced by IFNγ.[186] The effect of IL-1 on adhesion molecule expression is not exclusive to endothelial cells, since IL-1 , like TNF, promotes the expression of ICAM-1 by cardiac myocytes.[226]

The kinetics of IL-1 protein release follow a generally consistent pattern whether analyzing isolated muscle preparations, studying regional myocardial or cerebral ischemia, or examining global myocardial or hepatic ischemia. In each of these models, IL-1 protein is measurably elevated in the venous effluent within the first few minutes of reperfusion, peaks over the next 3 to 6 hours at levels up to tenfold higher than in control studies, and ultimately declines to baseline levels between 24 and 48 hours of reperfusion.[209,212,215,227–230] The kinetics of IL-1 mRNA expression follow a similar overall pattern, although upregulation of IL-1 mRNA has been detected even prior to the onset of reperfusion, and enhanced expression of either IL-1 mRNA or protein occurs strictly within the ischemic region.[215,229] In those few studies that have examined the relationship between IL-1 upregulation and either local or remote tissue damage, IL-1 correlates highly with several key indices of injury, including extent of tissue necrosis, leukocyte infiltration, vascular permeability, and mortality.[212,228] Finally, confirming a pathogenic role of IL-1 in reperfusion injury, both polyclonal IL-1 neutralizing antibodies and IL-1 receptor antagonists have been individually demonstrated to attenuate both the local and pulmonary injuries characteristic of the rat hind limb ischemia model.[209] It remains to be determined if IL-1 asserts a similar role in the pathogenesis of pulmonary reperfusion injury.

In a manner similar to that described for TNF, prior exposure to IL-1, as a prelude to oxidative stress, may also ameliorate myocardial ischemia-reperfusion injury. As with TNF, although perhaps better characterized, the mechanism appears to involve either the induction of, or the activation of, several enzymes critical to the management of oxidant injury including Cu/Zn-SOD. Mn-SOD, catalase, glutathione peroxidase, and glucose-6-phosphate dehydrogenase.[224,231,232] Since IL-1 fails to confer any beneficial effect on reperfused kidneys, the cytoprotective activity may be exclusively cardiac, and none have as yet reported studies on this phenomenon in the lung.[233]

Interleukin-2

Interleukin-2 (IL-2) is expressed only by T lymphocytes, and as such would be anticipated to be a relatively unimportant factor in the pathogenesis of early postischemic graft dysfunction. Nevertheless, IL-2 is significanly increased in the alveolar space within 4 hours of reperfusion following 4-hour hypothermic preservation of either pulmonary allografts or autografts, and declines to baseline levels within 24 hours.[221,222] The essentially equivalent response to both foreign and native tissue suggest the early elevation in IL-2 represents either one component of a generalized upregulation of the inflammatory process or a specific response to some factor intrinsic to the preservation scheme, rather than an initial arousal of specific immunity. Whatever mechanism pertains, the significance of an early elevation in IL-2 following pulmonary preservation remains obscure.

Interleukin-4

Like IL-2, interleukin-4 (IL-4) is primarily a product of T lymphocytes. IL-4 is not generally considered proinflammatory and, at this time, has no certain role in the pathogenesis of graft reperfusion injury. However, several studies suggest that IL-4 may assert a regulatory influence during acute inflammation, and in particular, may modulate the response of monocytes, eosinophils, and basophils. IL-4 promotes a rapid, dose-dependent tyrosine phosphorylation of the endothelial IL-4 receptor and, in concert with IL-1, promotes endothelial expression of the mRNA for MCP-1.[234,235] Conversely, IL-4 inhibits the IL-4 induced expression of the monocyte-derived chemoattractant MIP-1α, largely by promoting an accelerated degradation of the MIP-1α subunit mRNA.[236] In concert with TNF or PMA, IL-4 promotes the expression of endothelial VCAM-1 and an L-selectin ligand, but has no effect on E-selectin or ICAM-1 expression and, thus, promotes the VLA-4 mediated firm adhesion of monocytes, eosinophils, and basophils rather than neutrophils, which lack VLA-4 expression.[235,237–239] Since this specific pattern of adhesion molecule upregulation parallels the β-2 integrin mediated sequence which selectively effects neutrophil recruitment, the role of IL-4 during acute inflammation may be to regulate the late influx of monocytes. As of this writing, we are unaware of studies which have attempted to explore either the knetics of IL-4 production or the regulatory role of IL-4 in ischemia-reperfusion injury.

Interleukin-6

Interleukin-6 (IL-6) is expressed by numerous cell lines, including monocytes, macrophages, and endothelial cells, and several recent reports suggest a distinct role for IL-6 in the induction of the postischemic inflammatory response. Although IL-6 mRNA is not ordinarily detectable in cultured cardiac myocytes, short-term hypoxia increases both IL-6 mRNA expression and increased production of IL-6, and both mRNA expression and IL-6 protein production are further augmented by subsequent reoxygenation after the initial hypoxic exposure.[240] In anesthetized dogs, IL-6 mRNA is induced in ischemic myocardium, and expression is significantly enhanced during reperfusion, reaching a peak within 3 hours.[241] Similarly, when analyzed after reperfusion of pulmonary allografts, plasma IL-6 levels are elevated within 4 hours, and the clinical severity of postischemic lung injury was correlated with the peak detected IL-6 level.[242] Increased systemic levels of IL-6 have also been noted following experimental skeletal muscle ischemia and reperfusion and during clincial cardiopulmonary bypass and myocardial revascularization, and these increments have been related to assembly of the complement membrane attack complex, C5b-9.[209,243,244] The role of IL-6 is not unequivocally established, however, since some groups have been unable to detect any changes in IL-6 mRNA after shorter periods of coronary occlusion or during the very early stages of reperfusion, or while demonstrating an increase in epicardial venous IL-6 levels, have been unable to isolate the increased levels specifically to the ischemic or reperfused myocardial segments.[219,229] While the basis for these disparate findings is as yet uncertain, the biologic role of IL-6 in postischemic injury may be related to the induction of ICAM-1 expression. Cardiac-specific lymph collected during reperfusion after 1-hour coronary occlusion induces ICAM-1 expression by cultured cardiac myocytes; the capacity of reperfusion lymph to stimulate ICAM-1 expression was reduced by an IL-6 neutralizing mAb, and could be replicated by stimulation of cultured cardiac myocytes with exogenous IL-6.[245] These same workers also found that ICAM-1 mRNA colocalizes with IL-6 mRNA in ischemic and reperfused myocardial segments and, further, that peak IL-6 mRNA synthesis preceded that of ICAM-1 mRNA.[241] It has not yet been determined if IL-6 is capable of inducing a comparable upregulation of ICAM-1 in the reperfused lung.

Interleukin-8

Interleukin-8 (IL-8) is produced by activated neutrophils and monocytes, in part mediated by the binding of L-selectin; local production by surrounding nonimmune cells, including endothelium can, in turn, be induced by infiltrating inflammatory cells, further amplifying leukocyte recruitment.[122,127,246,247] IL-8 stimulates high-affinity glutamyl transpeptidase guanosine triphosphate (GTP) binding and GTPase activity in neutrophil plasma membranes, and its receptor, like those of the other CXC-chemokines, has been demonstrated to be a member of the seven transmembrane domain class of guanine nucleotide binding proteins required for neutrophil activation.[248,249] While still preliminary, evidence for a role of IL-8 in the induction of reperfusion injury continues to accumulate. In culture, anoxic preconditioning stimulates increased production of IL-8 mRNA and secretion of IL-8 protein by monocytes.[246] As previously noted, IL-8 rapidly increases surface expression of Mac-1 by neutrophils. Recombinant IL-8 increases neutrophil adhesion to and toxicity for isolated cardiac myocytes, and both effects can be abrogated by antibodies that neutralize IL-8 or interfere with β-2 integrin mediated adhesion.[250] In vivo, IL-8 mRNA in reperfused myocardium following 1-hour coronary occlusion peaks within 4 hours of reperfusion, and remains elevated for up to 24 hours; with ischemic intervals as long as 4 hours, only minimal IL-8 mRNA induction is detected in the absence of reperfusion, and none can be demonstrated in continuously perfused regions of myocardium.[250] In a comparable model, the induction of immunoreactive IL-8 in reperfused myocardium followed a similar temporal pattern, although it could be significantly attenuated by prior neutrophil depletion.[247] The increase in IL-8 occurred subsequent to the rapid (less than 5 minutes) induction of immunoreactive C5a, which was unaltered by neutrophil depletion. Increased IL-8 production has also been noted during postischemic reperfusion of the lung, and specific neutralization of IL-8 by antibody reduced neutrophil infiltration and parenchymal damage during reperfusion.[154,251] However, even though the above cited studies strongly suggest that IL-8 acts largely to promote leukocyte recruitment in acute inflammation, some groups have described anti-inflammatory effects. In vitro, IL-8 induced the loss of L-selectin and an increase in Mac-1 expression, but paradoxically inhibited neutrophil attachment to activated endothelium, promoted the rapid detachment of tightly adherent neutrophils from activated endothelium, and abolished neutrophil transendothelial migration.[122] Similarly, within minutes following intravenous administration of an IL-8 analog (Ser-IL-8), the number of rolling leukocytes in rabbit mesenteric venules was dramatically reduced, recovering to control levels over the ensuing 30 minutes; although L-selectin expression was unaltered, CD18 expression by circulating neutrophils was briefly upregulated.[252] In that same study, local extravascular application of Ser-IL-8 reduced adhesion and emigration of neutrophils. When given 10 minutes prior to reperfusion after 1.5-hour coronary artery occlusion in rabbits, an IL-8 derivative ([Ala-IL-8]77) reduced both the size of the necrotic zone, as well as myeloperoxidase activity in the necrotic zone, and preserved endothelium dependent vasodilation in postischemic coronary artery rings; because this effect was not found in isolated, perfused hearts, these workers suggested the derivative's modulatory effect was dependent on circulating leukocytes, rather than endothelium.[253] On balance, the role of IL-8 in the induction or perpetuation of reperfusion injury is unresolved, but the topic is sufficiently compelling to warrant additional inquiry.

Interferon-γ

IFNγ is produced by stimulated lymphocytes and pulmonary macrophages. IFNγ alone has no effect on endothelial E-selectin expression but, as previously noted, stimulates a redistribution of endothelial PECAM-1 away from intercellular junctions and induces a delayed upregulation of ICAM-1.[73,74,100,186] In addition to these isolated effects, IFNγ potentiates the TNF mediated upregulation of endothelial E-selectin and augments the TNF induced release of IL-1 by monocytes; these synergistic effects occur in the absence of any direct effects by IFNγ on the TNF receptor.[185,186,254] In association with either TNF or IL-1, IFNγ also increases endothelial nitric oxide (NO) synthase activity.[255] While these activities suggest that IFNγ may mediate some of the early pathophysiologic alterations of organ reperfusion injury, evidence for such a role in vivo is, thus far, largely unexplored and, indeed, those data which exist are in apparent conflict. Cardiac IFNγ mRNA is not altered during the initial 30 minutes of left anterior descending coronary occlusion in rats, while within this identical interval, the mRNA for TNF, IL-1, IL-2, and transforming growth factor-β-1 have already increased several fold.[229] Conversely, and perhaps reflecting the influence of pulmonary macrophages, the level of IFNγ in bronchoalveolar lavage fluid is significantly elevated within 1 hour of hypothermic pulmonary preservation and reperfusion, recovering to baseline within 24 hours, and in the absence of any detectable increment in the systemic levels.[221]

Complement

Knowledge of the role of complement in postischemic injury has been increasingly refined in recent years, and the capacity to arrest complement activation or moderate the effects of complement may soon be a clinical reality. Complement components, and in particular C5a, are potent chemotactic agents and leukocyte activators.[225,256] In vitro, C5a incites L-selectin shedding, Mac-1 upregulation, and PAF synthesis by neutrophils, and also promotes the production of IL-1 and TNF by monocytes.[23,87,90,182,257] Similarly, assembly of the membrane terminal attack complex C5b-9 promotes endothelial P-selectin expression both in vitro and in vivo.[37,258] Leukocyte recruitment is an obligate cofactor for the expression of lung injury induced by intravascular activation of the alternative pathway, since blocking antibodies that interfere with the function of P-selectin, LFA-1, Mac-1, or ICAM-1 each attenuate the development of such injury following administration of cobra venom factor.[258,259]

While the precise factors that activate complement following tissue ischemia are ill-defined, in at least one model, the generation of hydroxyl radicals during the initial moments of reperfusion has been directly correlated with activation of the alternative pathway, since pretreatment with the hydroxyl radical scavenger dimethylthiourea or the iron chelator deferoxamine prevented the initial generation of C5a during reperfusion.[256] Whatever the inciting mechanism, C5a can be detected in extracts of postischemic myocardial segments within 5 minutes of the onset of reperfusion, and measurable levels are evident in cardiac lymph within 1 hour.[247,260] Further verifying activation of the alternative pathway, Bb begins to increase in regional coronary venous plasma within 15 minutes of myocardial reperfusion.[261] In the absence of neutrophils, oxygen radicals are generated only momentarily after reperfusion in isolated hearts, and the full expression of contractile dysfunction and increased vascular permeability that occurs in this model is dependent on both neutrophil mediated cytotoxic effects, as well as the direct myocyte damage that follows the assembly of C5b-9.[261-263] Although the contribution of complement generation to postischemic dysfunction is well established in other organs, at present the notion that complement contributes to postischemic lung dysfunction is strictly inferential.

Although strategies to reduce the undesirable effects of complement during tissue reperfusion have generally proven elusive, at least one agent has recently shown promise. Recombinant complement receptor 1 (sCR1) is a genetically engineered molecule which lacks the cytoplasmic and transmembrane domains of the native receptor.[264] sCR1 binds and promotes the inactivation of C3b by 1 and, by interfering with C3 and C5 convertases, inhibits activation of both the classic and alternative pathways.[264,265] In experimental myocardial reperfusion injury, administration of sCR1 impaired membrane assembly of the C5b-9 attack complex, attenuated but did not eliminate neutrophil infiltration, curtailed oxygen radical production, and reduced infarct size, while enhancing recovery of postischemic coronary flow and ventricular function.[264–266] In experimental hypothermic cardiopulmonary bypass, sCR1 inhibited complement activation, and although the anticipated increase in postbypass pulmonary vascular resistance was reduced by sCR1 administration, there were no significant alterations in the extent of neutropenia, lung myeloperoxidase levels, lung edema, or respiratory gas exchange.[267] Similarly, beneficial local effects have been described when sCR1 was employed in experimental mesenteric or hind limb ischemia, and while sCR1 reduced the associated increase in lung permeability, it failed to influence either pulmonary neutrophil infiltration or lung myeloperoxidase activity.[268,269] No studies have examined the use of sCR1 during normothermic lung ischemia or as an adjunct to the management of reperfusion following hypothermic pulmonary preservation. While the cited studies suggest that sCR1 may be a useful adjunct in organ preservation, it should be remembered that one agent common to all organ preservation schemes has not eliminated postischemic organ dysfunction: heparin, as well as an N-desulfated, N-acetylated derivative lacking important anticoagulant activity, significantly inhibits complement activation both in vitro and in vivo.[270] However, it should be emphasized that the heparin required to effectively curtail complement activation is substantially higher than the dosage employed clinically.

Platelet-Activating Factor

PAF is a proinflammatory glycerophospholipid produced by deacylation of membrane ether lipids when leukocyte or endothelial phospholipase A2 is activated by oxygen radicals, thrombin, histamine, bradykinin, C5a, fMLP, TNF, and IL-1, among others.[39,113,257,271–274] Prior exposure to GM-CSF is a prerequisite for production of PAF by neutrophils in response to either C5a or fMLP; whether this is an obligate costimulus for all neutrophil agonists is uncertain.[257] The kinetics of PAF production are both rapid and brief, with peak activity generally occurring within 15 minutes of stimulation, and cessation of synthesis within 1 hour.[113,211,257]

When administered systemically, PAF rapidly causes bronchoconstriction, systemic hypotension, neutropenia, thrombocytopenia, and respiratory arrest.[275,276] Mediated in part by reductions in ventricular adenosine 3',5'-cyclic monophosphate (cAMP) levels, and in concert with the stimulated production of thromboxane A2, leukotriene C4, leukotriene D4, and leukotriene E4, exogenous PAF increases coronary vascular resistance, depresses myocardial contractility, and increases permeability of the coronary microcirculation.[277–281] Although PAF induces reductions in global cardiac performance, it has no significant direct effect on the viability of isolated cardiac myocytes subjected to 20-minute hypoxia and subsequent reoxygenation.[282] In addition to its role in promoting platelet aggregation and its indirect effects on smooth muscle, PAF is a potent cytokine with a pronounced influence on leukocyte recruitment and activation which is further enhanced by autocrine amplification.[257,283] Within minutes following exposure to PAF, endothelial cells coexpress both P-selectin and PAF.[39] Endothelial-associated PAF initiates the juxtacrine activation of neutrophils following the engagement of P-selectin by PSGL-1; this tandem interaction promotes disengagement of the P-selectin bond, phosphorylation of ICAM-3, L-selectin shedding, enhanced Mac-1 expression, and production of hydrogen peroxide.[48,81,87,91,113,128,130,284] In similar fashion, endothelial PAF, facilitated by the prior binding of PSGL-1 to P-selectin, stimulates tethered monocytes to elaborate MCP-1 and TNF and, transduced by engagement of the β-glucan receptor, the release of additional PAF.[126,285]

That PAF is an important intermediate in the pathogenesis of ischemia-reperfusion injury is no longer questioned, although its effects have largely been inferred as a consequence of injury attenuation by administration of PAF receptor antagonists, rather than by direct measurement. Despite remaining largely cell-associated, PAF levels in the coronary sinus rapidly increase with reperfusion following regional myocardial ischemia, and the administration of several different PAF antagonists (CV-6209, L-659,989, SDZ 63–675, TCV-309, WEB 2170) has substantially mitigated the development of the characteristic injury profile, with significant reductions in neutrophil chemotactic activity, neutrophil oxidative burst, neutrophil infiltration, myocardial myeloperoxidase levels, myocardial permeability, and myocardial infarct size.[211,281,284,286–289] Concomitant with reductions in tissue necrosis and myocardial inflammation, the administration of PAF receptor antagonists has been associated with relatively greater preservation of global ventricular function, a reduced incidence of bradycardia and systemic hypotension, and better recovery of coronary flow during reperfusion, the latter attributable to enhanced preservation of endothelium-dependent coronary artery relaxation. Studies examining the relative efficacy of myocardial preservation with different PAF receptor antagonists are lacking, while only modest differences were evident in the one protocol that attempted to compare the proportionate utility of a PAF receptor antagonist versus reperfusion with leukocyte depleted blood.[290]

Studies of the role of PAF in pulmonary preservation are still few. Following both short-term (45 minutes) and long-term hypothermic pulmonary (up to 22 hours) preservation, using either modified Euro-Collins or University of Wisconsin solutions for flushing and storage, and with provision of PAF receptor antagonists (BN 52021, CV-3988, or WEB 2170) to both donor and recipient, as well as in the storage solution, several groups have demonstrated improvements in experimental allograft function, employing the conventional criteria of respiratory gas exchange, static compliance, pulmonary vascular resistance, and tissue water content.[291–294] No groups have reported a direct comparison of the relative efficacy of different PAF receptor antagonists. In separate works contrasting deferoxamine with either CV-3988 or BN 52021 in experimental lung preservation, dramatic advantages could not be claimed with either strategy.[292,294]

Nitric Oxide and Endothelin

For some time, it has been recognized that alterations in blood vessel tone in response to many intrinsic neurohumoral transmitters (acetylcholine, catecholamines, histamine, vasopressin, serotonin, bradykinin, and thrombin, among others) were dependent on the functional integrity of the endothelium.[295] Other vasoactive substances directly influenced cGMP levels in the subjacent vascular smooth muscle and, thus, induced an endothelium independent response. In more recent years, it has been shown that the endothelium dependent mediators work by binding to specific membrane receptors, each of which is capable of influencing the release of a second messenger, NO, which in paracrine fashion modulates the activity of smooth muscle guanylate cyclase and, thereby, controls cGMP levels.[296] Although NO was initially characterized as a consequence of its function in endothelial cells, it has since been identified as a second messenger in cells of diverse lineage, including myeloid derivatives (Figure 4).[297]

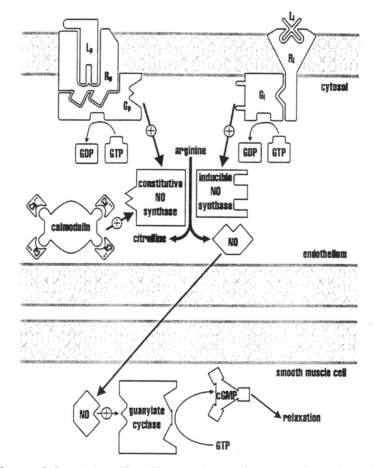

Figure 4. Scheme of the nitric oxide (NO) signal transduction pathway in endothelial cells. Binding of ligands (L_p) such as acetylcholine to specific membrane receptors (R_p) activates a membrane associated G protein (G_p). G_p stimulates the constitutively expressed NO synthase to convert arginine to NO and citrulline. NO diffuses across the ablumenal endothelial cell membrane, activating the soluable guanylate cyclase in subjacent smooth muscle cells. The guanylate cyclase dependent conversion of GTP to cGMP causes smooth muscle relaxation and vasodilation. Cytokines stimulate NO dependent signaling both by inducing an NO synthase isozyme and secondarily activating that isozyme through distinct receptor, G-protein linked pathways (L_1, R_1, G_1).

During the same interval in which the role of NO was defined, the endothelins were identified and characterized. The endothelins are a family of 21 amino acid peptides synthesized and released by endothelial cells in response to thrombin, angiotensin II, and epinephrine, among other agonists.[298,299] The endothelins are among the most potent endogenous vasoconstrictors identified, yet paradoxically, when administered, they elicit a preliminary vasodilator response through stimulation of endothelin-B receptors as a prelude to a slower developing, but sustained vasoconstriction mediated by endothelin-A receptors.[300] Endothelin promotes vasoconstriction by influencing the voltage sensitive calcium channels, and the response can be inhibited by the dihydropyridine class of calcium channel blockers, as well as by NO itself, which may dampen endothelin function both by displacing endothelin from its membrane receptor, as well as interfering with endothelin-induced calcium signaling.[301,302] In pace with this newer information on the physiologic mechanisms regulating vascular tone, the vasomotor response to ischemia has been the subject of increasing inquiry. Although the regulation of postischemic vasomotor tone has been explored most vigorously in the coronary circulation, by and large, the mechanisms demonstrated active in the heart have been verified in almost all other vascular systems.

In the absence of reperfusion, coronary occlusion for up to 6 hours in vivo results in scant morphologic evidence of endothelial injury, consisting primarily of subendothelial swelling.[303] Nevertheless, even within this interval, there is a progessive deterioration in the capacity of epicardial coronary arteries from within the ischemic region to relax in response to vasodilators which stimulate the release of N0, although there is minimal degradation of the endothelium independent response.[303,304] In stark contrast, NO mediated relaxation is significantly attenuated within the initial 2.5 minutes of reperfusion, and is essentially eliminated within 20 minutes; regeneration of the vasodilator response is, however, quite rapid and virtually complete by 2 hours of reperfusion.[305,306] While reperfusion after brief (less than 20 minutes) ischemia has no apparent morphologic consequences, ischemia of longer duration induces cytoplasmic vacuolation, swelling of cytoplasmic organelles, and partial detachment of the endothelium during the initial hours after the onset of reperfusion.[306]

The relatively slow degradation of endothelium dependent vasodilation during ischemia may be in large part attributable to the generation of superoxide, which rapidly inactivates NO and in the process generates hydroxyl radicals; this same reaction indicates why, in some studies, SOD helps to preserve the NO dependent vasomotor mechanism.[305,307,308] By analogy, the oxidant stress at the onset of reperfusion accounts for the rapid deterioration and early recovery in endothelium dependent vasodilation, which transpires well in advance and independently of neutrophil accumulation.[303,305,309] In part because the vasomotor response to membrane receptor transduced agonists is impaired, while the response to agonists which induce relaxation without transduction through a membrane receptor is not, some have alternatively proposed that a defect in NO release from the receptors accounts for the endothelial dysfunction.[310,311]

Even though neutrophils are not essential for the initial deterioration in NO mediated vasorelaxation in the coronary circulation, the subsequent influx of leukocytes is associated with a depressed vasomotor response which can be effectively restored by interfering with selectin or β-2 integrin mediated neutrophil adhesion.[148,158,162–164,167,312] When this same phenomenon was studied employing a model of cardiopulmonary bypass for circulatory support during the cardiac ischemic interval, leukocyte filtration had only limited effect on coronary artery relaxation; however, the conclusion that leukocytes do not alter vasomotor function may be untenable, since cardiopulmonary bypass may itself induce significant aberrations in vasomotor function.[267,313,314] While abnormal pulmonary artery vasomotor responses occur following hypothermic preservation and reperfusion, the relationship between the degradation of this control mechanism and leukocyte recruitment has not been specifically studied in the lung.[310]

Which comes first: the late reduction in vasomotor function or the late influx of leukocytes? At least in the heart, both responses may be correct, and both may be contingent on the initial degradation of NO in response to the oxidant stress of reperfusion. in vitro, exposure of endothelial cells to a NO synthase inhibitor (NG-nitro-L-arginine methyl ester [L-NAME]) induces ICAM-1 expression and β-2 integrin-lCAM-1 dependent neutrophil adhesion to endothelial cells by 4 hours; the upregulation of ICAM-1 could be prevented by administration of L-arginine (the natural precursor, via NO synthase, of NO), intracellular oxygen radical scavengers, the iron chelator deferoxamine, or a PAF receptor antagonist (WEB 2086), but not by the extracellular scavengers SOD and catalase.[78] In vivo, an infusion of NO during ischemia and throughout the reperfusion interval reduced myocardial infarct size and reduced cardiac myeloperoxidase activity; although comparable tissue salvage has been achieved with NO donors, leukocyte influx was not significantly curtailed.[315,316] In a companion study employing L-NAME as a probe to assess basal NO levels, endothelial dysfunction early after reperfusion could be completely reversed with L-arginine, which also reduced leukocyte adherence to postischemic epicardial vessels.[304]

In addition to the deterioration of the NO dependent vasoregulatory control mechanism, variations in endothelin expression and endothelin receptor activity may potentiate the postischemic changes in vascular resistance. Plasma endothelin levels are increased in the venous drainage during reperfusion after normothermic myocardial, hepatic, and mesenteric ischemia.[299,317–322] The kinetics of endothelin peptide release have varied significantly between studies, with peak levels noted at intervals ranging between 5 minutes and 1 hour after restoration of circulation.[318,323] Both endothelin-1 mRNA transcripts and immunoreactive protein are exclusively enhanced in the ischemic tissue, and increased levels of mRNA are found even in the absence of reperfusion.[324,325] Infusion of L-arginine during reperfusion, which enhances the production of NO, ameliorates the tissue accumulation of endothelin, while the release of peptide can be diminished by a variety of agonists, including adenosine, calcium channel blockers, and iloprost, the latter suggesting the cyclooxygenase derivative prostaglandin E_2 may contribute to the release of endothelin during ischemia.[318,321,324,326,327] Although it has not clearly been established whether the change is mediated by increased expression of endothelin receptors or by augmented activity of the endothelin-A receptor, the vasoconstrictor activity of all three endothelins is enhanced during reperfusion, and this response is dependent on the influx of activated neutrophiis.[300,317,328–330]

While NO has been validated as an important second messenger in the control of pulmonary vasomotor tone, some important variations have been uncovered even while ratifying the fundamental constructs. Using cGMP accumulation in vascular smooth muscle cells during coculture incubation to indirectly assay NO, both basal and receptor stimulated NO production by pulmonary endothelial cells decline as oxygen tension is reduced, even if excess L-arginine is provided, suggesting hypoxia alters intracellular calcium metabolism and, thus, inhibits NO release. Of note the dependence of NO metabolism on oxygen tension could not be demonstrated using endothelium from extrapulmonary sources.[331] Similarly, reperfusion after 30-minute normothermic ischemia in isolated, blood-perfused lungs significantly augments the NO dependent pulmonary pressor response to hypoxia.[332] Vasorelaxation in response to acetylcholine during sustained hypoxic vasoconstriction was no different than observed in control lungs never subjected to ischemia, suggesting that pulmonary ischemia and reperfusion may specifically enhance endothelin activity, as well as alter NO metabolism.[332] When changes in endothelin activity were specifically examined, it was noted that plasma endothelin-1 concentration increased significantly within 90 minutes of the onset of reperfusion following 60 minutes of normothermic lung ischemia. Endothelin-1 mRNA transcript levels were unchanged during ischemia, but increased in both the reperfused and the nonischemic lung during the reperfusion interval. In addition, prior administration of an endothelin-A receptor antagonist (FR139317) attenuated the development of lung injury, as defined by improved oxygenation, and a reduction in lung edema and neutrophil influx.[333]

It should also be noted that cytokines produced during reperfusion may also modulate NO production. IFNγ, TNF, and IL-1 increase NO production in cultured endothelial and pulmonary vascular smooth muscle cells; in pulmonary vascular smooth muscle cells, the incremental production was dependent on induction of NO synthase, and could be inhibited either by administration of the NO synthase inhibitor NG-monomethyl-L-arginine (NMMA) or by provision of an antisense oligodeoxynucleotide probe complementary to the NO synthase mRNA sequence which, thereby, inhibited transcription of NO synthase.[201,308,334–336] Paradoxically, the enhanced production of NO by endothelium occurs in spite of a pronounced reduction in steady-state NO synthase mRNA transcript levels, but this mechanism also requires transcriptional expression, and is associated with increased activity of GTP cyclohydrolase 1, the rate limiting step in the synthesis of tetrahydrobiopterin, which is an obligate cofactor in NO production.[201,255,337]

The novel appreciation of the role of NO and other second messengers has significant implications for organ preservation. Based on the observation that NO is depleted in hypothermically preserved (19 to 38 hours) rat hearts during the initial moments of reperfusion, and confirming the work of others that SOD could attenuate this depletion, promoters of the NO pathway (nitroglycerin, nitroprusside, L-arginine, 8-bromoguanosine 3',5'monophosphate) were added to either a simple balanced salt solution or to University of Wisconsin solution and were demonstrated to improve the initial function of heterotopically transplanted hearts even after 12-hour preservation.[309] Having previously shown that the addition of cAMP analogs (dibutyryl cAMP, 8-bromo-cAMP) or phosphodiesterase inhibitors (indolidan, rolipram) to a preservation solution extended rat cardiac graft survival in dose-dependent fashion, and that the most effective of these interventions (dibutyryl cAMP) improved postimplantation coronary flow and reduced leukocyte infiltration, both dibutyryl cAMP and nitroglycerin were employed as adjuncts to cardiac preservation.[338,339] In that summation study, the combined intervention dramatically improved early survival after long-term (24-hour) preservation of rat and baboon hearts, even while using University of Wisconsin solution as the benchmark for comparison.[339] Extending their inquiries to the lung, comparable reductions in postimplantation NO levels were identified, although in this model, SOD was less effective in restoring NO than in their cardiac model.[340] In this model, addition of a cGMP analog (8-Br-cGMP) to the base preservation solution (lactated Ringer's) improved recipient survival, gas exchange, and pulmonary flow while reducing neutrophil influx over the initial 30 minutes of reperfusion following 4-hour preservation.[340] This group has since demonstrated equivalent results in this model of experimental lung preservation when nitroglycerine was employed to stimulate NO production.[341] Only one other group has, thus far, explored the role of NO mediated responses in the context of pulmonary preservation. In that study, endothelium-independent relaxation of the pulmonary vascular bed was unaltered, while relaxation in response to the endothelium-dependent mediators acetylcholine and isoproterenol was depressed when these parameters were assessed at 1 hour of reperfusion following 4-hour preservation.[314] In that same work, the use of cardiopulmonary bypass during transplantation caused even greater degradation in the NO mediated response but, in addition, depressed the endothelium independent response to nitroprusside.

Oxygen Radicals

The consequences of short-term (1 to 6 hours) pulmonary ischemia include the depletion of adenosine triphosphate and dissipation of the purine nucleotide pool by conversion of nucleotides to nucleosides, inosine, and hypoxanthine.[342] Although the ultimate consequence is identical, the kinetics of purine catabolism in the ischemic lung are much slower than in heart, kidney, or brain. While this may reflect the intrinsically lower metabolic rate of lung tissue, and although it completely ignores the intrinsically higher metabolic rate of the endothelium, it is probable that retained alveolar oxygen stores contribute to the delayed onset of purine breakdown, since the rate of glycolysis in isolated, perfused lungs does not diminish until alveolar oxygen partial pressure approaches 1 mm Hg.[343,344] In contrast, even under hypothermic conditions, replacement of alveolar oxygen with nitrogen rapidly leads to lactate accumulation and purine nucleotide depletion.[345]

During ischemia or hypoxia, the nicotinamide adenine dinucleotide (NAD) reducing enzyme, xanthine dehydrogenase, in endothelial and alveolar type II cells is converted by proteases to xanthine oxidase, although the release of elastase by adherent activated neutrophils during reperfusion may also facilitate this conversion, and at least in cultured pulmonary endothelial cells, this conversion can be initiated by C5a, TNF, or fMLP.[346–352] With the reintroduction of oxygen during reperfusion, xanthine oxidase further degrades hypoxanthine to xanthine and, as a consequence, generates the toxic species superoxide radical and hydrogen peroxide.[353–357] Within cells, superoxide radical is degraded by superoxide dismutase, which catalyzes the conversion of superoxide to hydrogen peroxide. In the presence of catalase, hydrogen peroxide is detoxified to water and oxygen. In the presence of glutathione peroxidase and two molecules of glutathione, hydrogen peroxide is reduced to water, and the glutathione is converted to glutathione disulfide.

One additional source of superoxide generation during initial reperfusion phase is the synthesis of arachidonic acid derivatives, following the activation of phospholipase A2 by oxygen radicals, as well as a host of other substances, including thrombin, histamine, bradykinin, C5a, fMLP, TNF, and IL-1.[39,113,257,271–274,358] Not only are arachidonic acid derivatives released in response to oxygen radicals, the lipid peroxidations requisite for their synthesis produces superoxide and hydroxyl radicals as an intermediate in the production of the leukotrienes, thromboxane A_2, and prostacyclin.[358]

Neutrophils and other leukocytes also produce superoxide during the respiratory burst using an intrinsic membrane bound nicotinamide adenine dinucleotide phosphate (NADPH)-dependent oxidase.[359,360] The secondary product, hydrogen peroxide, is further converted, via myeloperoxidase, to hypochlorous acid, which can then react with endogenous amines to form a reactive class of compounds called chloramines.[361] The production of oxygen radicals by this process is a β-2 integrin adherence dependent event; it is also autocatalytic, since hydrogen peroxide induces upregulation of endothelial ICAM-1 by a mechanism contingent on PAF release.[272,362]

Two iron catalyzed reactions are important amplifying mechanisms for the additional generation of reactive oxygen species at the outset of reperfusion.[363,364] In the Haber-Weiss reaction, hydrogen peroxide is reduced by superoxide, producing the more highly toxic hydroxyl radical. In the Fenton reaction, which is considered to be the biologically more important process, ferric iron is reduced by superoxide, producing hydroxyl radical, as well as generating ferrous iron.[353] The possibility exists, however, that much of the tissue injury attributed to the hydroxyl radical is instead mediated by a perferryl radical.[346,353,363–365] If the initial burst of iron dependent radical formation is unconstrained, tissue injury ensues as a chain of redox reactions peroxidate polyunsaturated membrane lipids and oxidize the sulfhydryl side groups of proteins, with the subsequent creation of sulfide bridges. The concomitant DNA strand breakage may prevent the synthesis of proteins essential to cellular repair.[366] The net result is a loss of cellular integrity, inactivation of membrane associated proteins, and potentially cell death.[367,368]

In reperfused organs, the availability of ferrous iron may be the rate limiting factor for hydroxyl radical generation. In the lung, the iron catalyzed cytochrome P-450 enzymes, which generate superoxide as an intermediate during normal metabolism, may serve as the primary source of iron during oxidant stress, since inhibition of these enzymes, while failing to limit postischemic increases in superoxide radical generation, reduced the anticipated increase in microvascular permeability and associated lipid peroxidation.[369,370] Both the rapidity with which the Fenton reaction proceeds after the onset of reperfusion, and the extreme reactivity of the hydroxyl radical suggests that agents administered to quench this reaction or scavenge radicals must be in place at the immediate onset of reperfusion, with even minimal delays abrogating the beneficial effect of the iron chelator deferoxamine or the hydroxyl radical scavenger dimethylthiourea.[371–374] Although provision of deferoxamine during the ischemic interval does not reduce tissue oxygen radical content prior to reperfusion, it significantly attenuates the initial burst of reactive intermediates that immediately follows reperfusion.[372,375–379]

Surfactant

While neither a signal or a message, alterations in surfactant during preservation and reperfusion may have a substantial influence on the initial function of the pulmonary graft. A brief discussion of available work is presented for the sake of completeness.

The contribution of pulmonary surfactant to the immediate function of lung grafts was among the initial subjects examined by groups interested in prolonging the safe interval of pulmonary preservation. The first to examine this subject concluded that surfactant composition in preserved grafts was normal, and also that the capability of alveolar type II cells to synthesize new surfactant was unaltered by preservation and reperfusion, even with storage intervals as long as 48 hours.[380] More recent data suggests these initial results were erroneous. Although the amount of phospholipid does not change as reperfusion is prolonged following up to 2-hour lung preservation, the proportion of phosphatidylcholine is progressively reduced in proportion to the duration of storage, and these changes parallel reductions in both lung compliance and in vitro measures of surfactant function.[381] Because surfactant composition and function was constant during ischemia, and deteriorated only during reperfusion, these workers concluded that lipid peroxidation either during the initial burst of oxygen radicals, or subsequent to the neutrophil influx, accounted for the degradations observed. Others examining this subject have also noted reductions in surfactant function, and have isolated a component of this to a diminution of the dipalmitoyl-phosphatidylcholine fraction.[382] However, this group noted that the decline in dipalmitoyl-phosphatidylcholine occurred even during ischemia, that this declne could be reversed by provision of L-carnitine and, moreover, that L-carnitine supplementation improved the initial function of the graft.[382] This latter work suggests several possibilities for the mechanism of surfactant depletion, among which are impairment of alveolar type II cell metabolism, a failure of endogenous radical scavenging mechanisms during ischemia, or catabolism of phospholipid during ischemia, as well as any subsequent degradation that occurred as a consequence of reperfusion. When others have studied surfactant, equivalent reductions in both function and composition were observed after hypothermic preservation with either modified Euro-Collins or University of Wisconsin solution.[383] Based on that study, this same group examined the effect of exogenous surfactant administered immediately prior to reperfusion after long-term (37-hour) storage with modified Euro-Collins solution.[384] While dramatic improvements in respiratory gas exchange were observed in three of eight treated subjects, five failed to respond to this intervention. Interestingly, in subjects that responded to surfactant, graft pulmonary artery blood flow was well maintained, while flow in nonresponders progressively deteriorated. The improvement in flow in responders further implies that hypoxic pulmonary vasoconstriction, rather than microvascular obstruction by platelet-leukocyte aggregates, accounts for the major proportion of the abnormal pulmonary vasomotor response during reperfusion.

The Pathophysiology of Hypoxemia in Lung Reperfusion Injury

Although our recognition of the role of abnormal signal processing in the evolution of reperfusion injury has already stimulated experimental advances, for the most part, the molecular and cellular hallmarks of postischemic injury are inaccessible in clinical practice, and we must instead rely on the classic techniques of physiology to assess the performance of the pulmonary allograft. Within this segment, we propose to annotate the gross pathophysiology of lung reperfusion injury with specific references to certain aspects of this relatively newer information and, as far as possible, explore how it is that events that transpire at the cellular level may lead to postreperfusion lung dysfunction. Although our intent is to focus on the mechanisms by which arterial hypoxemia may develop, it should be recognized that alterations in pulmonary vascular resistance, pulmonary blood flow, lung compliance, airway resistance, and other commonly employed indices of lung function are fully amenable to an equivalent analysis; indeed, it is impossible to regard the reduction in arterial oxygenation that may occur during the hours following reperfusion as a phenomenon wholly independent of alteration in these other parameters.

In the perioperative period, arterial oxygen tension is the monitor most frequently employed to assess the performance of the pulmonary allograft and, with the possible exception of the cardiac dysfunction caused by idiopathic pulmonary hypertension, it might be argued that improving respiratory gas exchange is the sole indication for considering pulmonary replacement. In this context, it is worth recalling that the lung functions almost exclusively as an intermediary in respiratory gas exchange, and that arterial oxygen tension is sensitive not only to the intrinsic efficiency of the lung, but to variations in oxygen supply and utilization as well. Thus, if the arterial partial pressure of oxygen differs from the partial pressure of oxygen in alveolar gas by only a small factor, it is eminently reasonable to infer that the graft is performing satisfactorily, and conclude that minimal reperfusion injury has been incurred. The converse inference, that an abnormal arterial oxygen tension is solely indicative of preservation or reperfusion injury, is not as readily warranted, and therein lies a fundamental flaw in the manner in which we currently assess pulmonary preservation schemes. While it is difficult to envisage circumstances in which significant preservation or reperfusion injury could exist without influencing oxygenation, a concatenation of several extrinsic factors can readily degrade arterial oxygen tension, even in the face of good graft function. At the bedside and, more importantly, in the laboratory, it is pertinent to consider how these seemingly extraneous factors may interact to reduce arterial oxygenation and, thus, confound our attempt to employ respiratory gas exchange, not only as a marker of effective pulmonary preservation, but also as a gauge to assess the suitability of potential donors.

Briefly listed, the extrapulmonary determinants of arterial oxygenation are inspired oxygen fraction, alveolar ventilation, hemoglobin concentration, the P50 of the oxygen dissociation curve, pH, cardiac output, and systemic oxygen consumption.[385] The effects of these sundry factors on arterial oxygenation during steady-state gas exchange are asserted through their influence on the two parameters that specify the gradient for the mass transfer of oxygen within the alveolus, specifically alveolar and mixed venous oxygen tension. By definition, the partial pressure of oxygen in inspired gas imposes an absolute ceiling on alveolar oxygen tension. Since inspired oxygen fraction is externally regulated and generally augmented in the initial hours of reperfusion, it is almost never a significant factor when hypoxemia develops early after reperfusion, although in fact, once alveolar oxygen tension is actually estimated using any of the variants of the Bohr equation, the magnitude of the disparity between alveolar and arterial oxygen tensions may be surprisingly high. The safety margin afforded by an imposed elevation in inspired oxygen fraction during the early hours of reperfusion is unequivocal, yet the prudent clinician must remain vigilant to this potential deception. At the same time, it should be recalled that higher alveolar oxygen tensions can actually degrade arterial oxygenation by the mechanism of absorption atelectasis and the development of shunt in lung units with low ventilation-perfusion ratios.[386]

Alveolar ventilation, the product of tidal volume (less dead space) and respiratory frequency, is externally controlled and, thus, infrequently a significant consideration when hypoxemia is noted during the earliest hours following lung transplantation. With the resumption of spontaneous ventilation and the changes in ventilator management that ensue, this assertion is less tenable. Since alveolar ventilation during spontaneous breathing is autonomically controlled, the recipient with preoperative hypercapnia is vulnerable to a failure of this intrinsic regulatory mechanism and, thus, may limit ventilatory effort whenever arterial oxygen tension substantially exceeds preoperative levels.[387,388] Detection of alveolar hypoventilation may be problematic in such patients, since the usual test for this condition, an increase in arterial carbon dioxide tension, is at the outset abnormal. Respiratory drive may also be blunted by residual narcotic or inhalational anesthetics, and effort may be further impaired by unmetabolized neuromuscular blocking agents, particularly in the presence of hypothermia. Incisional discomfort, altered chest wall compliance and phrenic nerve injury may each impede effective tidal ventilation, and although an increase in respiratory frequency may be compensatory, alveolar ventilation may ultimately suffer from the disproportionate expansion of dead space ventilation at higher respiratory rates.[389–391]

Immediately after transplantation, some reduction in hemoglobin concentration is inevitable. If red cell mass and hemoglobin levels are repleted with banked blood, up to 24 hours may elapse before 2,3-diphosphoglycerate levels in the transfused cells are restored and the P50 of the oxyhemoglobin dissociation curve normalizes.[392–394] During this interval, the leftward shift in the oxyhemoglobin dissociation curve may limit peripheral oxygenation, and this effect can be further augmented by alkalosis, hypocapnia, or hypothermia. The net influence of reductions in hemoglobin level or changes in P50 on arterial oxygen tension may be nullified by concomitant reductions in blood viscosity, or by reflex increases in cardiac output and regional blood flow. If, however, these compensatory mechanisms fail, mixed venous oxygen tension will be reduced and arterial oxygen tension may accordingly decline.

Under usual circumstances, cardiac output and systemic oxygen consumption are properly regarded as extrapulmonary factors that may influence arterial oxygen tension, and both assert their effect through changes in mixed venous oxygen tension. Excluding heart-lung transplants, where cardiac performance may be limited as a consequence of poor preservation or reperfusion injury, the risk of primary cardiac dysfunction following unilateral or bilateral lung transplantation is largely eliminated by the preliminary recipient screening, and even in those candidates with significant right ventricular failure secondary to pulmonary hypertension, the decline in right ventricular afterload that initially accompanies reperfusion generally reduces the extent of cardiac dysfunction to a level readily managed with low-level inotropic support. Because pulmonary resistance tends to increase in the hours following reperfusion, however, cardiac output may again become a limiting factor in oxygen delivery, and this reduction may further compound any deterioration in arterial oxygenation strictly attributable to inefficient oxygen exchange by the graft.[395]

Systemic oxygen consumption is the final, and perhaps most infrequently considered extrinsic factor influencing arterial oxygen tension following pulmonary replacement, yet even casual reflection suggests it may be profoundly altered during the early hours of reperfusion. General anesthesia reduces oxygen consumption through hypothalamic depression and loss of central temperature regulation; neuromuscular blocking agents decrease resting muscle tone and the attendant thermogenesis. Radiant heat loss to the relatively cool operating room environment is enhanced by cutaneous vasodilation, and additional heat loss may occur by evaporative cooling from the operative field, topical hypothermia, and heat transfer to the graft during reperfusion. Following operation, oxygen consumption increases approximately 10% for each degree (Celsius) of temperature elevation during rewarming, but may double if shivering is not prevented.[396,397] With the resumption of spontaneous ventilation, the metabolic demands of the repiratory muscles may add as much as 20% to the increased oxygen utilization.[398] Even when anesthetic depth and neuromuscular blockade are maintained at constant levels, as in experimental preparations, lung reperfusion may precipitate significant elevations in core temperature and oxygen consumption, largely caused by the elaboration of pyrogenic cytokines, including TNF and IFNγ.[181,185,399,400] As with systemic blood flow, if mixed venous oxygen tension is not depressed, increments in oxygen utilization generally will not reduce arterial oxygen tension. However, the interval during which oxygen consumption is most variable is that identical period during which the most significant degradation in graft function is ordinarily encountered. Within that time frame, any increase in oxygen consumption may significantly aggravate a trend toward hypoxemia caused by a dysfunctioning graft.

If abnormalities in oxygenation attributable to any of the preceding extrapulmonary factors can either be excluded or accounted for, and if we momentarily discount what may be significant effects of the contralateral lung on respiratory gas exchange, than any increase in the alveolar to arterial oxygen tension gradient must be the result of inefficient oxygen transfer by the graft, and the possible mechanisms can be reduced to just three: shunt, ventilation-perfusion inequality, or diffusion impairment.[385,401–403] When the multiple inert gas elimination technique was used to study the evolution of abnormal respiratory gas exchange following either normothermic ischemia or hypothermic preservation and transplantation, a characteristic response was noted during the initial hours of unmodified reperfusion.[178,181,404] A universal finding was a progressive narrowing of a consistently unimodal distribution centered about a ventilation-perfusion ratio of 1.0. Regions of low or high ventilation-perfusion ratio were sporadically encountered; however, these regions never accounted for more than a token component of total ventilation or perfusion, and such regions were never identified in the same subject during successive measurement intervals. The net increase in ventilation-perfusion inequality was, thus, consistently small, and the aggregate effect on respiratory gas exchange was relatively inconsequential through the initial 6 hours of reperfusion. The analysis of multiple inert gas elimination also incorporates an indirect estimate for the failure of oxygen diffusion equilibration, since the tension of respiratory gases in arterial blood are estimated from the derived ventilation-perfusion distributions and experimental assay of the relevant parameters, including each of those described above. Inert gas equilibration is an order of magnitude more rapid than that required for diffusion equilibration of oxygen, and if a failure of inert gas equilibration occurred, the estimated respiratory gas tensions in arterial blood would accordingly deviate significantly from the gas tensions actually obtained.[405,406] By this measure, respiratory gas exchange in the initial hours of lung reperfusion was never altered by a failure of diffusion equilibration. Rather, the dominant finding during unmodified reperfusion was an increase in shunt, with this technique equivalent to that component of total perfusion distributed to gas exchange units with a ventilation-perfusion ratio less than 0.001. Dead space, with this method equivalent to that proportion of total ventilation distributed to gas exchange units with a ventilation-perfusion ratio greater than 1000 to 1, was also significantly increased within the initial 30 minutes of reperfusion. However, additional increments in dead space beyond that initial interval were limited and failed to influence respiratory gas exchange to any significant extent.

If we concede that shunt is the predominant physiologic mechanism of abnormal gas exchange in lung reperfusion injury, then our goal of discerning the molecular and cellular basis of hypoxemia is greatly simplified: we need only identify agents whose profile of action would culminate in an admittedly abstract alveolus to which perfusion, no matter how profoundly reduced, nevertheless exceeds ventilation by a factor of 1000 or more. Conceptually, this limits the potential agents to those which restrict the flow of gas in the conducting airways, and to those that promote alveolar flooding or collapse. However, any combination is theoretically permitted, and we should acknowledge that it may be impossible to discriminate between a single agent acting at several sites and multiple agents sharing a similar profile of activity based solely on these ideal physiologic possibilities. In this regard, both the modulating effect of agents that inhibit leukocyte adhesion and the pace at which shunt develops in both modified and unmodified reperfusion provide certain additional constraints on the allowed mechanisms. First, because interference with L- and E-selectin mediated adhesion does not eliminate the evolution of shunt, at least some of the causative factors must be expressed either prior to or simultaneously with the development of rolling and tethering.[178] Second, because interference with β-2 integrin mediated adhesion limits, but does not eliminate the development of shunt, at least one important mechanism for the development of shunt is contingent on firm leukocyte adherence and leukocyte activation.[181] Finally, because the shunt that does develop in the presence of an mAb that limits L- and E- selectin mediated adhesion is readily dissipated, the inciting agent(s) for that early component of shunt must be expressed for only a transient interval at the outset of reperfusion, and the effects must be equally ephemeral.[178] Taken together, these findings suggest that there are at least two discrete, albeit concurrently evolving, processes that contribute to the development of shunt triggered by reperfusion. Equally important, these data indicate that the development of shunt can occur by leukocyte-independent as well as leukocyte-dependent mechanisms.

Are these sufficient data with which to establish a direct causal relationship linking the development of hypoxemia to any single cellular event or inflammatory intermediate produced during ischemia or reperfusion? Disappointingly, the answer at the present time is a qualified no. There are both morphologic and physiologic correlates to each of the three postulated physical analogs of shunt (alveolar flooding, alveolar collapse, and airflow restriction) during reperfusion, so that none can be excluded from consideration a priori, and at present it is difficult to apportion the relative contribution to hypoxemia caused by gradations in any one. From the perspective of the present discussion, however, the most nettlesome problem is that shunt is a physical concept that has no clear definition at anatomic levels smaller than the alveolus. Thus, if we are to further our appreciation for the causes of hypoxemia during lung reperfusion, we must substitute a marker for shunt that transcends this anatomic constraint. Among the possible markers, endothelial permeability seems an ideal surrogate for a variety of reasons. First, even though a strict correlation between the quantity of shunt and the extent of capillary permeability is not readily available, the association of alveolar filling with the development of shunt is a common feature of many models of acute lung injury, and the development of alveolar flooding presumes the occurrence of some finite increment in endothelial permeability. Second, endothelial permeability can be studied over a broad range of interests, from the intact lung to confluent endothelial monolayers. Third, interventions that increase the permeability of endothelial monolayers assert comparable effects in intact lungs; as important, agents capable of reversing the permeability increase seem equipotent over that same structural range. Finally, if we focus on that component of injury intrinsic to the lung, incorporation of the amplifying effects of leukocytes into our general scheme becomes a rudimentary exercise.

When isolated lungs are subjected to ischemia and the reperfusion phase is monitored using isogravimetric techniques, protein and solute filtration increase within the initial hour of reperfusion.[149,176,407–418] Since the increase in filtration coefficient occurs even with acellular reperfusates, the preliminary phases of this response are not necessarily contingent on leukocyte adherence and activation.[149,409,416,418] However, because lung myeloperoxidase levels increase in isolated lungs even with acellular reperfusates, the possibility that leukocytes sequestered within the pulmonary vascular bed initiate the injury cannot wholly be excluded.[149] That leukocytes facilitate the increase in capillary filtration is unequivocal, since interference with β-2 integrin mediated adhesion attenuates the postischemic response.[143,176] Because agents that interfere with iron catalyzed oxygen radical formation or that inactivate the reaction products (dimethylthiourea, superoxide dismutase, catalase, transferrin, U74500A), as well as interventions that reduce xanthine oxidase activity (allopurinol, dietary tungsten supplementation) inhibit the postischemic increase in capillary permeability, reactive oxygen species generated by injured endothelial cells, activated leukocytes, or both, must mediate some major component of this response, and in fact, comparable increases in capillary permeability can be induced solely by superfusion with exogenous oxidants (hydrogen peroxide, t-butyl hydroperoxide, chlorinated amines).[176,407–410,419–22] In analogous fashion, reeoxygenation of confluent endothelial monolayers provokes a rapid increase in the permeability of the monolayers to both solute and macromolecules, and as is the case with whole lung preparations, this effect can be replicated either by xanthine oxidase generated oxygen radicals or direct oxidant challenge.[423–27] Even though oxidants directly reduce high energy phosphate stores, this depletion does not appear to be a primary factor in the reduction of endothelial barrier function, since depletion of ATP to equivalent levels using metabolic inhibitors does not change permeability in either confluent cultures or buffer perfused lungs.[428–430] Rather, the proximate cause of increased endothelial permeability following exposure to hydrogen peroxide appears to be an hydroxyl radical mediated activation of the phosphatidylinositol signal transduction pathway, which leads to alterations in endothelial calcium flux and activation of protein kinase C.[424,431–433] The broad details relating these signal transduction pathways to the maintenance of endothelial barrier function have been refined over the past decade; as will be seen, these and other second messenger systems are central to the promulgation of the inflammatory response during lung reperfusion and, ultimately, to the degradation in respiratory gas transfer that may ensue.

Although the mechanisms are in all instances not completely understood, oxidants and other substances variably present during inflammation (PAF, C5b-9, endothelin, thrombin, fibrin, histamine, bradykinin, thromboxane A_2, neutrophil cathepsin G) activate endothelial membrane phospholipases.[37,301,434–446] Phospholipase C activation by receptor specific G proteins promotes the hydrolysis of phosphatidylinositol 4,5-biphosphate, producing diacylglycerol and inositol 1,4,5-triphosphate.[436,437,447,448] Membrane-associated diacylglycerol causes translocation of inactive protein kinase C from the cytosol to the plasma membrane, thereby activating it, while inositol 1,4,5-triphosphate stimulates the rapid mobilization of calcium from the endoplasmic reticulum, increasing cytosolic free calcium.[423,425,433,435,439,449-452] The activation of protein kinase C stimulates phosphorylation of those linking protein (vinculin, catenins, α-actinin, talin) that indirectly couple actin to the plasma membrane cadherins and integrins that mediate homophilic intercellular adhesion, as well as adhesion to the interstitial matrix proteins, while the increase in free calcium promotes a calmodulin dependent activation of myosin light-chain kinase; this in turn facilitates an actin and myosin based contraction that results in the centripetal retraction of individual endothelial cells, resulting in the development of gaps between adjacent endothelial cells, and an increase in paracellular transport.[427,435,437,448,453-462] The ultimate reduction in endothelial barrier integrity, thus, depends in large part on a reorganization of the endothelial actin cytoskeleton, although the anatomic sites affected may vary considerably between different agonists, and their influence on capillary permeability may be further modulated by the discrete effects many of these substances assert on segmental vascular tone (Figures 5 and 6).[419,423,424,435-437,463-469]

As a general rule, biologic regulatory systems are rarely unopposed, and equally

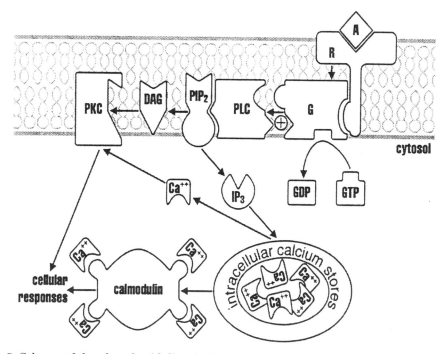

Figure 5. Scheme of the phosphatidylinositol signal transduction pathway in endothelial cells. The binding of an agonist (**A**) such as histamine or thrombin to its specific membrane receptor (**R**) activates a membrane associated G protein (**G**), which in turn stimulates phospholipase C (**PLC**). PLC mediated hydrolysis of phosphatidylinositol 4,5-biphosphate (PIP$_2$) produces diacylglycerol (DAG) and inositol 1,4,5-triphosphate (IP$_3$). DAG directly activates protein kinase C (PKC), while IP$_3$ increases cytosolic-free calcium. The flux in cytosolic calcium promotes calmodulin dependent cellular responses and independently activates PKC. The details of the mechanism by which oxygen radicals activate this pathway remain uncertain.

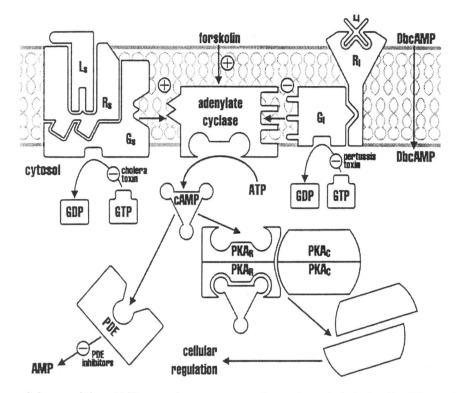

Figure 6. Scheme of the cAMP second messenger pathway in endothelial cells. When stimulatory ligands (L_S) bind to their specific membrane receptor (R_S), they activate a cholera toxin sensitive G protein (G_S). GS, in turn, activates membrane associated adenylate cyclas, and increases the conversion of ATP to cAMP. CAMP binds to the regulatory subunits of protein kinase A (PKA$_R$), activating the catalytic subunits (PKA$_C$) which, in turn, regulate cellular function by activating other cytosolic enzymes. Adenylate cyclase activity is reduced by receptor (R_I) specific ligand (L_I) mediated activation of pertussis toxin sensitive inhibitory G protein. (G_I). Phosphodiesterase (PDE) isozymes downregulate protein kinase A activity by accelerating the conversion of cAMP to AMP. Forskolin activates adenylate cyclase directly, while membrane permeant cAMP mimetics such as dibutyryl cAMP (DbcAMP) bypass adenylate cyclase and directly activate protein kinase A.

pertinent to this discussion is the recent recognition that agents that activate cAMP-dependent protein kinase A (isoproterenol, salmeterol, and salbutamol [selective β_1 adrenoreceptor agonists), adenosine, CGS-21680 [a selective adenosine-2-receptor agonist], prostacyclin, forskolin [an adenylate cyclase activator), dibutyryl cAMP, 8-bromo-cAMP, rolipram, zardaverine [a dual phosphodiesterase type III/IV inhibitor], 2-o-propoxyphenyl-8-azapurin-6-one [a phosphodiesterase type V inhibitor], cholera toxin [a stimulatory G-protein activator]) can suppress and even reverse the increase in endothelial and epithelial permeability and vascular tone induced by ischemia-reperfusion injury, oxidant challenge, and receptor specific agonists including PAF, thrombin, and histamine.[340,411–414,416,422,434,438,441,445,460,470–473] Similar effects have been demonstrated by provision of arginine, which, by augmenting NO synthesis, activates guanylate cyclase, increases intracellular cGMP and, thereby, reduces the activity of the cGMP-inhibitable cAMP phosphodiesterase; however, the extent to which this latter modulates other effects of the NO pathway in pulmonary reperfusion is as yet uncertain.[340,413] The precise site at which activation of cAMP-dependent protein kinase A interferes with the protein kinase C and calcium-calmodulin induced alterations in vascular homeostasis is not certain, although it is likely at a locus subsequent to the elevation in cytosolic calcium and prior to the activation of myosin light chain kinase.[457,458] Nor is protein kinase A activation the sole mechanism capable of inhibiting or reversing the increase in paracellular transport promoted by the phosphatidylinositol and protein kinase C signaling pathways; an equivalent and independent effect has been found by activation of ATP-sensitive potassium channels, as well as by inhibition of the sodium-hydrogen antiporter.[415,417,418]

The interdependence of these signaling pathways is substantial, although the myriad mechanisms by which they interact are still vague, and their concerted influence on respiratory gas exchange in lung reperfusion extends well beyond the regulatory control of alveolar permeability and vascular tone. Protein kinase C activation upregulates phospholipase A2 and phospholipase D activity in endothelial cells; among other effects, this amplifies the release of prostacyclin and PAF in response to the calcium flux promoted by other G protein mediated stimuli.[113,444,446,447,474–477] Protein kinase C activation, in turn, downregulates endothelial phospholipase C, thus tempering the response to agonists that increases intracellular calcium levels.[447,450,454,456,477,478] In tandem, the receptor dependent and independent mobilization of intracellular calcium and activation of protein kinase C promote a calmodulin facilitated phosphorylation essential to the exocytic expression of P-selectin, while cAMP downregulates the nuclear factor kappa B mediated transcriptional activation of E-selectin.[36,37,40,195,451,479–484] Endothelin-1 mRNA transcripts are increased by a calmodulin dependent activation of tyrosine kinase, while protein kinase C activation decreases surfactant production; not surprisingly, this latter effect is attenuated by agonists that stimulate protein kinase A.[349,485–488] The effect of hypoxia on vascular smooth muscle cells is primarily mediated by a reduction in cAMP levels, largely through enhanced phosphodiesterase activity rather than by reduced adenylate cyclase activity; these effects, in turn, may be altered by the regulatory influence of cAMP on calcium flux and ATP-insensitive potassium channels.[338,489–491]

Strategies in Lung Preservation

An abundant literature is readily available detailing the merits of various lung preservation solutions. Many have rigorously been compared in well-designed experimental trials, and if we overlook the occasional hyperbole, it is clear that substantial progress has been accomplished since the era in which heart-lung procurement was of necessity performed in an operating room immediately adjacent to that of the recipient. Autoperfusion and donor core cooling on cardiopulmonary bypass were the first methods that offered the prospect of safe, remote procurement, but both have been superseded by a static preservation technique which is less cumbersome, less demanding technically, and less expensive by any criteria.[492–494] Our purpose within this segment is not to provide a strict endorsement of one individual solution or additive, but rather to consider a general approach that will in each instance optimize the initial function of the implanted graft.

Brain death has many antecedents. The declaration of brain death is rarely pronounced within hours of hospital admission; all donors are of necessity mechanically ventilated, and rarely are circumstances as pristine as in the experimental model.[5] In preparation for lung procurement, the simple strategy of avoiding unnecessarily high inspired oxygen fractions will eliminate any tendency to hyperoxic lung injury, and will limit the development of absorption atelectasis.[385] Macroscopic atelectasis is a more urgent concern, since regional hypoxic pulmonary vasoconstriction as a consequence of atelectasis will promote a significant maldistribution of lung preservation solutions, thus reducing their efficacy.[495] While we do not espouse routine fiberoptic bronchoscopy in our own practice, in at least this circumstance, the procedure can be advocated with merit.

In many programs, the standard donor acceptance criteria will exclude those donors with arterial oxygen tension less than 300 mm Hg when ventilated at an inspired oxygen fraction of 1.0, a tidal volume and minute ventilation appropriate for the donor's size, and with positive end-expiratory pressure less than 5 cm H_2O. It should be noted that an arterial oxygen tension at this level already signals that a significant impairment in gas exchange has occurred in advance of preservation, with the estimated shunt in excess of 17% (assuming inspired oxygen fraction = 1.0; barometric pressure = 60 mm Hg; body temperature = 37°C; hemoglobin = 13.0 gm/dL; arterial carbon dioxide tension = 40 mm Hg: shunt = 17.52%). While lungs with preexisting impairment of this extent are successfully implanted, it is only prudent to be aware of the impairment and avoid maneuvers that might precipitate additional dysfunction.[496] Volume resuscitation is curtailed to the extent practical to maintain other organ function, recognizing that both in donor and recipient, fluid overload can provoke rapid deterioration in gas exchange in the face of otherwise modest lung dysfunction.[497,498]

Hypothermia is the single most important component in the pulmonary preservation scheme. Because the thermal conductivity of air is poor, hypothermia is more effectively induced by intravascular infusion of cold solutions than by topical measures, but acceptable clinical and experimental results have been achieved without intravascular flushing.[499,500] The ideal temperature for infusion and storage is still contested. Analysis of the disparate results obtained by different groups contrasting flushing and storage temperatures between 4°C and 23°C is confounded, since dramatically different outcomes occur even with the same preservation solutions when the species are varied or if reperfusion is conducted in isolation, rather than a transplant model.[344,501–503] In our own practice, we do not scrupulously monitor the temperature of either the flushing solution or the stored organ, preferring the simplicity afforded by this lack of rigor. We are not yet persuaded by the available data to deviate from this technique, and believe our clinical experience validates this approach.[504,505]

Heparin is the second critical component common to every current preservation regimen. Apart from its well-recognized anticoagulant activity, heparin and hepain derivatives without anticoagulant activity inhibit complement activation and interfere with both L- and P-selectin function.[270,506] In the recipient, both of these latter effects are theoretically advantageous; in the absence of significant hemorrhage, it may be preferable to avoid neutralization with protamine.

The rediscovery of the capacity of the ischemic lung to maintain aerobic metabolism with retained alveolar oxygen stores during hypothermic storage suggests that there are benefits to the provision of substrate in the base preservation solution.[343,344,507,508] Furthermore, we concede that there are both genuine and theoretical merits to tailoring the composition of the preservation solution to accommodate this capacity, and similar arguments can be advanced for each of the additives currently advocated. We are not yet persuaded that any of the clinically available solutions or adjuncts offer signal advantages and, in our own practice, continue to employ modified Euro-Collins solution, as initially described. [509]

The Future of Experimental Lung Preservation

Pulmonary transplantation is in its infancy, and while a safe and useful technique by almost any standard, much remains to be learned. This review of pulmonary preservation has, for us, posed more questions than answers, and we offer the following as a guide to the direction of future study.

The endothelium is the focal point for the graft's response to the oxidant stress of preservation and reperfusion. Oxygen radicals are formed by endothelial xanthine oxidase at the inception of reperfusion, and the self-inflicted injury incurred during those brief moments may well determine the fate of the graft over the ensuing hours and days. The signals initiated and propagated by the damaged endothelium inaugurate an autocatalytic sequence that may lead to increased microvascular permeability, alterations in regional blood flow, and ultimately a deterioration in respiratory gas exchange. As we have shown, many of the intermediates that promulgate and amplify this sequence have been characterized, and in the experimental setting, several strategies have proven successful in tempering this self-destructive process. Few modalities have found their way into the clinical arena on even a trial basis, and the disparity between experimental successes and clinical practice must be reduced. As a fundamental preliminary, a robust animal model in which to accumulate preclinical data should be defined.[5] The deficiencies of a uniform test platform are apparent to all; with prudence, it should be possible to devise a consensus model which can easily be adapted to accommodate future discoveries.

The economic burden entailed in the purchase, housing, and care of large animal subjects is significant, but the stunning achievements of solid organ transplantation could not have been accomplished without those investments. The administrative and regulatory burden of animal experimentation is progressively odious, as otherwise temperate and intelligent individuals compel increasing restrictions on the scope of animal work. The transplant community must be outspoken in safeguarding the capability to continue experimental work, since there are no available alternatives that can replicate the vast repertoire of the host in its response to foreign antigens. The transplant community has an equivalent ethical burden to demonstrate that it can husband this increasingly precious resource and restrict animal work to just that which is essential to validate concepts fully refined in vitro. In contrast to other organs, the endothelium accounts for a preponderance of metabolic activity in the lung. It seems eminently reasonable to infer that if we can protect the endothelium from ischemia, the parenchymal elements of the lung can scarcely do worse. If this concept can be validated and accepted, the biochemical and genetic engineering techniques enjoyed by our basic science colleagues can be employed to expeditiously characterize in each detail the cellular response to oxidative stress. As this new information is gleaned, novel interventions will assuredly be conceived, and this same platform can serve equally well to economically screen and characterize the efficacy of newer modalities, under conditions that can be rigorously controlled, and with freedom from the technical vagaries and individual subject variability inherent in animal work. Only if an advance can be demonstrated in vitro, should consideration be given to additional testing in vivo and, even then, only if the experimental conclusion would be one that would alter clinical practice. Although we herald our laboratory successes, how many would modify their current clinical routine if the interval of unequivocally safe lung preservation could be extended by 6, or 12, or even an additional 24 hours beyond what is currently available?

The questions to be answered are legion, and we close by offering a few that interest us. How hypoxic must an endothelial cell be, and for how long, before injury is incurred? Why and how does hypoxia signal intracellular proteases to make xanthine oxidase? If mRNA transcripts signaling cellular injury are already being produced even prior to reperfusion (lL-1, IL-6, endothelin-1), surely, some reserve metabolic capacity must be available to support this energy dependent process. Why aren't the intrinsic cellular repair mechanisms given priority instead? Consider one final experimental observation. As already indicated, sublethal concentrations of hydrogen peroxide cause the cells in confluent endothelial monolayers to retract, in a reversible process, in such a way that gaps develop between previously adjacent cells, and during this retraction ICAM-1, ICAM-2, PECAM-1, and the β-1 and β-3 integrins are redistributed about the surface membrane.[510] This is a process dependent on active metabolism, although not protein synthesis, and this mechanism is important in the development of abnormal capillary permeability during lung reperfusion. If this phenomenon is in fact occurring in reperfused tissue, when energy stores are at a premium, why do the endothelial cells engage in a behavior that allows the injury to be extended to the subjacent tissue? If this is in fact a reversible process, and a task that even a damaged cell can accomplish, why can't we?

References

1. Toledo-Pereyra LH, Hau T, Simmons RL, Najarian JS: Lung preservation techniques. *Ann Thorac Surg* 23:487–494, 1977.
2. Haverich A, Scott WC, Jamieson SW: Twenty years of lung preservation: a review. *J Heart Transplant* 4:234–240, 1985.
3. Novick RJ, Menkis AH, McKenzie FN: New trends in lung preservation: a collective review. *J Heart Lung Transplant* 11:377–392, 1992.
4. Egan TM: Lung preservation. *Semin Thorac Cardiovasc Surg* 4:83–89, 1992.
5. Cooper JD, Vreim CE: NHLBI workshop summary. Biology of lung preservation for transplantation. *Am Rev Respir Dis* 146:803–807, 1992.
6. Kirk AJ, Colquhoun IW, Dark JH: Lung preservation: a review of current practice and future directions. *Ann Thorac Surg* 56:990–1000, 1993.
7. Unruh HW: Lung preservation and lung injury. *Chest Surg Clin N Am* 5:91–106, 1995.
8. Vane JR, Anggard EE, Botting RM: Regulatory functions of the vascular endothelium. *N Engl J Med* 323:27–36, 1990.
9. Becker RC: Seminars in thrombosis, thrombolysis, and vascular biology. I. The vascular endothelium. *Cardiology* 78:13–22, 1991.
10. Springer TA: Adhesion receptors of the immune system. *Nature* 346:425–434, 1990.
11. Springer TA: Traffic signals for lymphocyte recirculation and leukocyte emigration: the multistep paradigm. *Cell* 76:301–314, 1994.
12. Suzuki M, Grisham MB, Granger DN: Leukocyte-endothelial cell adhesive interactions: role of xanthine oxidase-derived oxidants. *J Leukoc Biol* 50:488–494, 1991.

13. Oliver MG, Specian RD, Perry MA, Granger DN: Morphologic assessment of leukocyte-endothelial cell interactions in mesenteric venules subjected to ischemia and reperfusion. *Inflammation* 15:331–346, 1991.

14. Kurose I, Anderson DC, Miyasaka M, et al: Molecular determinants of reperfusion-induced leukocyte adhesion and vascular protein leakage. *Circ Res* 74:336–343, 1994.

15. von Andrian UH, Chambers JD, McEvoy LM, Bargatze RF, Arfors KE, Butcher EC: Two-step model of leukocyte-endothelial cell interaction in inflammation: distinct roles for LECAM-1 and the leukocyte beta 2 integrins in vivo. *Proc Natl Acad Sci USA* 88:7538–7542, 1991.

16. Moore KL, Varki A, McEver RP: GMP-140 binds to a glycoprotein receptor on human neutrophils: evidence for a lectin-like interaction. J Cell Biol 112:491–499, 1991.

17. Zhou Q, Moore KL, Smith DF, Varki A, McEver RP, Cummings RD: The selectin GMP-140 binds to sialylated, fucosylated lactosaminoglycans on both myeloid and nonmyeloid cells. *J Cell Biol* 115:557–564, 1991.

18. Bevilacqua MP, Stengelin S, Gimbrone MA Jr, Seed B: Endothelial leukocyte adhesion molecule 1: an inducible receptor for neutrophils related to complement regulatory poteins and lectins. *Science* 243:1160–1165, 1989.

19. Johnston GI, Cook RG, McEver RP: Cloning of GMP-140, a granule membrane protein of platelets and endothelium: sequence similarity to proteins involved in cell adhesion and inflammation. *Cell* 56:1033–1044, 1989.

20. Bowen BR, Nguyen T, Lasky LA: Characterization of a human homologue of the murine peripheral lymph node homing receptor. *J Cell Biol* 109:421–427, 1989.

21. Picker LJ, Warnock RA, Burns AR, Doerschuk CM, Berg EL, Butcher EC: The neutrophil selectin LECAM-1 presents carbohydrate ligands to the vascular selectins ELAM-1 and GMP-140. *Cell* 66:921 -933, 1991.

22. Jutila MA, Rott L, Berg EL, Butcher EC: Function and regulation of the neutrophil MEL-14 antigen in vivo: comparison with LFA-1 and MAC-1. J Immunol 143:3318–3324, 1989.

23. Jutila MA, Kishimoto TK, Butcter EC: Regulation and lectin activity of the human neutrophil peripheral lymph node homing receptor. *Blood* 76:178–183, 1990.

24. Griffin JD, Spertini 0, Ernst TJ, et al: Granulocyte-macrophage colony-stimulating factor and other cytokines regulate surface expression of the leukocyte adhesion molecule-1 on human neutrophils, monocytes, and their precursors. *J Immunol* 145:576–584, 1990.

25. Smith CW, Kishimoto TK, Abbassi 0, et al: Chemotactic factors regulate lectin adhesion molecule 1 (LECAM-1)-dependent neutrophil adhesion to cytokine-stimulated endothelial cells in vitro. *J Clin Invest* 87:609–618, 1991.

26. Palecanda A, Walcheck B, Bishop DK, Jutila MA: Rapid activation-independent shedding of leukocyte L-selectin induced by cross-linking of the surface antigen. *Eur J Immunol* 22:1279–1286, 1992.

27. Schleiffenbaum B, Spertini O, Tedder TF: Soluble L-selectin is present in human plasma at high levels and retains functional activity. *J Cell Biol* 119:229–238, 1992.

28. Kishimoto TK, Jutila MA, Berg EL, Butcher EC: Neutrophil Mac-1 and MEL-14 adhesion proteins inversely regulated by chemotactic factors. *Science* 245:1238–1241, 1989.

29. Imai Y, Lasky LA, Rosen SD: Sulphation requirement for GlyCAM-1, an endothelial ligand for L-selectin. *Nature* 361:555–557, 1993.

30. Baumheter S, Singer MS, Henzel W, et al: Binding of L-selectin to the vascular sialomucin CD34. *Science* 262:436–438, 1993.

31. Lawrence MB, Berg EL, Butcher EC, Springer TA: Rolling of lymphocytes and neutrophils on peripheral node addressin and subsequent arrest on ICAM-1 in shear flow. *Eur J Immunol* 25:1025–1031, 1995.

32. Baumhueter S, Dybdal N, Kyle C, Lasky LA:. Global vascular expression of murine CD34, a sialomucin-like endothelial ligand for L-selectin. *Blood* 84:2554–2565, 1994.

33. Munro JM, Lo SK, Corless C, et al: Expression of sialyl-Lewis X, an E-selectin ligand, in inflammation, immune processes, and lymphoid tissues. *Am J Pathol* 141:1397–1408, 1992.

34. von Andrian UH, Chambers JD, Berg EL, et al: L-selectin mediates neutrophil rolling in inflamed venules through sialyl LewisX-dependent and -independent recognition pathways. *Blood* 82:182–191, 1993.

35. Stenberg PE, McEver RP, Shuman MA, Jacques YV, Bainton DF: A platelet alpha-granule membrane protein (GMP-140) is expressed on the plasma membrane after activation. *J Cell Biol* 101:880–886, 1985.
36. McEver RP, Beckstead JH, Moore KL, Marshall-Carlson L, Bainton DF: GMP-140, a platelet alpha-granule membrane protein, is also synthesized by vascular endothelial cells and is localized in Weibel-Palade bodies. *J Clin Invest* 84:92–99, 1989.
37. Hattori R, Hamilton KK, McEver RP, Sims PJ: Complement proteins C5b-9 induce secretion of high molecular weight multimers of endothelial von Willebrand factor and translocation of granule membrane protein GMP-140 to the cell surface. *J Biol Chem* 264:9053–9060, 1989.
38. Patel KD, Zimmerman GA, Prescott SM, McEver RP, McIntyre TM: Oxygen radicals induce human endothelial cells to express GMP-140 and bind neutrophils. *J Cell Biol* 112:749–759, 1991.
39. Lorant DE, Patel KD, McIntyre TM, McEver RP, Prescott SM, Zimmerman GA: Coexpression of GMP-140 and PAF by endothelium stimulated by histamine or thrombin: a juxtacrine system for adhesion and activation of neutrophils. *J Cell Biol* 115:223–234, 1991.
40. Birch KA, Pober JS, Zavoico GB, Means AR, Ewenstein BM: Calcium/calmodulin transduces thrombin-stimulated secretion: studies in intact and minimally permeabilized human umbilical vein endothelial cells. *J Cell Biol* 118:1501–1510, 1992.
41. Smith CW: Endothelial adhesion molecules and their role in inflammation. *Can J Physiol Pharmacol* 71:76–87, 1993.
42. Dore M, Hawkins HK, Entman ML, Smith CW: Production of a monoclonal antibody against canine GMP-140 (P-selectin) and studies of its vascular distribution in canine tissues. *Vet Pathol* 30:213–222, 1993.
43. Smith CW: Leukocyte-endothelial cell interactions. *Semin Hematol* 30:45–53, 1993.
44. Green SA, Setiadi H, McEver RP, Kelly RB: The cytoplasmic domain of P-selectin contains a sorting determinant that mediates rapid degradation in lysosomes. *J Cell Biol* 124:435–448, 1994.
45. Moore KL, Stuits NL, Diaz S, et al: Identification of a specific glycoprotein ligand for P-selectin (CD62) on myeloid cells. *J Cell Biol* 118:445–456, 1992.
46. Norgard KE, Moore KL, Diaz S, et al: Characterization of a specific ligand for P-selection on myeloid cells: a minor glycoprotein with sialylated O-linked oligosaccharides. *J Biol Chem* 268:12764–4, 1993.
47. Moore KL, Patel KD, Bruehl RE, et al: P-selectin glycoprotein ligand-1 mediates rolling of human neutrophils on P-selectin. *J Cell Biol* 128:661–671, 1995.
48. Lorant DE, McEver RP, McIntyre TM, Moore KL, Prescott SM, Zimmerman GA: Activation of polymorphonuclear leukocytes reduces their adhesion to P-selectin and causes redistribution of ligands for P-selectin on their surfaces. *J Clin Invest* 96:171–182, 1995.
49. Pober JS, Bevilacqua MP, Mendrick DL, Lapierre LA, Fiers W, Gimbrone MA Jr: Two distinct monokines, interleukin 1 and tumor necrosis factor, each independently induce biosynthesis and transient expression of the same antigen on the surface of cultured human vascular endothelial cells. *J Immunol* 136:1680–1687, 1986.
50. Luscinskas FW, Brock AF, Arnaout MA, Gimbrone MA Jr: Endothelial-leukocyte adhesion molecule-1-dependent and leukocyte (CD11/CD18)-dependent mechanisms contribute to polymorphonuclear leukocyte adhesion to cytokine-activated human vascular endothelium. *J Immunol* 142:2257–2263, 1989.
51. Hakkert BC, Kuijpers TW, Leeuwenberg JF, Van Mourik JA, Roos D: Neutrophil and monocyte adherence to and migration across monolayers of cytokine-activated endothelial cells: the contribution of CD18, ELAM-1, and VLA-4. *Blood* 78:2721–2726, 1991.
52. Munro JM, Pober JS, Cotran RS: Recruitment of neutrophils in the local endotoxin response: association with de novo endothelial expression of endothelial leukocyte adhesion molecule-1. *Lab Invest* 64:295, 1991.
53. Kishimoto TK, Warnock RA, Jutila MA, et al: Antibodies against human neutrophil LECAM-1 (LAM-l/Leu-8/DREG-56 antigen) and endothelial cell ELAM-1 inhibit a common CD18-independent adhesion pathway in vitro. *Blood* 78:805–811, 1991.

54. Moore KL, Eaton SF, Lynns DE, Lichenstein HS, Cummings RD, McEver RP: The P-selectin glycoprotein ligand from human neutrophils displays sialylated, fucosylated, O-linked poly-N-acetyllactosamine. *J Biol Chem* 269:23318–23327, 1994.

55. Asa D, Raycroft L, Ma L, et al: The P-selectin glycoprotein ligand functions as a common human leukocyte ligand for P- and E-selectins. *J Biol Chem* 270:11662–11670, 1995.

56. Ruoslahti E: Integrins. *J Clin Invest* 87:1–5, 1991.

57. Penberthy TW, Jiang Y, Luscinskas FW, Graves DT: MCP-1-stimulated monocytes preferentially utilize beta 2-integrins to migrate on laminin and fibronectin. *Am J Physiol* 269:60–68, 1995.

58. Corbi AL, Garcia-Aguilar J, Springer TA: Genomic structure of an integrin alpha subunit, the leukocyte p150,95 molecule. *J Biol Chem* 265:2782, 1990.

59. Dustin ML, Garcia-Aguilar J, Hibbs ML, et al: Structure and regulation of the leukocyte adhesion receptor LFA-1 and its counterreceptors, ICAM-1 and ICAM-2. *Cold Spring Harb Symp Quant Biol* 542:753–765, 1989.

60. Albert RK, Embree LJ, McFeely JE, Hickstein DD: Expression and function of beta 2 integrins on alveolar macrophages from human and nonhuman primates. *Am J Respir Cell Mol Biol* 7:182–189, 1992.

61. Ross GD, Reed W, Dalzell JG, Becker SE, Hogg N: Macrophage cytoskeleton association with CR3 and CR4 regulates receptor mobility and phagocytosis of iC3b-opsonized erythrocytes. *J Leukoc Biol* 51:109–117, 1992.

62. Makgoba MW, Sanders ME, Ginther Luce GE, et al: ICAM-1 a ligand for LFA-1-dependent adhesion of B, T, and myeloid cells. *Nature* 331:86–88, 1988.

63. Staunton DE, Dustin ML, Springer TA: Functional cloning of ICAM-2, a cell adhesion ligand for LFA-1 homologous to ICAM-1. *Nature* 339:61–64, 1989.

64. de Fougerolles AR, Stacker SA, Schwarting R, Springer TA: Characterization of ICAM-2 and evidence for a third counter-receptor for LFA-1. *J Exp Med* 174:253–267, 1991.

65. de Fougerolles AR, Klickstein LB, Springer TA: Cloning and expression of intercellular adhesion molecule 3 reveals strong homology to other immunoglobulin family counter-receptors for lymphocyte function-associated antigen 1. *J Exp Med* 177:1187–1192, 1993.

66. Dustin ML, Rothlein R, Bhan AK, Dinarello CA, Springer TA: Induction by IL 1 and interferon-gamma: tissue distribution, biochemistry, and function of a natural adherence molecule (ICAM-1). *J Immunol* 137:245–254, 1986.

67. Diacovo TG, deFougerolles AR, Bainton DF, Springer TA: A functional integrin ligand on the surface of platelets: intercellular adhesion molecule-2. *J Clin Invest* 94:1243–1251, 1994.

68. de Fougerolles AR, Springer TA: Intercellular adhesion molecule-3, a third adhesion counter-receptor for lymphocyte function-associated molecule-1 on resting lymphocytes. *J Exp Med* 175:185–190, 1992.

69. Staunton DE, Marlin SD, Stratowa C, Dustin ML, Springer TA: Primary structure of ICAM-1 demonstrates interaction between members of the immunoglobulin and integrin supergene families. *Cell* 52:925–933, 1988.

70. Diamond MS, Staunton DE, de Fougerolles AR, et al: ICAM-1 (CD54): a counter-receptor for Mac-1 (CD11b/CD18). *J Cell Biol* 111:3129–3139, 1990.

71. de Fougerolles AR, Qin X, Springer TA: Characterization of the function of intercellular adhesion molecule (ICAM)-3 and comparison with ICAM-1 and ICAM-2 in immune responses. *J Exp Med* 179:619–629, 1994.

72. de Fougerolles AR, Diamond MS, Springer TA: Heterogenous glycosylation of ICAM-3 and lack of interaction with Mac-1 and p150,95. *Eur J Immunol* 25:1008–1012, 1995.

73. Pober JS, Gimbrone MA Jr, Lapierre LA, et al: Overlapping patterns of activation of human endothelial cells by interleukin 1, tumor necrosis factor, and immune interferon. *J Immunol* 137:1893–1896, 1986.

74. Dustin ML, Springer TA: Lymphocyte function-associated antigen-1 (LFA-1) interaction with intercellular adhesion molecule-1 (ICAM-1) is one of at least three mechanisms for lymphocyte adhesion to cultured endothelial cells. *J Cell Biol* 107:321–331, 1988.

75. Smith CW, Rothlein R, Hughes BJ, et al: Recognition of an endothelial determinant for CD 18-dependent human neutrophil adherence and transendothelial migration. *J Clin Invest* 82:1746–1756, 1988.

76. Smith CW, Marlin SD, Rothlein R, Toman C, Anderson DC: Cooperative interactions of LFA-1 and Mac-1 with intercellular adhesion molecule-1 in facilitating adherence and transendothelial migration of human neutrophils in vitro. *J Clin Invest* 83:2008-2017, 1989.

77. Bradley JR, Johnson DR, Pober JS: Endothelial activation by hydrogen peroxide. Selective increases of intercellular adhesion molecule-1 and major histocompatibility complex class I. *Am J Pathol* 142:1598–1609, 1993.

78. Niu XF, Smith CW, Kubes P: Intracellular oxidative stress induced by nitric oxide synthesis inhibition increases endothelial cell adhesion to neutrophils. *Circ Res* 74:1133–1140, 1994.

79. Essani NA, Fisher MA, Farhood A, Manning AM, Smith CW, Jaeschke H: Cytokine-induced upregulation of hepatic intercellular adhesion molecule-1 messenger RNA expression and its role in the pathophysiology of murine endotoxin shock and acute liver failure. *Hepatology* 21:1632–1639, 1995.

80. del Pozo MA, Pulido R, Munoz C, et al: Regulation of ICAM-3 (CD50) membrane expression on human neutrophils through a proteolytic shedding mechanism. *Eur J Immunol* 24:2586–2594, 1994.

81. Skubitz KM, Ahmed K, Campbell KD, Skubitz AP: CD50 (ICAM-3) is phosphorylated on tyrosine and is associated with tyrosine kinase activity in human neutrophils. *J Immunol* 154:2888–2895, 1995.

82. Diamond MS, Staunton DE, Marin SD, Springer TA: Binding of the integrin Mac-1 (CD11b/CD18) to the third immunoglobulin-like domain of ICAM-1 (CD54) and its regulation by glycosylation. *Cell* 65:961–971, 1991.

83. Dustin ML, Springer TA: T-cell receptor cross-linking transiently stimulates adhesiveness through LFA-1. *Nature* 341:619–624, 1989.

84. Hibbs ML, Xu H, Stacker SA, Springer TA: Regulation of adhesion of ICAM-1 by the cytoplasmic domain of LFA-1 integrin beta subunit. *Science* 251:1611-1613, 1991.

85. Hibbs ML, Jakes S, Stacker SA, Wallace RW, Springer TA: The cytoplasmic domain of the integrin lymphocyte function-associated antigen 1 beta subunit: sites required for binding to intercellular adhesion molecule 1 and the phorbol ester-stimulated phosphorylation site. *J Exp Med* 174 1227–1238, 1991.

86. Lo SK, Detmers PA, Levin SM, Wright SD: Transient adhesion of neutrophils to endothelium. *J Exp Med* 169:1779–1793, 1989.

87. Sengelov H, Kjeldsen L, Diamond MS, Springer TA, Borregaard N: Subcellular localization and dynamics of Mac-1 (alpha m beta 2) in human neutrophils. *J Clin Invest* 92:1467–1476, 1993.

88. Jones DH, Anderson DC, Burr BL, et al: Quantitation of intracellular Mac-1 (CD11b/CD18) pools in human neutrophils. *J Leukoc Biol* 44:535–544, 1988.

89. Hughes BJ, Hollers JC, Crockett-Torabi E, Smith CW: Recruitment of CD11b/CD18 to the neutrophil surface and adherence-dependent cell locomotion. *J Clin Invest* 90:1687–1696, 1992.

90. Witthaut R, Farhood A, Smith CW, Jaeschke H: Complement and tumor necrosis factor-alpha contribute to Mac-1 (CD11b/CD18) up-regulation and systemic neutrophil activation during endotoxemia in vivo. *J Leukoc Biol* 55:105–111, 1994.

91. Borregaard N, Kjeldsen L, Sengelov H, et al: Changes in subcellular localization and surface expression of L-selectin, alkaline phosphatase, and Mac-1 in human neutrophils during stimulation with inflammatory mediators. *J Leukoc Biol* 56:80–87, 1994.

92. Diamond MS, Springer TA: A subpopulation of Mac-1 (CD11b/CD18) molecules mediates neutrophil adhesion to ICAM-1 and fibrinogen. *J Cell Biol* 120:545–556, 1993.

93. Vaddi K, Newton RC: Regulation of monocyte integrin expression by beta-family chemokines. *J Immunol* 153:4721–4732, 1994.

94. Stacker SA, Springer TA: Leukocyte integrin P150,95 (CD11c/CD18) functions as an adhesion molecule binding to a counter-receptor on stimulated endothelium. *J Immunol* 146:648–655, 1991.

95. Bilsland CA, Diamond MS, Springer TA: The leukocyte integrin p150,95 (CD11c/CD18) as a receptor for iC3b. Activation by a heterologous beta subunit and localization of a ligand recognition site to the I domain. *J Immunol* 152:4582–4589, 1994.

96. Ingalls RR, Golenbock DT: CD11c/CD18, a transmembrane signaling receptor for lipopolysaccharide *J Exp Med* 181:1473–1479, 1995.

97. Li R, Xie J, Kantor C, et al: A peptide derived from the intercellular adhesion molecule-2 regulates the avidity of the leukocyte integrins CD11b/CD18 and CD11c/CD18. *J Cell Biol* 129:1143–1153, 1995.

98. Fallman M, Andersson R, Andersson T: Signaling properties of CR3 (CD11b/CD18) and CR1 (CD35) in relation to phagocytosis of complement-opsonized particles. J Immunol 151:330–338, 1993.

99. DeLisser HM, Chilkotowsky J, Yan HC, Daise ML, Buck CA, Albelda SM: Deletions in the cytoplasmic domain of platelet-endothelial cell adhesion molecule-1 (PECAM-1, CD31) result in changes in ligand binding properties. *J Cell Biol* 124:195–203, 1994.

100. Romer LH, McLean NV, Yan HC, Daise M, Sun J, DeLisser HM: IFN-gamma and TNF-alpha induce redistribution of PECAM-1 (CD31) on human endothelial cells. *J Immunol* 154:6582–6592, 1995.

101. Schimmenti LA, Yan HC, Madri JA, Albelda SM: Platelet endothelial cell adhesion molecule, PECAM-1, modulates cell migration. *J Cell Physiol* 153:417–428, 1992.

102. DeLisser HM, Yan HC, Newman PJ, Muller WA, Buck CA, Albelda SM: Platelet/endothelial cell adhesion molecule-1 (CD31)-mediated cellular aggregation involves cell surface glycosaminoglycans. *J Biol Chem* 268:16037-16046, 1993.

103. Newman PJ, Albelda SM: Cellular and molecular aspects of PECAM-1. *Nouv Rev Fr Hematol* 34:9–13, 1992.

104. Goldberger A, Middleton KA, Oliver JA, et al: Biosynthesis and processing of the cell adhesion molecule PECAM-1 includes production of a soluble form. *J Biol Chem* 269:17183–17191, 1994.

105. Muller WA, Weigl SA, Deng X, Phillips DM: PECAM-1 is required for transendothelial migration of leukocytes. *J Exp Med* 178:449–460, 1993.

106. Tanaka Y, Albelda SM, Horgan KJ, et al: CD31 expressed on distinctive T cell subsets is a preferential amplifier of beta 1 integrin-mediated adhesion. *J Exp Med* 176:245–253, 1992.

107. Chen W, Knapp W, Majdic O, Stockinger H, Bohmig GA, Zlabinger GJ: Co-ligation of CD31 and Fc gamma RII induces cytokine in human monocytes. *J Immunol* 152:3991–3997, 1994.

108. Berman ME, Muller WA: Ligation of platelet/endothelial cell adhesion molecule 1 (PECAM-1/CD31) on monocytes and neutrophils increases binding capacity of leukocyte CR3 (CD11b/CD18). *J Immunol* 154:299–307, 1995.

109. Lawrence MB, Springer TA: Leukocytes roll on a selectin at physiologic flow rates: distinction from and prerequisite for adhesion through integrins. *Cell* 65:859–873, 1991.

110. Lawrence MB, Springer TA: Neutrophils roll on E-selectin. *J Immunol* 151:6338–6346, 1993.

111. Abbassi O, Kishimoto TK, McIntire LV, Smith CW: Neutrophil adhesion to endothelial cells. *Blood Cells* 19:245–259, 1993.

112. Ley K, Zakrzewicz A, Hanski C, Stoolman LM, Kansas GS: Sialylated O-glycans and L-selectin sequentially mediate myeloid cell rolling in vivo. *Blood* 85:3727–3735, 1995.

113. McIntyre TM, Zimmerman GA, Satoh K, Prescott SM: Cultured endothelial cells synthesize both platelet-activating factor and prostacycin in response to histamine, bradykinin, and adenosine triphosphate. *J Clin Invest* 76:271–280, 1985.

114. Abbassi O, Lane CL, Krater S, et al: Canine neutrophil margination mediated by lectin adhesion molecule-1 in vitro. *J Immunol* 147:2107–2115, 1991.

115. Downey GP, Worthen GS, Henson PM, Hyde DM: Neutrophil sequestration and migration in localized pulmonary inflammation: capillary localization and migration across the interalveolar septum. *Am Rev Respir Dis* 147:168–176, 1993.

116. Dore M, Korthuis RJ, Granger DN, Entman ML, Smith CW: P-selectin mediates spontaneous leukocyte rolling in vivo. *Blood* 82:1308–1316, 1993.

117. Abbassi O, Kishimoto TK, McIntire LV, Anderson DC, Smith CW: E-selectin supports neutrophil rolling in vitro under conditions of flow. *J Clin Invest* 92:2719–2730, 1993.

118. Jones DA, Abbassi O, McIntire LV, McEver RP, Smith CW: P-selectin mediates neutrophil rolling on histamine-stimulated endothelial cells. *Biophys J* 65:1560–1569, 1993.

119. Bargatze RF, Kurk S, Watts G, Kishimoto TK, Speer CA, Jutila MA: In vivo and in vitro

functional examination of a conserved epitope of L- and E-selectin crucial for leukocyte-endothelial cell interactions. *J Immunol* 152:5814–5825, 1994.

120. Olofsson AM, Arfors KE, Ramezani L, Wolitzky BA, Butcher EC, von Andrian UH: E-selectin mediates leukocyte rolling in interleukin-1-treated rabbit mesentery venules. *Blood* 84:2749–2758, 1994.

121. Lehr HA, Olofsson AM, Carew TE, et al: P-selectin mediates the interaction of circulating leukocytes with platelets and microvascular endothelium in response to oxidized lipoprotein in vivo. *Lab invest* 71:380–386, 1994.

122. Luscinskas FW, Kiely JM, Ding H, et al: In vitro inhibitory effect of IL-8 and other chemoattractants on neutrophil-endothelial adhesive interactions. *J Immunol* 149:2163–2171, 1992.

123. Monk PN, Barker MD, Partridge LJ: Multiple signalling pathways in the C5a-induced expression of adhesion receptor Mac-1. *Biochim Biophys Acta* 1221:323–329, 1994.

124. Hazeki K, Seya T, Hazeki O, Ui M: Involvement of the pertussis toxin-sensitive GTP-binding protein in regulation of expression and function of granulocyte complement receptor type 1 and type 3. *Mol Immunol* 31:511-518, 1994.

125. Crockett-Torabi E, Sulenbarger B, Smith CW, Fantone JC: Activation of human neutrophils through L-selectin and Mac-1 molecules. *J Immunol* 154:2291–2302, 1995.

126. Weyrich AS, McIntyre TM, McEver RP, Prescott SM, Zimmerman GA: Monocyte tethering by P-selectin regulates monocyte chemotactic protein-1 and tumor necrosis factor-alpha secretion: Signal integration and NF-kappa B translocation. *J Clin Invest* 95:2297–2303, 1995.

127. Simon SI, Burns AR, Taylor AD, et al: L-selectin (CD62L) cross-linking signals neutrophil adhesive functions via the Mac-1 (CD11b/CD18) beta 2-integrin. *J Immunol* 155:1502–1514, 1995.

128. Lorant DE, Topham MK, Whatley RE, et al: Inflammatory roles of P-selectin. *J Clin Invest* 92:559–570, 1993.

129. von Andrian UH, Hansell P, Chambers JD, et al: L-selectin function is required for beta 2-integrin-mediated neutrophil adhesion at physiological shear rates in vivo. *Am J Physiol* 263:1034–1044, 1992.

130. Lehr HA, Krombach F, Munzing S, et al: In vitro effects of oxidized low density lipoprotein on CD11b/CD18 and L-selectin presentation on neutrophils and monocytes with relevance for the in vivo situation. *Am J Pathol* 146:218–227, 1995.

131. Lawrence MB, Bainton DF, Springer TA: Neutrophil tethering to and rolling on E-selectin are separable by requirement for L-selectin. Immunity 1:137–145, 1994.

132. Kansas GS, Ley K, Munro JM, Tedder TF: Regulation of leukocyte rolling and adhesion to high endothelial venules through the cytoplasmic domain of L-selectin. *J Exp Med* 177:833-838, 1993.

133. Lawrence MB, Smith CW, Eskin SG, McIntire LV: Effect of venous shear stress on CD18-mediated neutrophil adhesion to cultured endothelium. *Blood* 75:227–237, 1990.

134. Argenbright LW, Letts LG, Rothlein R: Monoclonal antibodies to the leukocyte membrane CD18 glycoprotein complex and to intercellular adhesion molecule-1 inhibit leukocyte-endothelial adhesion in rabbits. *J Leukoc Biol* 49:253–257, 1991.

135. Furie MB, Tancinco MC, Smith CW: Monoclonal antibodies to leukocyte integrins CD11a/CD18 and CD11b/CD18 or intercellular adhesion molecule-1 inhibit chemoattractant-stimulated neutrophil transendothelial migration in vitro. *Blood* 78:2089–2097, 1991.

136. Robinson MK, Andrew D, Rosen H, et al: Antibody against the Leu-CAM beta-chain (CD18) promotes both LFA-1- and CR3-dependent adhesion events. *J Immunol* 148:1080–1085, 1992.

137. Vaporciyan AA, DeLisser HM, Yan HC, et al: Involvement of platelet-endothelial cell adhesion molecule-1 in neutrophil recruitment in vivo. *Science* 262:1580–1582, 1993.

138. Petruzzelli L, Maduzia L, Springer TA: Activation of lymphocyte function-associated molecule-1 (CD11a/CD18) and Mac-1 (CD11b/CD18) mimicked by an antibody directed against CD18. *J Immunol* 155:854–866, 1995.

139. Hernandez LA, Grisham MB, Twohig B, Arfors KE, Harlan JM, Granger DN: Role of neutrophils in ischemia-reperfusion-induced microvascular injury. *Am J Physiol* 253:699–703, 1987.

140. Simpson PJ, Todd RF 3d, Fantone JC, Mickelson JK, Griffin JD, Lucchesi BR: Reduction of experimental canine myocardial reperfusion injury by a monoclonal antibody (anti-Mol, anti-CD11b) that inhibits leukocyte adhesion. *J Clin Invest* 81:624–629, 1988.

141. Bishop MJ, Chi EY, Su M, Cheney FW: Dimethylthiourea does not ameliorate reperfusion lung injury in dogs or rabbits. *J Appl Physiol* 65:2051–2056, 1988.

142. Deeb GM, Grum CM, Lynch MJ: et al. Neutrophils are not necessary for induction of ischemia-reperfusion lung injury. *J Appi Physiol* 68:374–381, 1990.

143. Horgan MJ, Wright SD, Malik AB: Antibody against leukocyte integrin (CD18) prevents reperfusion-induced lung vascular injury. *Am J Physiol* 259:315–319, 1990.

144. Horgan MJ, Ge M, Gu J, Rothlein R, Malik AB: Role of ICAM-1 in neutrophil-mediated lung vascular injury after occlusion and reperfusion. *Am J Physiol* 261:1578–1584, 1991.

145. Steimle CN, Guynn TP, Morganroth ML, Bolling SF, Carr K, Deeb GM: Neutrophils are not necessary for ischemia-reperfusion lung injury. *Ann Thorac Surg* 53:64–72, 1992.

146. Wickersham NE, Johnson JJ, Meyrick BO, Gilroy RJ, Loyd JE: Lung ischemia-reperfusion injury in awake sheep: protection with verapamil. *J Appl Physiol* 71:1554–1562, 1991.

147. Palace GP, Horgan MJ, Malik AB: Generation of 5-lipoxygenase metabolites following pulmonary reperfusion in isolated rabbit lungs. *Prostaglandins* 43:339–349, 1992

148. Ma XL, Lefer DJ, Lefer AM: Rothlein R: Coronary endothelial and cardiac protective effects of a monoclonal antibody to intercellular adhesion molecule-1 in myocardial ischemia and reperfusion. *Circulation* 86:937–946, 1992.

149. Seibert AF, Haynes J, Taylor A: Ischemia-reperfusion injury in the isolated rat lung: role of flow and endogenous leukocytes. *Am Rev Respir Dis* 147:270–275, 1993.

150. Horiguchi T, Harada Y: The effect of protease inhibitor on reperfusion injury after unilateral pulmonary ischemia. *Transplantation* 55:254–258, 1993.

151. Yamazaki T, Seko Y, Tamatani T, et al: Expression of intercellular adhesion molecule-1 in rat heart with ischemia/reperfusion and limitation of infarct size by treatment with antibodies against cell adhesion molecules. *Am J Pathol* 143:410–418, 1993.

152. Kukielka GL, Hawkins HK, Michael L, et al: Regulation of intercellular adhesion molecule-1 (ICAM-1) in ischemic and reperfused canine myocardium. *J Clin Invest* 92:1504–1516, 1993.

153. Lefer DJ, Shandelya SM, Serrano CV Jr, Becker LC, Kuppusamy P, Zweier JL: Cardioprotective actions of a monoclonal antibody against CD-18 in myocardial ischemia-reperfusion injury. *Circulation* 88:1779–1787, 1993.

154. Sekido N, Mukaida N, Harada A, Nakanishi I, Watanabe Y, Matsushima K: Prevention of lung reperfusion injury in rabbits by a monoclonal antibody against interleukin-8. *Nature* 365:654–657, 1993.

155. Youker KA, Hawkins HK, Kukielka GL: et al. Molecular evidence for induction of intracellular adhesion molecule-1 in the viable border zone associated with ischemia-reperfusion injury of the dog heart. *Circulation* 89:2736–2746, 1994.

156. Youker KA, Hawkins HK, Kukielka GL, et al: Molecular evidence for a border zone vulnerable to inflammatory reperfusion injury. *Trans Assoc Am Physicians* 106:145–154, 1993.

157. Thomas DD, Sharar SR, Winn RK, et al: CD18-independent mechanism of neutrophil emigration in the rabbit lung after ischemia-reperfusion. *Ann Thorac Surg* 60:1360–1366, 1995.

158. Weyrich AS, Ma XY, Lefer DJ, Albertine KH, Lefer AM: In vivo neutralization of P-selectin protects feline heart and endothelium in myocardial ischemia and reperfusion injury. *J Clin Invest* 91:2620–2629, 1993.

159. Shen I, Verrier ED: Expression of E-selectin on coronary endothelium after myocardial ischemia and reperfusion. *J Card Surg* 9:437–441, 1994.

160. Weyrich AS, Buerke M, Albertine KH, Lefer AM: Time course of coronary vascular endothelial adhesion molecule expression during reperfusion of the ischemic feline myocardium. *J Leukoc Biol* 57:45–55, 1995.

161. Billups KL, Palladino MA, Hinton BT, Sherley JL: Expression of E-selectin mRNA during ischemia/reperfusion injury. *J Lab Clin Med* 125:626–633, 1995.

162. Ma XL, Weyrich AS, Lefer DJ, et al: Monoclonal antibody to L-selectin attenuates neutrophil accumulation and protects ischemic reperfused cat myocardium. *Circulation* 88:649–658, 1993

163. Buerke M, Weyrich AS, Zheng Z, Gaeta FC, Forrest MJ, Lefer AM: Sialyl Lewisx-containing oligosaccharide attenuates myocardial reperfusion injury in cats. *J Clin Invest* 93:1140–1148, 1994.

164. Chen LY, Nichols WW, Hendricks JB, Yang BC, Mehta JL: Monoclonal antibody to P-selectin (PB1.3) protects against myocardial reperfusion injury in the dog. *Cardiovasc Res* 28:1414–1422, 1994.

165. Buerke M, Weyrich AS, Murohara T, et al: Humanized monoclonal antibody DREG-200 directed against I-selectin protects in feline myocardial reperfusion injury. *J Pharmacol Exp Ther* 271:134–142, 1994.

166. Silver MJ, Sutton JM, Hook S, et al: Adjunctive selectin blockade successfully reduces infarct size beyond thrombolysis in the electrolytic canine coronary artery model. *Circulation* 92:492–499, 1995.

167. Kawata H, Aoki M, Hickey PR, Mayer JE, Jr: Effect of antibody to leukocyte adhesion molecule CD18 on recovery of neonatal lamb hearts after 2 hours of cold ischemia. *Circulation* 86:364–370, 1992.

168. Gomoll AW, Lekich RF, Grove RI: Efficacy of a monoclonal antibody (MoAb 60.3) in reducing myocardial injury resulting from ischemia/reperfusion in the ferret. *J Cardiovasc Pharmacol* 17:873–887, 1991.

169. Ide H, Ino T, Hasegawa T, Matsumoto H: The role of leukocyte depletion by in vivo use of leukocyte filter in lung preservation after warm ischemia. *Angiology* 41:318–327, 1990.

170. Breda MA, Hall TS, Stuart RS, et al: Twenty-four hour lung preservation by hypothermia and leukocyte depletion. *J Heart Transplant* 4:325–329, 1985.

171. Pillai R, Bando K, Schueler S, Zebly M, Reitz BA, Baumgartner WA: Leukocyte depletion results in excellent heart-lung function after 12 hours of storage. *Ann Thorac Surg* 50:211–214, 1990.

172. Bando K, Schueler S, Cameron DE, et al: Twelve-hour cardiopulmonary preservation using donor core cooling, leukocyte depletion, and liposomal superoxide dismutase. *J Heart Lung Transplant* 10:304–309, 1991.

173. Schueler S, De Valeria PA, Hatanaka M, et al: Successful twenty four-hour lung preservation with donor core cooling and leukocyte depletion in an orthotopic double lung transplantation model. *J Thorac Cardiovasc Surg* 104:73–82, 1992

174. Shimizu N, Miyai Y, Aoe M, Nakata M, Date H, Teramoto S: The effects of radical scavengers and leukocyte-depleted blood on reperfusion injury of extirpated rabbit lung. *Tohoku J Exp Med* 166:321–329, 1992.

175. Bishop MJ, Kowalski TF, Guidotti SM, Harlan JM: Antibody against neutrophil adhesion improves reperfusion and limits alveolar infiltrate following unilateral pulmonary artery occlusion. *J Surg Res* 52:199–204, 1992.

176. Adkins WK, Taylor AE: Role of xanthine oxidase and neutrophils in ischemia-reperfusion injury in rabbit lung. *J Appl Physiol* 69:2012–2018, 1990.

177. Moore TM, Khimenko P, Adkins WK, Miyasaka M, Taylor AE: Adhesion molecules contribute to ischemia and reperfusion-induced injury in the isolated rat lung. *J Appl Physiol* 78:2245–2252, 1995.

178. Steinberg JB, Mao HZ, Niles SD, Jutila MA, Kapelanski DP: Survival in lung reperfusion injury is improved by an antibody that binds and inhibits L- and E-selectin. *J Heart Lung Transplant* 13:306–318, 1994.

179. Uthoff K, Zehr KJ, Lee PC, et al: Neutrophil modulation results in improved pulmonary function after 12 and 24 hours of preservation. *Ann Thorac Surg* 59:7–12, 1995.

180. Smith RJ, Justen JM, Bleasdale JE, Sly LM: NPC 15669-modulated human polymorphonuclear neutrophil functional responsiveness: effects on receptor-coupled signal transduction. *Br J Pharmacol* 114:1694–1702, 1995.

181. Kapelanski DP, Iguchi A, Niles SD, Mao HZ: Lung reperfusion injury is reduced by inhibiting a CD18-dependent mechanism. *J Heart Lung Transplant* 12:294–306, 1993.

182. Okusawa S, Yancey KB, van der Meer JW, et al: C5a stimulates secretion of tumor necrosis factor from human mononuclear cells in vitro: comparison with secretion of interleukin 1 beta and interleukin 1 alpha. *J Exp Med* 168:443–448, 1988.

183. Mulligan MS, Varani J, Warren JS, et al: Roles of beta 2 integrins of rat neutrophils in complement- and oxygen radical-mediated acute inflammatory injury. *J Immunol* 148:1847–1857, 1992.

184. Schwartz MD, Repine JE, Abraham E: Xanthine oxidase-derived oxygen radicals increase lung cytokine expression in mice subjected to hemorrhagic shock. *Am J Respir Cell Mol Biol* 12:434–440, 1995.

185. Dinarello CA, Cannon JG, Wolff SM, et al: Tumor necrosis factor (cachectin) is an endogenous pyrogen and induces production of interleukin 1. *J Exp Med* 163:1433–1450, 1986.

186. Doukas J, Pober JS: IFN-gamma enhances endothelial activation induced by tumor necrosis factor but not IL-1. *J Immunol* 145:1727–1733, 1990.

187. Smith CW, Entman ML, Lane CL, et al: Adherence of neutrophiis to canine cardiac myocytes in vitro is dependent on intercellular adhesion molecule-1. *J Clin Invest* 88:1216–1223, 1991.

188. Mulligan MS, Varani J, Dame MK, et al: Role of endothelial-leukocyte adhesion molecule 1 (ELAM-1) in neutrophil-mediated lung injury in rats. *J Clin Invest* 88:1396–1406, 1991.

189. Bradley JR, Johnson DR, Pober JS: Four different classes of inhibitors of receptor-mediated endocytosis decrease tumor necrosis factor-induced gene expression in human endothelial cells. *J Immunol* 150:5544–5545, 1993.

190. Slowik MR, De Luca LG, Fiers W, Pober JS: Tumor necrosis factor activates human endothelial cells through the p55 tumor necrosis factor receptor, but the p75 receptor contributes to activation at low tumor necrosis factor concentration. *Am J Pathol* 143:1724–1730, 1993.

191. Read MA, Whitley MZ, Williams AJ, Collins T: NF-kappa B and I kappa B alpha: an inducible regulatory system in endothelial activation. *J Exp Med* 179:503–512, 1994.

192. Whitley MZ, Thanos D, Read MA, Maniatis T, Collins T: A striking similarity in the organization of the E-selectin and beta interferon gene promoters. *Mol Cell Biol* 14:6464–6475, 1994.

193. Read MA, Neish AS, Luscinskas FW, Palombella VJ, Maniatis T, Collins T: The proteasome pathway is required for cytokine-induced endothelial-leukocyte adhesion molecule expression. *Immunity* 2:493–506, 1995.

194. Rollins BJ, Yoshimura T, Leonard EJ, Pober JS: Cytokine-activated human endothelial cells synthesize and secrete a monocyte chemoattractant, MCP-1/JE. *Am J Pathol* 136:1229–1233, 1990.

195. Pober JS, Slowik MR, De Luca LG, Ritchie AJ: Elevated cyclic AMP inhibits endothelial cell synthesis and expression of TNF-induced endothelial leukocyte adhesion molecule-1, and vascular cell adhesion molecule-1, but not intercellular adhesion molecule-1. *J Immunol* 150:5114–5123, 1993.

196. Satriano JA, Shuldiner M, Hora K, Xing Y, Shan Z, Schlondorff D. Oxygen radicals as second messengers for expression of the monocyte chemoattractant protein, JE/MCP-1, and the monocyte colony-stimulating factor, CSF-1, in response to tumor necrosis factor-alpha and immunoglobulin G: evidence for involvement of reduced nicotinamide adenine dinucleotide phosphate (NADPH)-dependent oxidase. *J Ciin Invest* 92:1564–1571, 1993.

197. Hanasaki K, Varki A, Stamenkovic I, Bevilacqua MP: Cytokine-induced beta-galactoside alpha-2,6-sialyltransferase in human endothelial cells mediates alpha 2,6-sialylation of adhesion molecules and CD22 ligands. *J Biol Chem* 269:10637–10643, 1994.

198. Brown JM Anderson BO, Repine JE, et al: Neutrophils contribute to TNF induced myocardial tolerance to ischaemia. *J Mol Cell Cardiol* 24:485–495, 1992.

199. Eddy LJ, Goeddel DV, Wong GH: Tumor necrosis factor-alpha pretreatment is protective in a rat model of myocardial ischemia-reperfusion injury. *Biochem Biophys Res Commun* 184:1056–1059, 1992.

200. Nelson SK, Wong GH, McCord JM: Leukemia inhibitory factor and tumor necrosis factor induce manganese superoxide dismutase and protect rabbit hearts from reperfusion injury. *J Mol Cell Cardiol* 27:223–229, 1995.

201. Aoki N, Siegfried M, Lefer AM: Anti-EDRF effect of tumor necrosis factor in isolated, perfused cat carotid arteries. *Am J Physiol* 256:1509–1512, 1989.

202. Colletti LM, Burtch GD, Remick DG, et al: The production of tumor necrosis factor alpha

and the development of a pulmonary capillary injury following hepatic ischemia/reperfusion. *Transplantation* 49:268–272, 1990.

203. Colletti LM, Remick DG, Burtch GD, Kunkel SL, Strieter RM, Campbell DA Jr: Role of tumor necrosis factor-alpha in the pathophysiologic alterations after hepatic ischemia/reperfusion injury in the rat. *J Clin Invest* 85:1936–1943, 1990.

204. Caty MG, Guice KS, Oldham KT, Remick DG, Kunkel SI: Evidence for tumor necrosis factor-induced pulmonary microvascular injury after intestinal ischemia-reperfusion injury. *Ann Surg* 212:694–700, 1990.

205. Welbourn R, Goldman G, O'Riordain M, et al: Role for tumor necrosis factor as mediator of lung injury following lower torso ischemia. *J Appl Physiol* 70:2645–2649, 1991.

206. Jansen NJ, van Oeveren W, van den Broek L, et al: Inhibition by dexamethasone of the reperfusion phenomena in cardiopulmonary bypass. *J Thorac Cardiovasc Surg* 102:515–525, 1991.

207. Palace GP, Del Vecchio PJ, Horgan MJ, Malik AB: Release of tumor necrosis factor after pulmonary artery occlusion and reperfusion. *Am Rev Respir Dis* 147:143–147, 1993.

208. Squadrito F, Altavilla D, Zingarelli B, et al: The effect of cloricromene, a coumarine derivative, on leukocyte accumulation, myocardial necrosis, and TNF-alpha production in myocardial ischaemia-reperfusion injury. *Life Sci* 53:341–355, 1993.

209. Seekamp A, Warren JS, Remick DG, Till GO, Ward PA: Requirements for tumor necrosis factor-alpha and interleukin-1 in limb ischemia/reperfusion injury and associated lung injury. *Am J Pathol* 143:453–463, 1993.

210. Squadrito F, Altavilla D, Zingarelli B, et al: Tumor necrosis factor involvement in myocardial ischaemia-reperfusion injury. *Eur J Pharmacol* 237:223–230, 1993.

211. Squadrito F, Ioculano M, Altavilla D, et al: Platelet activating factor in myocardial ischaemia-reperfusion injury. *J Lipid Mediat* 8:53–65, 1993.

212. Suzuki S, Toledo-Pereyra LH: Interleukin 1 and tumor necrosis factor production as the initial stimulants of liver ischemia and reperfusion injury. *J Surg Res* 57:253–258, 1994.

213. Sternbergh WC 3rd, Tuttle TM, Makhoul RG, Bear HD, Sobel M, Fowler AA 3rd: Postischemic extremities exhibit immediate release of tumor necrosis factor. *J Vasc Surg* 20:474–481, 1994.

214. Canale P, Squadrito F, Altavilla D, et al: TCV-309, a novel platelet activating factor antagonist, inhibits leukocyte accumulation and protects against splanchnic artery occlusion shock. *Agents Actions* 42:128–34, 1994.

215. Wang X, Yue TL, Barone FC, White RF, Gagnon RC, Feuerstein GZ: Concomitant cortical expression of TNF-alpha and IL-1 beta mRNAs follows early response gene expression in transient focal ischemia. *Mol Chem Neuropathol* 23:103–114, 1994.

216. Sorkine P, Setton A, Halpern P, et al: Soluble tumor necrosis factor receptors reduce bowel ischemia-induced lung permeability and neutrophil sequestration. *Crit Care Med* 23:1377–1381, 1995.

217. Ascer E, Gennaro M, Cupo S, Mohan C: Do cytokines play a role in skeletal muscle ischemia and reperfusion? *J Cardiovasc Surg* 33:588–592, 1992.

218. Chazouilleres O, Guechot J, Balladur P, et al: Tumor necrosis factor-alpha in liver transplantation and resection: no evidence for a key role in ischemia-reperfusion injury. *J Hepatol* 16:376–379, 1992.

219. Field G, Conn CA, McClanahan TB, Nao BS, Kluger MJ, Gallagher KP: Tumor necrosis factor and interleukin-6 are not elevated in venous blood from ischemic canine myocardium. *Proc Soc Exp Biol Med* 206:384–391, 1994.

220. Scales WE, Campbell DA Jr, Green ME, Remick DG: Hepatic ischemia/reperfusion injury: importance of oxidant/tumor necrosis factor interactions. *Am J Physiol* 267:1122–1127, 1994.

221. Serrick C, Adoumie R, Giaid A, Shennib H: The early release of interleukin-2, tumor necrosis factor-alpha, and interferon-gamma after ischemia reperfusion injury in the lung allograft. *Transplantation* 58:1158–1162, 1994.

222. Serrick C, La Franchesca S, Giaid A, Shennib H: Cytokine interleukin-2, tumor necrosis factor-alpha, and interferon-gamma release after ischemia/reperfusion injury in a novel lung autograft animal model. *Am J Respir Crit Care Med* 152:277–282, 1995.

223. Saklatvala J, Guesdon F: Interleukin 1 and tumor necrosis factor signal transduction mechanisms: potential targets for pharmacological control of inflammation. *J Rheumatol Suppl* 32:65–69, 1992.

224. Maulik N, Engelman RM, Wei Z, Lu D, Rousou JA, Das DK: Interleukin-1 alpha preconditioning reduces myocardial ischemia reperfusion injury. *Circulation* 88:387–394, 1993.

225. Issekutz AC, Chuluyan HE, Lopes N: CD11/CD18-independent transendothelial migration of human polymorphonuclear leukocytes and monocytes: involvement of distinct and unique mechanisms. *J Leukoc Biol* 57:553–561, 1995.

226. Entman ML, Youker K, Shappell SB, et al: Neutrophil adherence to isolated adult canine myocytes: evidence for a CD18-dependent mechanism. *J Clin Invest* 85:1497–1506, 1990.

227. Ascer E, Mohan C, Gennaro M, Cupo S: Interleukin-1 and thromboxane release after skeletal muscle ischemia and reperfusion. *Ann Vasc Surg* 6:69–73, 1992.

228. Suzuki S, Toledo-Pereyra LH, Rodriguez F, Lopez F: Role of Kupffer cells in neutrophil activation and infiltration following total hepatic ischemia and reperfusion. *Circ Shock* 42:204–209, 1994.

229. Herskowitz A, Choi S, Ansari AA, Wesselingh S: Cytokine mRNA expression in postischemic/reperfused myocardium. *Am J Pathol* 146:419–428, 1995.

230. Kamikubo Y, Murakami M, Imamura M, Murashita T, Yasuda K, Uede T: Neutrophil-independent myocardial dysfunction during an early stage of global ischemia and reperfusion of isolated hearts. *Immunopharmacology* 29:261–271, 1995.

231. Brown JM, White CW, Terada LS, et al: Interleukin 1 pretreatment decreases ischemia/reperfusion injury. *Proc Natl Acad Sci U S A* 87:5026–5030, 1990.

232. Repine JE: Oxidant-antioxidant balance: some observations from studies of ischemia-reperfusion in isolated perfused rat hearts. *Am J Med* 91:45–53, 1991.

233. Guidot DM, Linas SL, Repine MJ, Shanley PF, Fisher HS, Repine JE: Interleukin-1 treatment increases neutrophils, but not antioxidant enzyme activity or resistance to ischemia-reperfusion injury in rat kidneys. *Inflammation* 18:537–545, 1994.

234. Rollins BJ, Pober JS: Interleukin-4 induces the synthesis and secretion of MCP-1/JE by human endothelial cells. *Am J Pathol* 138:1315–1319, 1991.

235. Palmer-Crocker RL, Pober JS: IL-4 induction of VCAM-1 on endothelial cells involves activation of a protein tyrosine kinase. *J Immunol* 154:2838–2845; 1995.

236. Standiford TJ, Kunkel SL, Liebler JM, Burdick MD, Gilbert AR, Strieter RM: Gene expression of macrophage inflammatory protein-1 alpha from human blood monocytes and alveolar macrophages is inhibited by interleukin-4. *Am J Respir Cell Mol Biol* 9:192–198, 1993.

237. Schleimer RP, Sterbinsky SA, Kaiser J, et al: IL-4 induces adherence of human eosinophils and basophils but not neutrophils to endothelium: association with expression of VCAM-1. *J Immunol* 148:1086–1092, 1992.

238. Briscoe DM, Cotran RS, Pober JS: Effects of tumor necrosis factor, lipopolysaccharide, and IL-4 on the expression of vascular cell adhesion molecule-1 in vivo: correlation with CD3+ T cell infiltration. *J Immunol* 149:2954–2960, 1992.

239. Luscinskas FW, Kansas GS, Ding H, et al: Monocyte rolling, arrest, and spreading on IL-4-activated vascular endothelium under flow is mediated via sequential action of L-selectin, beta 1-integrins, and beta 2-integrins. *J Cell Biol* 125:1417–1427, 1994.

240. Yamauchi-Takihara K, Ihara Y, Ogata A, Yoshizaki K, Azuma J, Kishimoto T: Hypoxic stress induces cardiac myocyte-derived interleukin-6. *Circulation* 91:1520–1524, 1995.

241. Kukielka GL, Smith CW, Manning AM, Youker KA, Michael LH, Entman ML: Induction of interleukin-6 synthesis in the myocardium: potential role in postreperfusion inflammatory injury. *Circulation* 92:1866–1875, 1995.

242. Pham SM, Yoshida Y, Aeba R, et al: Interleukin-6, a marker of preservation injury in clinical lung transplantation. *J Heart Lung Transplant* 11:1017–1024, 1992.

243. Steinberg JB, Kapelanski DP, Olson JD, Weiler JM: Cytokine and complement levels in patients undergoing cardiopulmonary bypass. *J Thorac Cardiovasc Surg* 106:1008–1016, 1993.

244. Kawamura T, Wakusawa R, Okada K, Inada S: Elevation of cytokines during open-heart surgery with cardiopulmonary bypass: participation of interleukin 8 and 6 in reperfusion injury. *Can J Anaesth* 40:1016–1021, 1993.

245. Youker K, Smith CW, Anderson DC, et al: Neutrophil adherence to isolated adult cardiac myocytes: induction by cardiac lymph collected during ischemia and reperfusion. *J Clin Invest* 89:602–609, 1992.

246. Metinko AP, Kunkel SL, Standiford TJ, Strieter RM: Anoxia-hyperoxia induces monocyte-derived interleukin-8. *J Clin Invest* 90:791–798, 1992.

247. Ivey CL, Williams FM, Collins PD, Jose PJ, Williams TJ: Neutrophil chemoattractants generated in two phases during reperfusion of ischemic myocardium in the rabbit: evidence for a role for C5a and interleukin-8. *J Clin Invest* 95:2720–2728, 1995.

248. Kupper RW, Dewald B, Jakobs KH, Baggiolini M, Gierschik P: G-protein activation by interleukin 8 and related cytokines in human neutrophil plasma membranes. *Biochem J* 282:429–434, 1992.

249. Federsppiel B, Melhado IG, Duncan AM, et al: Molecular cloning of the cDNA and chromosomal localization of the gene for a putative seven-transmembrane segment (7-TMS) receptor isolated from human spleen. *Genomics* 16:707–712, 1993.

250. Kukielka GL, Smith CW, LaRosa GJ, et al: Interleukin-8 gene induction in the myocardium after ischemia and reperfusion in vivo. *J Clin Invest* 95:89–103, 1995.

251. Harada A, Sekido N, Akahoshi T, Wada T, Mukaida N, Matsushima K: Essential involvement of interleukin-8 (IL-8) in acute inflammation. *J Leukoc Biol* 56:559–564, 1994.

252. Ley K, Baker JB, Cybulsky MI, Gimbrone MA Jr, Luscinskas FW: Intravenous interleukin-8 inhibits granulocyte emigration from rabbit mesenteric venules witbut altering L-selectin expression or leukocyte rolling. *J Immunol* 151:6347–6357, 1993.

253. Lefer AM, Johnson G 3d, Ma XL, Tsao PS Thomas GR: Cardioprotective and endothelial protective effects of [Ala-IL8]77 in a rabbit model of myocardial ischaemia and reperfusion. *Br J Pharmacol* 103:1153–1159, 1991.

254. Johnson DR, Pober JS: Tumor necrosis factor and immune interferon synergistically increase transcription of HLA class I heavy- and light-chain genes in vascular endothelium. *Proc Natl Acad Sci U S A* 87:5183–5187, 1990.

255. Rosenkranz-Weiss P, Sessa WC, Milstien S Kaufman S, Watson CA, Pober JS: Regulation of nitric oxide synthesis by proinflammatory cytokines in human umbilical vein endothelial cells: elevations in tetrahydrobiopterin levels enhance endothelial nitric oxide synthase specific activity. *J Clin Invest* 93:2236–2243, 1994.

256. Turnage RH, Magee JC, Guice KS, Myers SI, Oldham KT: Complement activation by the hydroxyl radical during intestinal reperfusion. *Shock* 2:445–450, 1994.

257. Dahinden CA, Kurimoto Y, Wirthmuller U: Growth factors, lipid mediators, and effector cells. *J Lipid Mediat* 2:129–136, 1990.

258. Mulligan MS, Polley MJ, Bayer RJ, Nunn MF, Paulson JC, Ward PA: Neutrophil-dependent acute lung injury: requirement for P-selectin (GMP-140) *J Clin Invest* 90:1600–1607, 1992.

259. Mulligan MS, Smith CW, Anderson DC, et al: Role of leukocyte adhesion molecules in complement-induced lung injury. *J Immunol* 150:2401–2406, 1993.

260. Dreyer WJ, Michael LH, Nguyen T, et al: Kinetics of C5a release cardiac lymph of dogs experiencing coronary artery ischemia-reperfusion injury. *Circ Res* 71:1518–1524, 1992.

261. Amsterdam EA, Stahl GL, Pan HL, Rendig SV, Fletcher MP, Longhurst JC: Limitation of reperfusion injury by a monoclonal antibody to C5a during myocardial infarction in pigs. *Am J Physiol* 268:448–457, 1995.

262. Shandelya SM, Kuppusamy P, VVeisfeldt ML Zweier JL: Evaluation of the role of polymorphonuclear leukocytes on contractile function in myocardial reperfusion injury: Evidence for plasma-mediated leukocyte activation. *Circulation* 87:536–546, 1993.

263. Buerke M, Murohara T, Lefer AM: Cardioprotective effects of a C1 esterase inhibitor in myocardial ischemia and reperfusion. *Circulation* 91:393–402, 1995.

264. Weisman HF, Bartow T, Leppo MK, et al: Soluble human complement receptor type 1: in vivo inhibitor of complement suppressing post-ischemic myocardial inflammation and necrosis. *Science* 249:146–151, 1990.

265. Weisman HF, Bartow T, Leppo MK, et al: Recombinant soluble CR1 suppressed complement activation, inflammation, and necrosis associated with reperfusion of ischemic myocardium. *Trans Assoc Am Physicians* 103:64–72, 1990.

266. Shandelya SM, Kuppusamy P, Kerskowitz A, Weisfeldt ML, Zweier JL: Soluble complement receptor type 1 inhibits the complement pathway and prevents contractile failure in the postischemic heart: evidence that complement activation is required for neutrophil-mediated reperfusion injury. *Circulation* 88:2812–2826, 1993.
267. Gillinov AM, DeValeria PA, Winkelstein JA, et al: Complement inhibition with soluble complement receptor type 1 in cardiopulmonary bypass. *Ann Thorac Surg* 55:619– 624, 1993.
268. Hill J, Lindsay TF, Ortiz F, Yeh CG, Hechtman HB, Moore FD Jr: Soluble complement receptor type 1 ameliorates the local and remote organ injury after intestinal ischemia-reperfusion in the rat. *J Immunol* 149:1723–1728, 1992.
269. Lindsay TF, Hill J, Ortiz F, et al: Blockade of complement activation prevents local and pulmonary albumin leak after lower torso ischemia-reperfusion. *Ann Surg* 216:677–683, 1992.
270. Weiler JM, Edens RE, Linhardt RJ, Kapelanski DP: Heparin and modified heparin inhibit complement activation in vivo. *J Immunol* 148:3210–3215, 1992.
271. Lefer AM: Induction of tissue injury and altered cardiovascular performance by platelet-activating factor: relevance to multiple systems organ failure. *Crit Care Clin* 5:331–352, 1989.
272. Gasic AC, McGuire G, Krater S, et al: Hydrogen peroxide pretreatment of perfused canine vessels induces ICAM-1 and CD18-dependent neutrophil adherence. *Circulation* 84:2154–2166, 1991.
273. Zhou W, McCollum MO, Levine BA, Olson MS: Inflammation and platelet-activating factor production during hepatic ischemia/reperfusion. *Hepatology* 16:1236–1240, 1992.
274. Vernon LP, Bell JD: Membrane structure, toxins and phospholipase A2 activity. *Pharmacol Ther* 54:269–295, 1992.
275. Darius H, Lefer DJ, Smith JB, Lefer AM: Role of platelet-activating factor-acether in mediating guinea pig anaphylaxis. *Science* 232:58–60, 1986.
276. Darius H, Smith JB, Lefer AM: Inhibtion of the platelet activating factor mediated component of guinea pig anaphylaxis by receptor antagonists. *Int Arch Allergy Appl Immunol* 80:369–375, 1986.
277. Lepran I, Lefer AM: Ischemia aggravating effeds of platelet-activating factor in acute myocardial ischemia. *Basic Res Cardiol* 80:135–141, 1985.
278. Stahl GL, Lefer AM: Mechanisms of platelet-activating factor-induced cardiac depression in the isolated perfused rat heart. *Circ Shock* 23:165–177, 1987.
279. Stahl GL, Lefer DJ, Lefer AM: PAF-acether induced cardiac dysfunction in the isolated perfused guinea pig heart. *Naunyn Schmiedebergs Arch Pharmacol* 336:459–463, 1987.
280. Terashita Z, Stahl GL, Lefer AM: Protective action of prostaglandin E1 (PGE1) against constrictor mediators in isolated rat heart and lung. *Biochem Pharmacol* 37:2659, 1988.
281. Stahl GL, Terashita Z, Lefer AM: Role of platelet activating factor in propagation of cardiac damage during myocardial ischemia. *J Pharmacol Exp Ther* 244:898–904, 1988.
282. Buerke M, Weyrich AS, Lefer AM: Isolated cardiac myocytes are sensitized by hypoxia-reoxygenation to neutrophil-released mediators. *Am J Physiol* 266:128–136, 1994.
283. Darius H, Smith JB, Lefer AM: Beneficial effects of a new potent and specific thromboxane receptor antagonist (SQ-29,548) in vitro and in vivo. *J Pharmacol Exp Ther* 235:274–281, 1985.
284. Ko W, Hawes AS, Lazenby WD, et al: Myocardial reperfusion injury: Platelet-activating factor stimulates polymorphonuclear leukocyte hydrogen peroxide production during myocardial reperfusion. *J Thorac Cardiovasc Surg* 102:297–308, 1991.
285. Elstad MR, La Pine TR, Cowley FS, et al: P-selectin regulates platelet-activating factor synthesis and phagocytosis by monocytes. *J Immunol* 155:2109–2122, 1995.
286. Ma XL, Weyrich AS, Krantz S, Lefer AM: Mechanisms of the cardioprotective actions of WEB-2170, bepafant, a platelet activating factor antagonist, in myocardial ischemia and reperfusion. *J Pharmacol Exp Ther* 260:1229–1236, 1992.
287. Montrucchio G, Alloatti G, Mariano F, et al: Role of platelet-activating factor in polymorphonuclear neutrophil recruitment in reperfused ischemic rabbit heart. *Am J Pathol* 142:471–480, 1993.

288. Ko W, Lang D, Hawes AS, Zelano JA, Isom OW, Krieger KH: Platelet-activating factor antagonism attenuates platelet and neutrophil activation and reduces myocardial injury during coronary reperfusion. *J Surg Res* 5:504–515, 1993.

289. Senoh M, Aosaki N, Ohsuzu F, et al: Early release of neutrophil chemotactic factor from isolated rat heart subjected to regional ischaemia followed by reperfusion. *Cardiovasc Res* 27:2194–2199, 1993.

290. Kawata H, Sawatari K, Mayer JE Jr: Evidence for the role of neutrophils in reperfusion injury after cold cardioplegic ischemia in neonatal lambs. *J Thorac Cardiovasc Surg* 103:908–917, 1992.

291. Conte JV Jr, Katz NM, Wallace RB, Foegh ML: Long-term lung preservation with the PAF antagonist BN 52021. *Transplantation* 51:1152–1156, 1991.

292. Qayumi AK, Jamieson WR, Poostizadeh A: Effects of platelet-activating factor antagonist CV-3988 in preservation of heart and lung for transplantation. *Ann Thorac Surg* 52:1026–1032, 1991.

293. Corcoran PC, Wang Y, Katz NM, et al: Platelet activating factor antagonist enhances lung preservation. *J Surg Res* 52:615–620, 1992.

294. Corcoran PC, Wang Y, Katz NM, et al: Platelet activating factor antagonist enhances lung preservation in a canine model of single lung allotransplantation. *J Thorac Cardiovasc Surg* 104:66–72, 1992.

295. Furchgott RF, Zawadzki JV: The obligatory role of endothelial cells in the relaxation of arterial smooth muscle by acetylcholine. *Nature* 288:373–376, 1980.

296. Moncada S, Palmer RM, Higgs EA: Nitric oxide: physiology, pathophysiology, and pharmacology. *Pharmacol Rev* 43:109–142, 1991.

297. Gross SS, Stuehr DJ, Aisaka K, Jaffe EA, Levi R, Griffith OW: Macrophage and endothelial cell nitric oxide synthesis: cell-type selective inhibition by NG-aminoarginine, NG-nitroarginine and NG-methylarginine. *Biochem Biophys Res Commun* 170:96–103, 1990.

298. Reid JL, Dawson D, Macrae IM: Endothelin, cerebral ischaemia and infarction. *Clin Exp Hypertens* 17:399–407, 1995.

299. Brunner F: Tissue endothelin-1 levels in perfused rat heart following stimulation with agonists and in ischaemia and reperfusion. *J Mol Cell Cardiol* 27:1953–1963, 1995.

300. Thompson M, Westwick J, Woodward B: Responses to endothelins-1, -2, and -3 and sarafotoxin 6c after ischemia/reperfusion in isolated perfused rat heart: role of vasodilator loss. *J Cardiovasc Pharmacol* 25:156–162, 1995.

301. Nayler WG, Liu JJ, Panagiotopoulos S: Nifedipine and experimental cardioprotection. *Cardiovasc Drugs Ther* 45:879–885, 1990.

302. Goligorsky MS, Tsukahara H, Magazine H, Andersen TT, Malik AB, Bahou WF: Termination of endothelin signaling: role of nitric oxide. *J Cell Physiol* 158:485–494, 1994.

303. Viehman GE, Ma XL, Lefer DJ, Lefer AM: Time course of endothelial dysfunction and myocardial injury during coronary arterial occlusion. *Am J Physiol* 261:874–881, 1991.

304. Ma XL, Weyrich AS, Lefer DJ, Lefer AM: Diminished basal nitric oxide release after myocardial ischemia and reperfusion promotes neutrophil adherence to coronary endothelium. *Circ Res* 72:403–412, 1993.

305. Lefer AM, Lefer DJ: Endothelial dysfunction in myocardial ischemia and reperfusion: role of oxygen-derived free radicals. *Basic Res Cardiol* 862:109–116, 1991.

306. Kim YD, Fomsgaard J5, Heim KF, et al: Brief ischemia-reperfusion induces stunning of endothelium in canine coronary artery. *Circulation* 85:1473–1482, 1992.

307. Wennmalm A, Lanne B, Petersson AS: Detection of endothelial-derived relaxing factor in human plasma in the basal state and following ischemia using electron paramagnetic resonance spectrometry. *Anal Biochem* 187:359–363, 1990.

308. Lefer AM, Aoki N: Leukocyte-dependent and leukocyte-indepenent mechanisms of impairment of endothelium-mediated vasodilation. *Blood Vessels* 27:162–168, 1990.

309. Pinsky DJ, Oz MC, Koga S, et al: Cardiac preservation is enhanced in a heterotopic rat transplant model by supplementing the nitric oxide pathway. *J Clin Invest* 93:2291–2297, 1994.

310. Fullerton DA, Mitchell MB, McIntyre RC Jr, et al: Cold ischemia and reperfusion each produce pulmonary vasomotor dysfunction in the transplanted lung. *J Thorac Cardiovasc Surg* 106:1213–1217, 1993.

311. Evora PR, Pearson PJ, Schaff HV: Impaired endothelium-dependent relaxation after coronary reperfusion injury: evidence for G-protein dysfunction. *Ann Thorac Surg* 57:1550–1556, 1994.
312. Ma XL, Tsao PS, Lefer AM: Antibody to CD-18 exerts endothelial and cardiac protective effects in myocardial ischemia and reperfusion. *J Clin Invest* 88:1237–1243, 1991.
313. Sheridan FM, Dauber IM, McMurtry IF, Lesnefsky EJ, Horwitz LD: Role of leukocytes in coronary vascular endothelial injury due to ischemia and reperfusion. *Circ Res* 69:1566–1574, 1991.
314. Fullerton DA, McIntyre RC Jr, Mitchell MB, Campbell DN, Grover FL: Lung transplantation with cardiopulmonary bypass exaggerates pulmonary vasomotor dysfunction in the transplanted lung. *J Thorac Cardiovasc Surg* 109:212–216, 1995.
315. Johnson G 3d, Tsao PS, Lefer AM: Cardioprotective effects of authentic nitric oxide in myocardial ischemia with reperfusion. *Crit Care Med* 19:244–252, 1991.
316. Siegfried MR, Erhardt J, Rider T, Ma XL, Lefer AM: Cardioprotection and attenuation of endothelial dysfunction by organic nitric oxide donors in myocardial ischemia-reperfusion. *J Pharmacol Exp Ther* 260:668–675, 1992.
317. Nambi P, Pullen M, Egan JW, Smith EF 3d: Identification of cardiac endothelin binding sites in rats: downregulation of left atrial endothelin binding sites in response to myocardial infarction. *Pharmacology* 43:84–89, 1991.
318. Maulik N, Liu X, Subramanian R, Das DK: Release of endothelin during reperfusion of ischemic myocardium. ET-1 release from reperfused heart. *Am J Cardiovasc Pathol* 4:133–144, 1992.
319. Brunner F, du Toit EF, Opie LH: Endothelin release during ischaemia and reperfusion of isolated perfused rat hearts. *J Mol Cell Cardiol* 24:1291–1305, 1992.
320. Goto M, Takei Y, Kawano S, et al: Endothelin-1 is involved in the pathogenesis of ischemia/reperfusion liver injury by hepatic microcirculatory disturbances. *Hepatology* 19:675–681, 1994.
321. Aktan AO, Buyukgebiz O, Yegen C, et al: Does PGE2 act as a mediator for endothelin release? *Prostaglandins Leukot Essent Fatty Acids* 50:37–41, 1994.
322. Kawamura E, Yamanaka N, Okamoto E, Tomoda F, Furukawa K: Response of plasma and tissue endothelin-1 to liver ischemia and its implication in ischemia-reperfusion injury. *Hepatology* 21:1138–1143, 1995.
323. Krause SM, Lynch JJ Jr, Stabilito II, Woltmann RF: Intravenous administration of the endothelin-1 antagonist BQ-123 does not ameliorate myocardial ischaemic injury following acute coronary artery occlusion in the dog. *Cardiovasc Res* 28:1672–1678, 1994.
324. Wang QD, Hemsen A, Li XS, Lundberg JM, Uriuda Y, Pernow J: Local overflow and enhanced tissue content of endothelin following myocardial ischaemia and reperfusion in the pig: modulation by L-arginine. *Cardiovasc Res* 29:44–49, 1995.
325. Tonnessen T, Giaid A, Saleh D, Naess PA, Yanagisawa M, Christensen G: Increased in vivo expression and production of endothelin-1 by porcine cardiomyocytes subjected to ischemia. *Circ Res* 76:767–772, 1995.
326. Velasco CE, Jackson EK, Morrow JA, Vitola JV, Inagami T, Forman MB: Intravenous adenosine suppresses cardiac release of endothelin after myocardial ischaemia and reperfusion. *Cardiovasc Res* 27:121–128, 1993
327. Yegen C, Aktan AO, Buyukgebiz O, et al: Effect of verapamil and iloprost (ZK 36374) on endothelin release after mesenteric ischemia-reperfusion injury. *Eur Surg Res* 26:69–75, 1994.
328. Neubauer S, Zimmermann S, Hirsch A, et al: Effects of endothelin-1 in the isolated heart in ischemia/reperfusion and hypoxia/reoxygenation injury. *J Mol Cell Cardiol* 23:1397–1409, 1991.
329. Saito T, Fushimi E, Abe T, et al: Augmented contractile response to endothelin and blunted endothelium-dependent relaxation in post-ischemic reperfused coronary arteries. *Jpn Circ J* 56:657–670, 1992.
330. Nayler WG, Ou RC, Gu XH, Casley DJ: Effect of amlodipine pretreatment on ischaemia-reperfusion-induced increase in cardiac endothelin-1 binding site density. *J Cardiovasc Pharmacol* 20:416–420, 1992.

331. Shaul PW, Wells LB: Oxygen modulates nitric oxide production selectively in fetal pulmonary endothelial cells. *Am J Respir Cell Mol Biol* 11:432–438, 1994.

332. Evans TW, Griffiths MJ, Messent M: Pulmonary vascular reactivity and ischaemia-reperfusion injury in the rat. *Clin Sci* 85:71–75, 1993

333. Okada M, Yamashita C, Okada M, Okada K: Contribution of endothelin-1 to warm ischemia/reperfusion injury of the rat lung. *Am J Respir Crit Care Med* 152:2105–2110, 1995.

334. Thomae KR, Geller DA, Billiar TR, et al: Antisense oligodeoxynucleotide to inducible nitric oxide synthase inhibits nitric oxide synthesis in rat pulmonary artery smooth muscle cells in culture. *Surgery* 114:272, 1993.

335. Nakayama DK, Geller DA, Di Silvio M, et al: Tetrahydrobiopterin synthesis and inducible nitric oxide production in pulmonary artery smooth muscle. *Am J Physiol* 266:455–460, 1994.

336. Johnson BA, Lowenstein CJ, Schwarz MA, Nakayama DK, Pitt BR, Davies P: Culture of pulmonary microvascular smooth muscle cells from intraacinar arteries of the rat: characterization and inducible production of nitric oxide. *Am J Respir Cell Mol Biol* 10:604–612, 1994.

337. Werner-Felmayer G, Werner ER, Fuchs D, et al: Pteridine biosynthesis in human endothelial cells: impact on nitric oxide-mediated formation of cyclic GMP. *J Biol Chem* 268:1842–1846, 1993.

338. Pinsky D, Oz M, Liao H, et al: Restoration of the cAMP second messenger pathway enhances cardiac preservation for transplantation in a heterotopic rat model. *J Clin Invest* 92:2994–3002, 1993.

339. Oz MC, Pinsky DJ, Koga S, et al: Novel preservation solution permits 24-hour preservation in rat and baboon cardiac transplant models. *Circulation* 88:291–297, 1993.

340. Pinsky DJ, Naka Y, Chowdhury NC, et al: The nitric oxide/cyclic GMP pathway in organ transplanation: critical role in successful lung preservation. *Proc Natl Acad Sci USA* 91:12086–12090, 1994.

341. Naka Y, Chowdhury NC, Oz MC, et al: Nitroglycerin maintains graft vascular homeostasis and enhances preservation in an orthotopic rat lung transplant model. *J Thorac Cardiovasc Surg* 109:206–210, 1995.

342. Wichert P von, Bieling C, Busch EW: The catabolism of purin nucleotides in lung tissue ischemia. *Klin Wochenschr* 50:885–887, 1972.

343. Weber KC, Visscher MB: Metabolism of the isolated canine lung. *Am J Physiol* 217:1044–1052, 1969.

344. Date H, Lima O, Matsumura A, Tsuji H, d'Avignon DA, Cooper JD: In a canine model, lung preservation at 10°C is superior to that at 4°C: a comparison of two preservation temperatures on lung function and on adenosine triphosphate level measured by phosphorus 31-nuclear magnetic resonance. *J Thorac Cardiovasc Surg* 103:773–780, 1992.

345. Date H, Matsumura A, Manchester JK, Cooper JM, Lowry OH, Cooper JD: Changes in alveolar oxygen and carbon dioxide concentration and oxygen consumption during lung preservation: the maintenance of aerobic metabolism during lung preservation. *J Thorac Cardiovasc Surg* 105:492–501, 1993.

346. Zimmerman BJ, Grisham MB, Granger DN: Mechanisms of oxidant-mediated microvascular injury following reperfusion of the ischemic intestine. *Basic Life Sci* 49:881–886, 1988.

347. Friedl HP, Till GO, Ryan US, Ward PA: Mediator-induced activation of xanthine oxidase in endothelial cells. *FASEB J* 3:2512–2518, 1989.

348. Thompson-Gorman SL, Zweier JL: Evaluation of the role of xanthine oxidase in myocardial reperfusion injury. *J Biol Chem* 265:6656–63, 1990.

349. Baker RR, Panus PC, Holm BA, Engstrom PC, Freeman BA, Matalon S: Endogenous xanthine oxidase-derived O_2 metabolites inhibit surfactant metabolism. *Am J Physiol* 259:328–334, 1990.

350. Terada LS, Rubinstein JD, Lesnefsky EJ, Horwitz LD, Leff JA, Repine JE: Existence and participation of xanthine oxidase in reperfusion injury of ischemic rabbit myocardium. *Am J Physiol* 260:805–810, 1991.

351. Phan SH, Gannon DE, Ward PA, Karmiol S: Mechanism of neutrophil-induced xanthine dehydrogenase to xanthine oxidase conversion in endothelial cells: evidence of a role for elastase. *Am J Respir Cell Mol Biol* 6:270–278, 1992.

252. Hassoun PM, Yu FS, Zulueta JJ, White AC, Lanzillo JJ: Effect of nitric oxide and cell redox status on the regulation of endothelial cell xanthine dehydrogenase. *Am J Physiol* 268:809–817, 1995.

353. Freeman BA, Crapo JD: Biology of disease: free radicals and tissue injury. *Lab Invest* 47:412–426, 1982.

354. Ratych RE, Chuknyiska RS, Bulkley GB: The primary localization of free radical generation after anoxia/reoxygenation in isolated endothelial cells. *Surgery* 102:122–131, 1987.

355. Hamvas A, Palazzo R, Kaiser L, et al: Inflammation and oxygen free radical formation during pulmonary ischemia-reperfusion injury. *J Appl Physiol* 72:621–628, 1992.

356. Korthuis RJ, Granger DN: Reactive oxygen metabolites, neutrophils, and the pathogenesis of ischemic-tissue/reperfusion. *Clin Cardiol* 16:19–26, 1993.

357. Ashraf M, Samra ZQ: Subcellular distribution of xanthine oxidase during cardiac ischemia and reperfusion: an immunocytochemical study. *J Submicrosc Cytol Pathol* 25:193–201, 1993.

358. Kukreja RC, Kontos HA, Hess ML, Ellis EF: PGH synthase and lipoxygenase generate superoxide in the presence of NADH or NADPH. *Circ Res* 59:612–619, 1986.

359. Babior BM: Oxygen-dependent microbial killing by phagocytes (first of two parts). *N Engl J Med* 298:659–668, 1978.

360. Babior BM: Oxygen-dependent microbial killing by phagocytes (second of two parts). *N Engl J Med* 298:721–725, 1978.

361. Grisham MB, Jefferson MM, Thomas EL: Role of monochloramine in the oxidation of erythrocyte hemoglobin by stimulated neutrophils. *J Biol Chem* 259:6757–6765, 1984.

362. Shappell SB, Toman C, Anderson DC, Taybr AA, Entman ML, Smith CW: Mac-1 (CD11b/CD18) mediates adherence-dependent hydrogen peroxide production by human and canine neutrophils. *J Immunol* 144:2702–2711, 1990.

363. Koppenol WH. The reaction of ferrous EDTA with hydrogen peroxide: evidence against hydroxyl radical formation. *J Free Radic Biol Med* 1:281–285, 1985.

364. Minotti G, Aust SD: The role of iron in the initiation of lipid peroxidation. *Chem Phys Lipids* 44:191–208, 1987.

365. Rush JD, Koppenol WH: The reaction between ferrous polyaminocarboxylate complexes and hydrogen peroxide: an investigation of the reaction intermediates by stopped flow spectrophotometry. *J Inorg Biochem* 29:199–215, 1987.

366. Spragg RG: DNA strand break formation following exposure of bovine pulmonary artery and aortic endothelial cells to reactive oxygen products. *Am J Respir Cell Mol Biol* 4:4–10, 1991.

367. Parks DA, Granger DN: Ischemia-induced vascular changes: role of xanthine oxidase and hydroxyl radicals. *Am J Physiol* 245:285–289, 1983.

368. Lesnefsky EJ, Allen KG, Carrea FP, Horwitz LD. Iron-catalyzed reactions cause lipid peroxidation in the intact heart. *J Mol Cell Cardiol* 24:1031–1038, 1992.

369. Rush JD, Koppenol WH: Oxidizing intermediates in the reaction of ferrous EDTA with hydrogen peroxide: reactions with organic molecules and ferrocytochrome c. *J Biol Chem* 261:6730–6733, 1986.

370. Bysani GK, Kennedy TP, Ky N, Rao NV, Blaze CA, Hoidal JR: Role of cytochrome P-450 in reperfusion injury of the rabbit lung. *J Clin Invest* 86:1434–41, 1990.

371. Bolli R, Patel BA, Jeroudi MO, et al: Iron-mediated radical reactions upon reperfusion contribute to myocardial stunning. *Am J Physiol* 259:1901–1911, 1990.

372. Williams RE, Zweier JL, Flaherty JT: Treatment with deferoxamine during ischemia improves functional and metabolic recovery and reduces reperfusion-induced oxygen radical generation in rabbit hearts. *Circulation* 83:1006–1014, 1991.

373. Lambert CJ Jr, Egan TM: Optimal timing of administration of a free radical scavenger in lung preservation. *Transplantation* 54:205–209, 1992.

374. Karwatowska-Prokopczuk E, Czarnowska E, Beresewicz A: Iron availability and free radical induced injury in the isolated ischaemic/reperfused rat heart. *Cardiovasc Res* 26:58–66, 1992.

375. Flaherty JT, Zweier JL: Role of oxygen radicals in myocardial reperfusion injury: experimental and clinical evidence. *Klin Wochenschr* 69:1061–1065, 1991.

376. Takemura G, Onodera T, Ashraf M: Quantification of hydroxyl radical and its lack of relevance to myocardial injury during early reperfusion after graded ischemia in rat hearts. *Circ Res* 71:96–105, 1992.

377. Nakamura H, del Nido PJ, Jimenez E, Sarin M, Feinberg H, Levitsky S: Age-related differences in cardiac susceptibility to ischemia/reperfusion injury: response to deferoxamine. *J Thorac Cardiovasc Surg* 104:165–172, 1992.

378. Katoh S, Toyama J, Kodama I, Akita T, Abe T: Deferoxamine, an iron chelator, reduces myocardial injury and free radical generation in isolated neonatal rabbit hearts subjected to global ischaemia-reperfusion. *J Mol Cell Cardiol* 24:1267–1275, 1992.

379. Katoh S, Toyama J, Kodama I, Kamiya K, Akita T, Abe T: Protective action of iron-chelating agents (catechol, mimosine, deferoxamine, and kojic acid) against ischemia-reperfusion injury of isolated neonatal rabbit hearts. *Eur Surg Res* 24:349–355, 1992.

380. Prevost MC, Berthoumieux F, Douste-Blazy L, Eschapasse H: Pulmonary surfactant and dog lung transplant. *Biomedicine* 27:78–81, 1977.

381. Erasmus ME, Petersen AH, Oetomo SB, Prop J: The function of surfactant is impaired during the reimplantation response in rat lung transplants. *J Heart Lung Transplant* 13:791–802, 1994.

382. Klepetko W, Lohninger A, Wisser W, et al: Pulmonary surfactant in bronchoalveolar lavage after canine lung transplantation: effect of L-carnitine application. *J Thorac Cardiovasc Surg* 99:1048–1058, 1990.

383. Veldhuizen RA, Lee J, Sandler D, et al: Alterations in pulmonary surfactant composition and activity after experimental lung transplantation. *Am Rev Respir Dis* 148:208–215, 1993.

384. Novick RJ, Veldhuizen RA, Possmayer F, Lee J, Sandler D, Lewis JF: Exogenous surfactant therapy in thirty-eight hour lung graft preservation for transplantation. *J Thorac Cardiovasc Surg* 108:259–268, 1994.

385. Rodriguez-Roisin R, Wagner PD: Clinical relevance of ventilation-perfusion inequality determined by inert gas elimination. *Eur Respir J* 3:469–482, 1990.

386. Dantzker DR, Wagner PD, West JB: Instability of lung units with low Va / Q ratios during O2 breathing. *J Appl Physiol* 38:886–895, 1975.

387. Palecek F: Control of breathing in diseases of the respiratory system. *Int Rev Physiol* 14:255–290, 1977.

388. Irsigler GB, Severinghaus JW: Clinical problems of ventilatory control. *Annu Rev Med* 31:109–126, 1980.

389. Roussos C, Macklem PT: The respiratory muscles. *N Engl J Med* 307:786–797, 1982.

390. Downs JB, Mitchell LA: Pulmonary effects of ventilatory pattern following cardiopulmonary bypass. *Crit Care Med* 4:295–300, 1976.

391. Egan TM, Westerman JH, Lambert CJ Jr, et al: Isolated lung transplantation for end-stage lung disease: a viable therapy. *Ann Thorac Surg* 53:590–595, 1992.

392. Bunn HF, May MH, Kocholaty WF, Shields CE: Hemoglobin function in stored blood. *J Clin Invest* 48:311–321, 1969.

393. Collins JA: Problems associated with the massive transfusion of stored blood. *Surgery* 75:274–295, 1974.

394. Adamson JW, Finch CA: Hemoglobin function, oxygen affinity, and erythropoietin. *Annu Rev Physiol* 37:351–369, 1975.

395. Bonser RS, Fragomeni LS, Harris K, et al: Acute physiologic changes after extended pulmonary preservation. *J Heart Transplant* 9:220–229, 1990.

396. Waxman K, Lazrove S, Shoemaker WC: Physiologic responses to operation in high-risk surgical patients. *Surg Gynecol Obstet* 152:633–638, 1981.

397. Rodriguez JL, Weissman C, Damask MC, Askanazi J, Hyman AI, Kinney JM: Physiologic requirements during rewarming: suppression of the shivering response. *Crit Care Med* 11:490–497, 1983.

398. Manthous CA, Hall JB, Kushner R, Schmidt GA, Russo G, Wood LD: The effect of mechanical ventilation on oxygen consumption in critically ill patients. *Am J Respir Crit Care Med* 151:210–214, 1995.

399. Dinarello CA, Bernheim HA, Duff GW, et al: Mechanisms of fever induced by recombinant human interferon. *J Clin Invest* 74:906–913, 1984.

400. Bishop MJ, Chi EY, Cheney FW Jr: Lung reperfusion in dogs causes bilateral lung injury. _J Appl Physiol_ 63:942–950, 1987.
401. Wagner PD, Dantzker DR, Dueck R, Clausen JL, West JB: Ventilation-perfusion inequality in chronic obstructive pulmonary disease. _J Clin Invest_ 59:203–216, 1977.
402. Dantzker DR, Bower JS: Pulmonary vascular tone improves VA/Q matching in obliterative pulmonary hypertension. _J Appl Physiol_ 51:607–613, 1981.
403. D'Alonzo GE, Bower JS, DeHart P, Dantzker DR: The mechanisms of abnormal gas exchange in acute massive pulmonary embolism. _Am Rev Respir Dis_ 128:170–172, 1983.
404. Wagner PD, Saltzman HA, West JB. Measurement of continuous distributions of ventilation-perfusian ratios: theory. _J Appl Physiol_ 36:588–599, 1974.
405. Wagner PD, West JB. Effects of diffusion impairment on O_2 and CO_2 time courses in pulmonary capillaries. _J Appl Physiol_ 33:62–71, 1972.
406. Wagner PD: Diffusion and chemical reaction in pulmonary gas exchange. _Physiol Rev_ 57:257–312, 1977.
407. Paull DE, Keagy BA, Kron EJ, Wilcox BR: Improved lung preservation using a dimethylthiourea flush. _J Surg Res_ 46:333–338, 1989.
408. Horgan MJ, Lum H, Malik AB: Pulmonary edema after pulmonary artery occlusion and reperfusion. _Am Rev Respir Dis_ 140:1421–1428, 1989.
409. Haynes J Jr, Seibert A, Bass JB, Taylor AE: U74500A inhibition of oxidant-mediated lung injury. _Am J Physiol_ 259:144–148, 1990.
410. Allison RC, Kyle J, Adkins WK, Prasad VR, McCord JM, Taylor AE: Effect of ischemia reperfusion or hypoxia reoxygenation on lung vascular permeability and resistance. _J Appl Physiol_ 69:597–603, 1990.
411. Seibert AF, Thompson WJ, Taylor A, Wilborn WH, Barnard J, Haynes J: Reversal of increased microvascular permeability associated with ischemia-reperfusion: role of cAMP. _J Appl Physiol_ 72:389–395, 1992.
412. Adkins WK, Barnard JW, May S, Seibert AF, Haynes J, Taylor AE: Compounds that increase cAMP prevent ischemia-reperfusion pulmonary capillary injury. _J Appl Physiol_ 72:492–497, 1992.
413. Xiong L, Mazmanian M, Chapelier AR, et al: Lung preservation with Euro-Collins, University of Wisconsin, Wallwork, and low-potassium-dextran soiution. Universite++ Paris-Sud Lung Transplant Group. _Ann Thorac Surg_ 58:845–850, 1994.
414. Barnard JW, Seibert AF, Prasad VR, et al: Reversal of pulmonary capillary ischemia-reperfusion injury by rolipram, a cAMP phosphodiesterase inhibitor. _J Appl Physiol_ 77:774–781, 1994.
415. Khimenko PL, Barnard JW, Moore TM, Wilson PS, Baliard ST, Taylor AE: Vascular permeability and epithelial transport effects on lung edema formation in ischemia and reperfusion. _J Appl Physiol_ 77:1116–1121, 1994.
416. Khimenko PL, Moore TM, Hill LW, et al: Adenosine A_2 receptors reverse ischemia-reperfusion lung injury independent of beta-receptors. _J Appl Physiol_ 78:990–996, 1995.
417. Khimenko PL, Moore TM, Taylor AE. ATP-sensitive K+ channels are not involved in ischemia-reperfusion lung endothelial injury. _J Appl Physiol_ 79:554–559, 1995.
418. Moore TM, Khimenko PL, Taylor AE: Restoration of normal pH triggers ischemia-reperfusion injury in lung by Na+/H+ exchange activation. _Am J Physiol_ 269:1501–1505, 1995.
419. Johnson A, Phillips P, Hocking D, Tsan MF, Ferro T: Protein kinase inhibitor prevents pulmonary edema in response to H_2O_2. _Am J Physiol_ 256:1012–1022, 1989.
420. Shasby DM, Hampson F: Effects of chlorinated amines on endothelial and epithelial barriers in vitro and ex vivo. _Exp Lung Res_ 15:345–357, 1989.
421. Habib MP, Clements NC: Effects of low-dose hydrogen peroxide in the isolated perfused rat lung. _Exp Lung Res_ 21:95–112, 1995.
422. Seeger W, Hansen T, Rossig R, et al: Hydrogen peroxide-induced increase in lung endothelial and epithelial permeability: effect of adenylate cyclase stimulation and phosphodiesterase inhibition. _Microvasc Res_ 50:1–17, 1995.
423. Shasby DM, Lind SE, Shasby SS, Goldsmith JC, Hunninghake GW: Reversible oxidant-induced increases in albumin transfer across cultured endothelium: alterations in cell shape and calcium homeostasis. _Blood_ 65:605–614, 1985.

424. Lum H, Barr DA, Shaffer JR, Gordon RJ, Ezrin AM, Malik AB: Reoxygenation of endothelial cells increases permeability by oxidant-dependent mechanisms. *Circ Res* 70:991–998, 1992.

425. Siflinger-Birnboim A, Goligorsky MS, Del Vecchio PJ, Malik AB: Activation of protein kinase C pathway contributes to hydrogen peroxide-induced increase in endothelial permeability. *Lab Invest* 67:24–30, 1992.

426. Berman RS, Martin W: Arterial endothelial barrier dysfunction: actions of homocysteine and the hypoxanthine-xanthine oxidase free radical generating system. *Br J Pharmacol* 108:920–926, 1993.

427. Liu SM, Sundqvist T: Effects of hydrogen peroxide and phorbol myristate acetate on endothelial transport and F-actin distribution. *Exp Cell Res* 217:1–7, 1995.

428. Bolin R, Guest RJ, Albert RK: Glycolysis is not required for fluid homeostasis in isolated rabbit lungs. *J Appl Physiol* 64:2517–2521, 1988.

429. Wilson J, Winter M, Shasby DM: Oxidants, ATP depletion, and endothelial permeability to macromolecules. *Blood* 76:2578–2582, 1990.

430. Corretti MC, Koretsune Y, Kusuoka H, Chacko VP, Zweier JL, Marban E: Glycolytic inhibition and calcium overload as consequences of exogenously generated free radicals in rabbit hearts. *J Clin Invest* 88:1014–1025, 1991.

431. Britigan BE, Roeder TL, Shasby DM: Insight into the nature and site of oxygen-centered free radical generation by endothelial cell monolayers using a novel spin trapping technique. *Blood* 79:699–707, 1992.

432. Siflinger-Birnboim A, Malik AB: Neutrophil adhesion to endothelial cells impairs the effects of catalase and glutathione in preventing endothelial injury. *J Cell Physiol* 155:234–239, 1993.

433. Dreher D, Junod AF: Differential effects of superoxide, hydrogen peroxide, and hydroxyl radical on intracellular calcium in human endothelial cells. *J Cell Physiol* 162:147–153, 1995.

434. Killackey JJ, Johnston MG, Movat HZ: Increased permeability of microcarrier-cultured endothelial monolayers in response to histamine and thrombin: a model for the in vitro study of increased vasopermeability. *Am J Pathol* 122:50–61, 1986.

435. Rotrosen D, Gallin JI: Histamine type I receptor occupancy increases endothelial cytosolic calcium, reduces F-actin, and promotes albumin diffusion across cultured endothelial monolayers. *J Cell Biol* 103:2379–2387, 1986.

436. Shasby DM, Yorek M, Shasby SS: Exogenous oxidants initiate hydrolysis of endothelial cell inositol phospholipids. *Blood* 72:491, 1988.

437. Peterson MW, Gruenhaupt D, Shasby DM: Neutrophil cathepsin G increases calcium flux and inositol polyphosphate production in cultured endothelial cells. *J Immunol* 143:609–616, 1989.

438. Carson MR, Shasby SS, Shasby DM: Histamine and inositol phosphate accumulation in endothelium: cAMP and a G protein. *Am J Physiol* 257:259–264, 1989.

439. Lynch JJ, Ferro TJ, Blumenstock FA, Brockenauer AM, Malik AB: Increased endothelial albumin permeability mediated by protein kinase C activation. *J Clin Invest* 85:1991–1998, 1990.

440. Lo SK, Del Vecchio PJ, Lum H, Malik AB: Fibrin contact increases endothelial permeability to albumin. *J Cell Physiol* 151:63–70, 1992.

441. Tiruppathi C, Malik AB, Del Vecchio PJ, Keese CR, Giaever I: Electrical method for detection of endothelial cell shape change in real time: assessment of endothelial barrier function. *Proc Natl Acad Sci U S A* 89:7919–7923, 1992.

442. Jones RM, Prasad MR: Enhanced responses to endothelin during perfusion of ischemic myocardium: myocardial response to endothelin. *Am J Cardiovasc Pathol* 4:145–156, 1992.

443. Su M, Chi EY, Bishop MJ, Henderson WR Jr: Lung mast cells increase in number and degranulate during pulmonary artery occlusion/reperfusion injury in dogs. *Am Rev Respir Dis* 147:448–456, 1993.

444. Ricupero D, Taylor L, Polgar P: Interactions of bradykinin, calcium, G-protein, and protein kinase in the activation of phospholipase A_2 in bovine pulmonary artery endothelial cells. *Agents Actions* 40:110–118, 1993.

445. Noel PE, Fletcher JR, Thompson WJ: Rolipram and isoproterenol reverse platelet activating factor-induced increases in pulmonary microvascular permeability and vascular resistance. *J Surg Res* 59:159–164, 1995.

446. Boyer CS, Bannenberg GL, Neve EP, Ryrfeldt A, Moldeus P: Evidence for the activation of the signal-responsive phospholipase A$_2$ by exogenous hydrogen peroxide. *Biochem Pharmacol* 50:753–761, 1995.

447. Stasek JE Jr, Garcia JG: The role of protein kinase C in alpha-thrombin-mediated endothelial cell activation. *Semin Thromb Hemost* 18:117–125, 1992.

448. Carson MR, Shasby SS, Lind SE, Shasby DM: Histamine, actin-gelsolin binding, and polyphosphoinositides in human umbilical vein endothelial cells. *Am J Physiol* 263:664–669, 1992.

449. Lum H, Aschner JL, Phillips PG, Fletcher PW, Malik AB: Time course of thrombin-induced increase in endothelial permeability: relationship to Ca$_2$+ and inositol polyphosphates. *Am J Physiol* 263:219–225, 1992.

450. Wesson DE, Elliott SJ: Xanthine oxidase inhibits transmembrane signal transduction in vascular endothelial cells. *J Pharmacol Exp Ther* 270:1197–1207, 1994.

451. Vischer UM, Jornot L, Wollheim CB, Theler JM: Reactive oxygen intermediates induce regulated secretion of von Willebrand factor from cultured human vascular endothelial cells. *Blood* 85:3164–3172, 1995.

452. Wesson DE, Elliott SJ: The H$_2$O$_2$-generating enzyme, xanthine oxidase, decreases luminal Ca$_2$+ content of the IP3-sensitive Ca$_2$+ store in vascular endothelial cells. *Microcirculation* 2:195–203, 1995.

453. Wysolmerski RB, Lagunoff D: Involvement of myosin light-chain kinase in endothelial cell retraction. *Proc Natl Acad Sci U S A* 87:16–20, 1990.

454. Morel NM, Petruzzo PP, Hechtman HB, Shepro D: Inflammatory agonists that increase microvascular permeability in vivo stimulate cultured pulmonary microvessel endothelial cell contraction. *Inflammation* 14:571–583, 1990.

455. Wysolmerski RB, Lagunoff D: Regulation of permeabilized endothelial cell retraction by myosin phosphorylation. *Am J Physiol* 261:32–40, 1991.

456. Jacobson BC, Pober JS, Fenton JW 2d, Ewenstein BM: Thrombin and histamine rapidly stimulate the phosphorylation of the myristoylated alanine-rich C-kinase substrate in human umbilical vein endothelial cells: evidence for distinct patterns of protein kinase activation. *J Cell Physiol* 152:166–176, 1992.

457. Moy AB, Shasby SS, Scott BD, Shasby DM: The effect of histamine and cyclic adenosine monophosphate on myosin light chain phosphorylation in human umbilical vein endothelial cells. *J Clin Invest* 92:1198–1206, 1993.

458. Sheldon R, Moy A, Lindsley K, Shasby S, Shasby DM: Role of myosin light-chain phosphorylation in endothelial cell retraction. *Am J Physiol* 265:606–612, 1993.

459. Lum H, Malik AB: Regulation of vascular endothelial barrier function. *Am J Physiol* 267:223–241, 1994.

460. Patterson CE, Stasek JE, Schaphorst KL, Davis HW, Garcia JG: Mechanisms of pertussis toxin-induced barrier dysfunction in bovine pulmonary artery endothelial cell monolayers. *Am J Physiol* 268:926–934, 1995.

461. Goeckeler ZM, Wysolmerski RB. Myosin light chain kinase-regulated endothelial cell contraction: the relationship between isometric tension, actin polymerization, and myosin phosphorylation. *J Cell Biol* 130:613–627, 1995.

462. Qiao RL, Yan W, Lum H, Malik AB: Arg-Gly-Asp peptide increases endothelial hydraulic conductivity: comparison with thrombin response. *Am J Physiol* 269:110–117, 1995.

463. Rippe B, Allison RC, Parker JC, Taylor AE: Effects of histamine, serotonin, and norepinephrine on circulation of dog lungs. *J Appl Physiol* 57:223–232, 1984.

464. Lamm WJ, Luchtel D, Albert RK: Sites of leakage in three models of acute lung injury. *J Appl Physiol* 64:1079–1083, 1988.

465. Pedersen KE, Rigby PJ, Golde RG. Quantitative assessment of increased airway microvascular permeability to 125I-labelled plasma fibrinogen induced by platelet activating factor and bradykinin. *Br J Pharmacol* 104:128–132, 1991.

466. Tanabe S, Tamaki T, Wada Y: Sphingosine inhibits factor Xa-catalyzed prothrombin activation on the surface of cultured calf pulmonary artery endothelium perturbed by hydrogen peroxide. *Thromb Res* 67:115–122, 1992.

467. Arakawa H, Tokuyama K, Yokoyama T, et al: Effect of maturation on histamine-induced airflow obstruction and airway microvascular leakage in guinea pig airways. *Eur J Pharmacol* 215:51–56, 1992.
468. Sirois MG, de Lima WT, de Brum Fernandes AJ, Johnson RJ, Plante GE, Sirois P: Effect of PAF on rat lung vascular permeability: role of platelets and polymorphonuclear leucocytes. *Br J Pharmacol* 111:1111–1116, 1994
469. de Lima WT, Kwasniewski FH, Sirois P, Jancar S: Studies on the mechanism of PAF-induced vasopermeability in rat lungs. *Prostaglandins Leukot Essent Fatty Acids* 52:245–249, 1995.
470. Allison RC, Hernandez EM, Prasad VR, Grisham MB, Taylor AE: Protective effects of O_2 radical scavengers and adenosine in PMA-induced lung injury. *J Appl Physiol* 64:2175–2182, 1988.
471. Siflinger-Birnboim A, Bode DC, Malik AB: Adenosine 3',5'-cyclic monophosphate attenuates neutrophil-mediated increase in endothelial permeability. *Am J Physiol* 264:370–375, 1993.
472. Adkins WK, Barnard JW, Moore TM, Allison RC, Prasad VR, Taylor AE: Adenosine prevents PMA-induced lung injury via an A_2 receptor mechanism. *J Appl Physiol* 74:982, 1993.
473. Allen MJ, Coleman RA: Beta 2-adrenoceptors mediate a reduction in endothelial permeability in vitro. *Eur J Pharmacol* 274:7–15, 1995.
474. Lefer AM: Platelet activating factor (PAF) and its role in cardiac injury. *Prog Clin Biol Res* 301:53–60, 1989.
475. Zavoico GB, Hrbolich JK, Gimbrone MA Jr, Schafer AI: Enhancement of thrombin- and ionomycin-stimulated prostacyclin and platelet-activating factor production in cultured endothelial cells by a tumor-promoting phorbol ester. *J Cell Physiol* 143:596–605, 1990.
476. Chakraborti S, Michael JR, Sanyal T: Defining the role of protein kinase c in calcium-ionophore-(A23187)-mediated activation of phospholipase A2 in pulmonary endothelium. *Eur J Biochem* 206:965–972, 1992.
477. Exton JH: Phosphatidylcholine breakdown and signal transduction. *Biochim Biophys Acta* 1212:26–42, 1994.
478. Lum H, Andersen TT, Siflinger-Birnboim A, et al: Thrombin receptor peptide inhibits thrombin-induced increase in endothelial permeability by receptor desensitization. *J Cell Biol* 120:1491, 1993.
479. Hattori R, Hamilton KK, Fugate RD, McEver RP, Sims PJ: Stimulated secretion of endothelial von Willebrand factor is accompanied by rapid redistribution to the cell surface of the intracellular granule membrane protein GMP-140. *J Biol Chem* 264:7768–71, 1989.
480. Parhami F, Fang ZT, Fogelman AM, Andalibi A, Territo MC, Beriner JA: Minimally modified low density lipoprotein-induced inflammatory responses in endothelial cells are mediated by cyclic adenosine monophosphate. *J Clin Invest* 92:471–478, 1993.
481. Fujimoto T, McEver RP: The cytoplasmic domain of P-selectin is phosphorylated on serine and threonine residues. *Blood* 82:1758–1766, 1993.
482. Kaszubska W, van Huijsduijnen RH, Ghersa P, et al: Cyclic AMP-independent ATF family members interact with NF-kappa B and function in the activation of the E-selectin promoter in response to cytokines. *Mol Cell Biol* 13:7180–7190, 1993.
483. De Luca LG, Johnson DR, Whitley MZ, Collins T, Pober JS: cAMP and tumor necrosis factor competitively regulate transcriptional activation through and nuclear factor binding to the cAMP-responsive element/activating transcription factor element of the endothelial leukocyte adhesion molecule-1 (E-selectin) promoter. *J Biol Chem* 269:193–196, 1994.
484. Birch KA, Ewenstein BM, Golan DE, Pober JS: Prolonged peak elevations in cytoplasmic free calcium ions, derived from intracellular stores, correlate with the extent of thrombin-stimulated exocytosis in single human umbilical vein endothelial celis. *J Cell Physiol* 160:545–554, 1994.
485. Brown LA, Wood LH: Stimulation of surfactant secretion by vasopressin in primary cultures of adult rat type II pneumocytes. *Biochim Biophys Acta* 1001:76–81, 1989.
486. Chander A: Regulation of lung surfactant secretion by intracellular pH. *Am J Physiol* 257:354–360, 1989.
487. Fisher AB, Arad I, Dodia C, Chander A, Feinstein SI: cAMP increases synthesis of surfactant-associated protein A by perfused rat lung. *Am J Physiol* 260:226–233, 1991.
488. Marsen TA, Simonson MS, Dunn MJ: Thrombin-mediated ET-1 gene regulation involves CaM kinases and calcineurin in human endothelial cells. *J Cardiovasc Pharmacol* 263:1–4, 1995.

489. Lincoln TM, Cornwell TL, Taylor AE: cGMP-dependent protein kinase mediates the reduction of Ca2+ by cAMP in vascular smooth muscle cells. *Am J Physiol* 258:399–407, 1990.

490. Haynes J Jr, Kithas PA, Taybr AE, Strada SJ: Selective inhibition of cGMP-inhibitable cAMP phosphodiesterase decreases pulmonary vasoreactivity. *Am J Physiol* 261:487–492, 1991.

491. Haynes J Jr, Robinson J, Saunders L, Taylor AE, Strada SJ: Role of cAMP-dependent protein kinase in cAMP-mediated vasodilation. *Am J Physiol* 262:511–516, 1992.

492. Feeley TW, Mihm FG, Downing TP, et al: Hypothermic preservation of the heart and lungs with Collins solution: effect on cardiorespiratory function following heart-lung allotransplantation in dogs. *Ann Thorac Surg* 41:301–306, 1986.

493. Hardesty RL, Griffith BP: Autoperfusion of the heart and lungs for preservation during distant procurement. *J Thorac Cardiovasc Surg* 93:11–18, 1987.

494. Fraser CD Jr, Tamura F, Adachi H, et al: Donor core-cooling provides improved static preservation for heart-lung transplantation. *Ann Thorac Surg* 45:253–257, 1988.

495. Baretti R, Bitu-Moreno J, Beyersdorf F, Matheis G, Francischetti I, Kreitmayr B: Distribution of lung preservation solutions in parenchyma and airways: influence of atelectasis and route of delivery. *J Heart Lung Transplant* 14:80–91, 1995.

496. Sundaresan S, Trachiotis GD, Aoe M, Patterson GA, Cooper JD: Donor lung procurement: assessment and operative technique. *Ann Thorac Surg* 56:1409–1413, 1993.

497. Patterson CE, Barnard JW, Lafuze JE, Hull MT, Baldwin SJ, Rhoades RA: The role of activation of neutrophils and microvascular pressure in acute pulmonary edema. *Am Rev Respir Dis* 140:1052–1062, 1989.

498. Pennefather SH, Bullock F, Dark JH: The effect of fluid therapy on alveolar arterial oxygen gradient in brain-dead organ donors. *Transplantation* 56:1418–1422, 1993.

499. The Toronto Lung Transplant Group: Experience with single-lung transplantation for pulmonary fibrosis. *JAMA* 259:2258–2262, 1988.

500. Steen S, Sjoberg T, Ingemansson R, Lindberg L: Efficacy of topical cooling in lung preservation: is a reappraisal due? *Ann Thorac Surg* 58:1657–63, 1994.

501. Ueno T, Yokomise H, Oka T, et al: The effect of PGE$_1$ and temperature on lung function following preservation. *Transplantation* 52:626–630, 1991.

502. Mayer E, Puskas JD, Cardoso PF, Shi S, Slutsky AS, Patterson GA: Reliable eighteen-hour lung preservation at 4°C and 10°C by pulmonary artery flush after high-dose prostaglandin E$_1$ administration. *J Thorac Cardiovasc Surg* 103:1136–1142, 1992.

503. Wang LS, Nakamoto K, Hsieh CM, Miyoshi S, Cooper JD: Influence of temperature of flushing solution on lung preservation. *Ann Thorac Surg* 55:711–715, 1993.

504. Starkey TD, Sakakibara N, Hagberg RC, Tazelaar HD, Baldwin JC, Jamieson SW: Successful six-hour cardiopulmonary preservation with simple hypothermic crystalloid flush. *J Heart Transplant* 5:291–297, 1986.

505. Kriett JM, Smith CM, Hayden AM, et al: Lung transplantation without the use of antilymphocyte antibody preparations. *J Heart Lung Transplant* 12:915–922, 1993.

506. Nelson RM, Cecconi O, Roberts WG, Aruffo A, Linhardt RJ, Bevilacqua MP: Heparin oligosaccharides bind L- and P-selectin and inhibit acute inflammation. *Blood* 82:3253–8, 1993.

507. Shimada K, Davidson WD, Benfield JR: Metabolic changes in ischemic lungs for evaluation of graft viability. *J Thorac Cardiovasc Surg* 66:137–144, 1973.

508. Wagner FM, Jamieson SW, Fung J, Wolf P, Reichenspurner H, Kaye MP: A new concept for successful long-term pulmonary preservation in a dog model. *Transplantation* 59:1530–1536, 1995.

509. Haverich A, Aziz S, Scott WC, Jamieson SW, Shumway NE: Improved lung preservation using Euro-Collins solution for flush-perfusion. *Thorac Cardiovasc Surg* 34:368–376, 1986.

510. Bradley JR, Thiru S, Pober JS: Hydrogen peroxide-induced endothelial retraction is accompanied by a loss of the normai spatial organization of endothelial cell adhesion molecules. *Am J Pathol* 147:627–641, 1995.

Chapter 12

Routine Immediate Direct Bronchial Artery Revascularization for Single Lung Transplantation

Richard C. Daly, MD,
Christopher G.A. McGregor, MB, FRCS

Introduction

The techniques and indications for single lung transplantation (SLT) have evolved considerably over the last decade.[1] However, SLT remains the only solid organ transplanted without a systemic arterial blood supply. Impaired healing of the bronchial anastomosis, which is almost always due to ischemia of the donor bronchus, has been a significant source of morbidity and mortality for patients undergoing SLT. Bronchial ischemia may result in early (granulation tissue, mucosal sloughing, or bronchial dehiscence) or late (stricture) complications of airway healing.

In the initial era following the first SLT in humans by Hardy et al in 1963[2] and extending through 1978, approximately 38 SLTs were performed. Of these, 12 patients survived more than 2 weeks, and 7 of these 12 (58%) died of bronchial leak.[3] From this initial experience, it was clear that healing of the airway would be a pivotal challenge in the evolution of lung transplantation.

The Toronto Lung Transplant Group substantially improved the results of SLT after a series of laboratory studies led them to: optimize perioperative condition and nutrition; eliminate early postoperative steroids; and wrap the bronchial anastomosis with a vascularized pedicle of omentum.[1,4] These pioneering efforts resulted in lung transplantation becoming a clinical reality and an accepted form of therapy for patients with end-stage lung disease.

With current techniques, serious complications of bronchial healing occur in 5% to 14% of patients.[5-7] This is the incidence of airway dehiscence or late stricture requiring therapy. Usually, stricture can be treated endoscopically, but it often requires stent placement.[8] While frequently successful in treating strictures, stents require regular

From: Franco KL (ed). *Pediatric Cardiopulmonary Transplantation.* Armonk, NY: Futura Publishing Company, Inc.; © 1997.

bronchoscopic evaluation. Therapy for ischemia-related complications of bronchial healing can be challenging and prolonged.[7] A number of techniques have been employed as an adjunct to bronchial healing at the time of SLT.

Adjuncts to Healing

Without a systemic arterial blood supply, the donor bronchus is dependent on collateral flow from the pulmonary circulation. This collateral flow is affected by reperfusion injury, rejection, infection, and donor bronchial length. Thus, measures to maximize allograft preservation, optimize therapy and surveillance for infection and rejection, and shortening the donor bronchial stump are important. Furthermore, many centers "telescope," or intussuscept the donor and recipient bronchi. Early use of corticosteroids is controversial, but may improve donor bronchial blood flow.[9]

Most centers embarking on programs in SLT in the current era initially followed the lead of the Toronto Lung Transplant Group, and wrapped the bronchial anastomosis with omentum or other vascularized tissue. Omentopexy provides a systemic blood supply to the distal airway,[10–13] but this takes time to develop and is provided only via small collaterals. Ischemic changes in the bronchial anastomosis have been observed in as little as 4 days.[14] Many centers have stopped using omentopexy as a routine component of SLT. A prospective, randomized trial at Harefield Hospital in London found no difference in bronchial complications among 36 recipients of SLT randomized to omentopexy, internal thoracic artery (ITA) pedicle wrap, and no wrap.[15] We used omentopexy for the initial recipients of SLT at our institution; however, among a series of nine patients, two had airway complications. One developed bronchial stenosis requiring early revision of the anastomosis, but the second patient developed a late stricture requiring stent placement. It would seem that, while helpful, omentopexy does not reduce bronchial ischemia enough to eliminate early or late complications of airway healing.

Bronchial Artery Revascularization

The importance of restoring the systemic bronchial circulation for improved airway healing was recognized by Metras, who implanted the bronchial artery orifice on a button of donor aorta into the descending thoracic aorta of dogs undergoing SLT in 1950.[16,17] In 1970, after a significant number of SLTs, Mills et al predicted that division of bronchial circulation would result in bronchial anastomotic complications.[18] They also performed SLT in dogs with bronchial artery revascularization (BAR) by anastomosing a button of donor aorta containing the bronchial artery orifice to the recipient descending thoracic aorta, and showed that bronchial healing is improved with this technique. Mills et al were concerned that the anatomic variability of the bronchial arteries would limit the usefulness of direct BAR. In 1973, Haglin et al revascularized the left bronchial artery in a patient undergoing sequential bilateral SLT by implanting the donor aortic button into the recipient descending thoracic aorta; bronchial healing on the left side was normal, while the right developed necrosis.[19]

The importance of the bronchial artery circulation to airway healing is apparent when the experience of heart-lung and en-bloc double lung transplantation are examined. Tracheal healing after heart-lung transplantation was less problematic than bronchial healing in the early era of SLT, when airway healing was a major cause of mortality.[20] Collateral perfusion of the bronchial arteries from the coronary circulation in the heart-lung bloc reduced donor tracheal ischemia.[21] On the other hand, the experience with en-bloc double lung transplant was poor. En-bloc double lung transplant involves a tracheal anastomosis, but excludes the heart, and, thus, any source of systemic flow to the bronchial arteries; the procedure has been abandoned due to the development of tracheal dehiscence in half of patients, and half of these died from the complication.[22–24]

Potential Benefits

Bronchial artery revascularization would be expected to result in excellent early airway healing, and to prevent the development of late anastomotic strictures. Our and others' experiences have confirmed these expectations. In addition to affecting airway healing, prevention of bronchial ischemia may have a positive impact on early pneumonia, reperfusion injury, and late obliterative bronchiolitis (OB). Mills et al found that pneumonia developed in 50% of transplanted lungs in dogs that had bronchial mucosal ulceration, while none of those without mucosal ulceration developed pneumonia.[18] Aeba et al recently reported that interruption of the bronchial artery circulation contributes to increased severity of pneumonia in rats, with or without lung transplantation.[25] Mucociliary clearance has been shown to be compromised by interruption of the bronchial arteries and nerves,[26] which may contribute to the development of pneumonia.

There is some evidence that "reperfusion injury," or the development of pulmonary edema in the pulmonary allograft early postoperatively may be aggravated by bronchial ischemia. Experimental induction of bronchial ischemia has been shown to result in transient impairment in gas exchange[27] and pulmonary edema.[28] After transplantation, reperfusion injury will increase donor bronchial ischemia in the absence of BAR.

A final potential benefit of BAR with SLT is the possibility of favorably influencing the incidence of late OB. OB develops in 25% to 30% of patients after SLT and is the most significant long-term complication after lung transplantation.[29] The cause of OB is likely multifactorial, and may be related to rejection, infection, ischemia, preservation, and other factors. BAR may impact infection, as already noted.[18,25] The development of OB has been considered to represent chronic rejection,[30] and may be related to repeated episodes of acute rejection.[31] Reduced mucosal blood flow has been reported to occur with pulmonary rejection,[32–34] and has been postulated as a mechanism for the role of rejection in the development of late OB. It is conceivable that BAR could limit the degree of mucosal ischemia related to rejection and, thus, modify the contribution of rejection to the development of late OB. In a recent review of the experience at the University of Pittsburgh, Bando and associates found that risk factors associated with the development of OB were postoperative airway ischemia, recurrent acute rejection, and cytomegalovirus (CMV) infection.[29]

Challenges

If BAR is to be applied routinely to SLT, several challenges must be met. First, the small size and variable anatomy of the bronchial arteries requires the use of special techniques for organ procurement (without compromising procurement of other organs), and the ability to identify the bronchial artery origins on the descending thoracic aorta. Second, the ischemic time and the recipient operative time must not be unduly prolonged. Third, an optimal technique for BAR must be selected; that is, a good method that protects the small bronchial arteries and employs a proper conduit.

Bronchial Artery Anatomy

One of Mills et al's concerns in 1970 was that the anatomic variability of the bronchial artery circulation would limit the usefulness of BAR in lung transplantation.[18] Fortunately, the human bronchial circulation has proven to be predictable enough so that BAR can often be accomplished.[24,35,36] Schreinemakers and the group at Washington University in St. Louis studied the anatomic pattern of human bronchial arteries in 30 autopsy cases.[37] They found that the pattern in humans was reasonably predictable, with a consistent left bronchial artery in 93.3% and a consistent right bronchial artery in 83.3% of cases. In our experience, identification of the orifice of the bronchial arteries can be accomplished quickly in the majority of donors.

The anatomy of the bronchial arteries has been well described by other investigators,[18,37] and techniques for harvest of the double lung bloc that preserve the bronchial arteries have been previously described.[24,36–38] The bronchial arteries originate from the descending thoracic aorta (Figure 1). Usually, a right bronchial artery arises as a branch of the first or second intercostal artery. This right intercostal bronchial artery passes posterior to the esophagus (Figures 1 and 2); the right bronchial artery then passes anteriorly between the esophagus and azygos vein. The left bronchial artery, which may be multiple, arises from the descending thoracic aorta anterior to the left intercostal branches and passes directly anteriorly to the tracheobronchial tree (Figure 1). Thus, the bronchial arteries pass on either side of the esophagus (Figure 2). Occasionally, both right and left bronchial arteries arise from a common trunk on the anterior aspect of the aorta. There is always a network of collateral vessels in the mediastinal tissue around the carina which should be preserved with the lung during organ procurement. Dissection of individual bronchial arteries is not advisable in view of their small and delicate nature. Thus, protection of the mediastinal collaterals helps ensure protection of the bronchial arteries themselves, as well as numerous collateral vessels that can improve the chances of successful revascularization in the event that some vessels are injured during procurement.

Initially, we confirmed the identity of a bronchial artery orifice in the lumen of the donor descending thoracic aorta by passing a probe down the vessel. However, this risks injury to these very fragile arteries. Recently, we have relied on the presence of backbleeding from the vessel orifice on the donor thoracic aorta after reestablishing the pulmonary circulation. We have since abandoned the probe in most cases. The combination of inspection of the lumen of the donor aorta for the expected orifice, based on knowledge of the usual anatomy and back bleeding from the orifice are usually

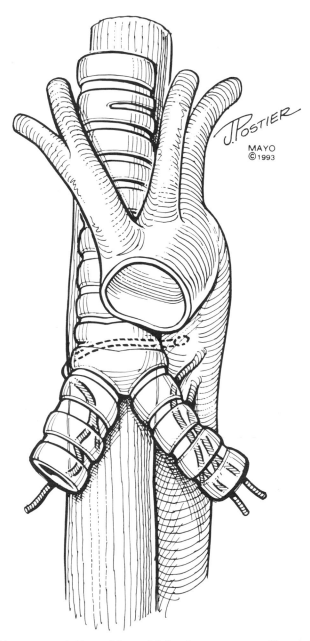

Figure 1. Schematic representation of bronchial artery anatomy. The right bronchial artery passes behind the esophagus and is a branch of the first or second right intercostal artery; the left brachial artery arises from the anterior aspect of the descending thoracic aorta. The intercostal vessels are not shown in this view. Variations occur (see text).

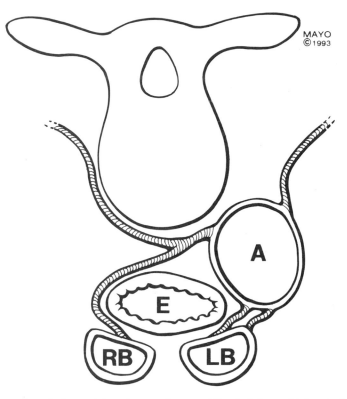

Figure 2. Cross-sectional view with spine at the **top.** The left bronchial arteries usually arise anterior to the left intercostal arteries. The right bronchial artery usually arises as a branch of the first or second right intercostal artery, passing behind the esophagus. A = aorta; E = esophagus; RB = right mainstem bronchus; LB = left mainstem bronchus.

sufficient to accomplish BAR. Nevertheless, the variability of bronchial arteries is a limiting factor in universal application of this technique.

Ischemic and Operative Time

Routine BAR for SLT depends on performing the procedure in a timely manner. The technique prolongs harvesting of the double lung bloc by about 5 minutes; basically the time needed to staple across the esophagus at its cranial and caudal ends. The heart can be harvested, while the double lung bloc is in situ or later on the back table. This technique does not interfere with the interests of the other harvesting teams at the time of multiorgan donation. The ischemic time of the lungs will be minimally prolonged by the back table dissection of the double-lung bloc. Subadventitial stripping of the esophagus, opening and trimming of the donor descending thoracic aorta, inspection of the donor aorta for the bronchial artery origins, and division of the bronchi with preservation of adjacent mediastinal tissues all must be performed. This process requires 10 to 15 minutes. Nothing additional is required until after the donor lung is implanted and the pulmonary circulation reestablished. Thus, the total ischemic time may be prolonged by about 15 to 20 minutes to accomplish BAR.[36]

The recipient operation is prolonged in order to allow BAR. The recipient ITA is mobilized from its bed prior to the anticipated arrival of the donor lung. Preparation of the ITA, performing the ITA to bronchial artery anastomosis, and achieving hemostasis in the revascularized donor mediastinal tissue adds 30 to 45 minutes to the recipient operation. This, of course, is not additional ischemic time. Further, these estimates of prolonged ischemic and recipient operative time are generous, and the time is reduced with experience.

Organ Procurement and Preservation of the Bronchial Arteries

Our technique has been previously reported.[36,39] A median sternotomy is performed and the organs examined. Prior to organ harvesting, the donor is given 1 g of intravenous methylprednisolone, and an intravenous infusion of prostaglandin E_1 is titrated to produce a 25% decrease in the systolic blood pressure. The nasogastric tube is withdrawn into the esophagus (confirmed by palpation through the left pleural space) into which 10 mL of betadine solution is injected.

After aortic cross-clamping, University of Wisconsin solution (60 mL/kg at 4°C) is administered directly into the pulmonary trunk while the lungs are gently ventilated with room air. The tip of the left atrial appendage is excised to decompress the left heart. Simultaneously, cardioplegia is administered into the aortic root. The heart can be excised prior to excision of the double lung bloc, or it can be separated on the back table at a later time. The nasogastric tube is removed, and ventilation is stopped for the dissection.

Protection of the bronchial arteries during excision of the double lung bloc requires en-bloc removal of the esophagus and descending thoracic aorta. The distal esophagus is mobilized bluntly and divided with a stapling device. The distal descending thoracic aorta is divided and the parietal pleural is incised, caudal to cranial, lateral to azygous vein on the right, and lateral to the aorta on the left. The aorta and esophagus are dissected off the anterior vertebral ligament with the double lung bloc. The branches of the aortic arch vessels are divided, and the cranial aspect of the esophagus divided with a stapling device. The lungs are gently inflated to a normal tidal volume with room air, and the trachea divided with the stapler. The double lung bloc is transferred to a cold (4°C) saline bath.

On the back table, the esophagus is stripped subadventially from the donor mediastinal tissue. This is done by grasping the esophagus at one end and retracting as the attachments of the esophagus to the surrounding donor mediastinal tissue are divided near the muscularis of the esophagus. The aortic arch, which was removed with the lung bloc to facilitate exposure of the proximal esophagus, is excised. The descending thoracic aorta is opened longitudinally along its pleural surface, just anterior to the left intercostal branches; this incision will pass between the left intercostal arteries and the left bronchial arteries, and extents to the left subclavian artery. The opened, donor descending thoracic aorta is examined. The bronchial artery orifices can usually be identified by inspection and knowledge of the bronchial artery anatomy. This may be confirmed by gently passing a probe through them to the tracheobronchial tree, and they may be marked with a suture.[24] We have stopped passing a probe and simply observed the orifices for backbleeding after the pulmonary circulation is reestablished in the recipient. Backbleeding from an orifice on the donor descending thoracic aorta after reestablishing the pulmonary circulation is due to pulmonary-bronchial collateral vessels, and implies that the orifice on the aorta leads to a bronchial artery.

The lungs are separated by dividing the left atrium and pulmonary arteries in the usual manner. The main stem bronchi are divided at the carina with a stapler. When dividing the airway, the remaining aortic patch is kept with the desired lung, along with adjacent mediastinal tissue containing the bronchial arteries.

It is possible, depending on the individual anatomy, to separate the bronchial arteries to both lungs from a single donor for transplant in separate recipients ("twinning"). The aortic patch is divided between the bronchial arteries to be preserved for each lung. It is necessary to gently pass a probe to identify the bronchial arteries while dividing the aortic patch and adjacent donor mediastinal tissue to avoid injuring the bronchial arteries. The bronchial arteries are separated prior to dividing the airway. Variability of the bronchial artery anatomy will limit the number of donors in whom this is possible.

We do not attempt to dissect the bronchial arteries out of the surrounding mediastinal tissue. The back table dissection of the double lung bloc is relatively brief. Stripping the esophagus, opening the aorta, and excising excess aorta take little time. Care is required when separating the main stem bronchi to protect and preserve the mediastinal tissue between the airway and the donor descending thoracic aorta.

The Recipient Procedure

Several techniques have been suggested for BAR at lung transplant including direct implantation of a donor aortic button (with the bronchial artery orifice) onto the recipient aorta,[14,18,37] use of a conduit of tailored donor aorta,[38,40] use of a saphenous vein graft,[35] and use of the ITA.[24] Direct implantation of the donor aortic button containing a bronchial artery orifice into the recipient aorta often requires dissection of the bronchial artery out of the donor mediastinal tissue, risking injury. Further, there is risk of morbidity from manipulating the recipient descending thoracic aorta. Conduits consisting of tailored donor aorta may be affected by stasis or embolus. The ITA is a proven conduit in coronary artery bypass grafting and has superior long-term patency, even in the presence of limited run-off. Small bronchial vessels and vasoconstriction from ischemia or cold preservation may result in very slow run-off after BAR.

The patient is placed in the lateral decubitus position. The ipsilateral groin is included in the field for cannulation should cardiopulmonary bypass be required. A standard posterolateral thoracotomy is performed. The ipsilateral ITA is dissected from its bed prior to anticipated arrival of the donor lung. Pneumonectomy and standard SLT is performed.[39] The bronchial anastomosis is performed with 4–0 polypropylene suture; the membranous portion is continuous, and the cartilaginous portion is interrupted. The donor and recipient bronchi are allowed to telescope as their relative sizes permit.

When the pulmonary circulation has been reestablished, the donor aortic cuff is inspected. Backbleeding will be noted from the orifice of the bronchial arteries on the patch of donor descending thoracic aorta due to pulmonary-bronchial collaterals. We choose the largest vessel with good backbleeding for revascularization, and avoid probing or further dissection of the bronchial arteries. Heparin, 5000 units intravenously, is administered at this time. The ITA is divided distally; it is left attached to the subclavian artery proximally.

The ITA is prepared by incising the distal aspect longitudinally for 0.5 to 1.0 cm, and anastomosing it to the chosen orifice of the bronchial artery on the opened patch of donor descending thoracic aorta with running 8–0 polypropylene suture. Bleeding from collateral branches in the donor mediastinal tissue and backbleeding from other orifices on the donor aorta are common. Hemostasis is carefully achieved with suture or clips to avoid injury to adjacent vessels in the donor mediastinal tissue, which may be important bronchial arteries or collaterals.

Limitations

BAR is not always technically feasible. The variable anatomy and delicate nature of the bronchial arteries will limit the number of patients who can benefit from direct BAR with SLT; however, we have found that it is usually possible. We have attempted to preserve and separate the bronchial arteries to both lungs, from a single donor, for implantation into separate recipients ("twinning"), with BAR of both lungs. Again, the variable anatomy will limit this for lungs from all donors, but it is occasionally possible. The procedure should not significantly prolong the allograft ischemic time or the recipient operative time, and procurement should not interfere with other teams. We have not found these issues to be a problem. The short-term benefit to airway healing seems undeniable. Any long-term benefits or effects remain unproven.

Results

We obtained angiograms, postoperatively, to document perfusion of the bronchial arteries in 13 consecutive patients in whom we performed BAR as a routine part of SLT. This was a consecutive series of patients, excluding one perioperative death (did not survive to angiography), and three transplants for which we did not procure the organs and, therefore, could not perform BAR. There were eight males and five females, with a mean age of 52.6 years (range 40 to 59 years). Eleven patients had left, and two, right SLT. Median donor age was 36 years (mean 28.9, range 16 to 47 years). Median ischemic time was 250 minutes (mean 236.2, range 132 to 373 minutes). Ischemic time was estimated to be prolonged by a maximum of about 15 to 20 minutes for BAR: 5 additional minutes for organ harvesting and 10 to 15 additional minutes to prepare the lung for implantation. Recipient operative time (not additional ischemic time), was estimated to be prolonged by a maximum of 30 to 45 minutes (takedown of ITA, preparation for and performance of ITA to bronchial artery anastomosis, and additional hemostasis).

Median follow-up was 28 months (range 1 to 37 months). There have been three late deaths. All 13 patients underwent angiography of the ITA 7 to 10 days after SLT. Bronchoscopic examination of the anastomoses was performed in the operating room immediately after SLT and just prior to extubation (1 to 4 days, postoperatively). Subsequent bronchoscopy was performed for clinical indications only; suspicion of rejection or infection, or unexplained changes on the chest x-ray.

Immunosuppression

Standard triple immunosuppressive therapy is employed with OKT3 induction (14-day course, 2.5 mg/d, intravenously). Intravenous methylprednisone is administered in the operating room (500 mg) and for three subsequent doses (125 mg) at

8-hour intervals. Steroids are then withheld for the remainder of the first 14 days, after which a standard course is administered (prednisone 1 mg/kg/d tapered to 0.3 mg/kg/d maintenance by day 28, postoperatively). Azathioprine (4 mg/kg) is administered preoperatively, and continued postoperatively, adjusting the dose to maintain a leukocyte count of 4000 to 6000 per cubic mm. Cyclosporin A is started during the first 14 days postoperatively, after renal function is stable. The dose is adjusted to achieve therapeutic levels by the end of the course of OKT3 (200 to 300 ng/mL serum by EIA); the levels are decreased to 75 to 150 ng/mL after 6 weeks.

Angiography

Angiography of the ITA was performed in all patients 7 to 10 days, postoperatively. All patients had patent ITAs. Excellent perfusion of the bronchial arteries was demonstrated in 11 of these 13 patients. The angiogram showed good perfusion of the entire distal bronchial artery distribution, as well as perfusion of the area of the bronchial anastomosis (Figures 3A–D). The two patients who had poor perfusion of the bronchial arteries had patent ITAs, but no flow was seen beyond the ITA, with the exception of an occasional small donor mediastinal vessel.

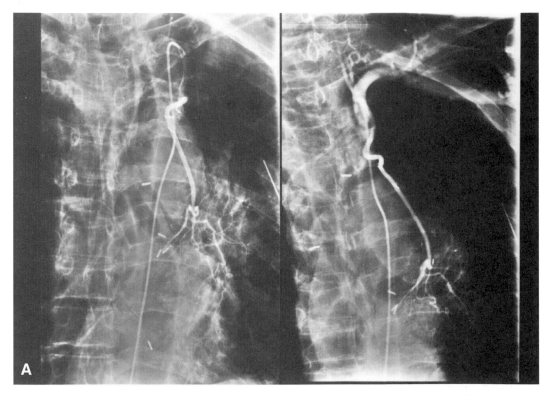

Figure 3. Four examples of postoperative internal thoracic arteriograms performed 7 days after SLT with direct, immediate bronchial artery revascularization (BAR). The recipient internal thoracic artery has been anastomosed to the origin of the bronchial artery on the donor descending thoracic aorta. Good perfusion of the bronchial arteries and the distal bronchial tree is demonstrated.

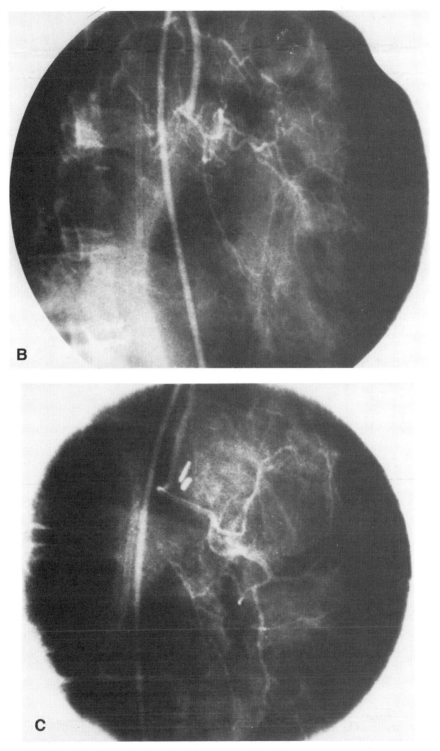

Figures 3B–C.

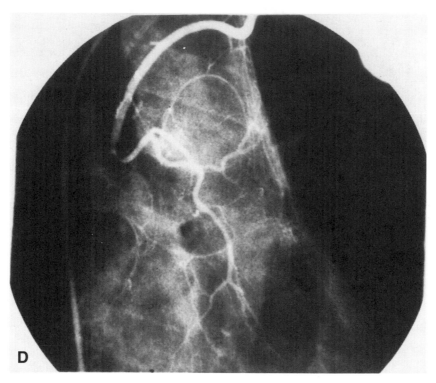

Figure 3D.

Bronchoscopy and Airway Healing

The distal bronchial mucosa of the transplanted lung looked pink and healthy at the initial perioperative bronchoscopic exam and throughout the follow-up period in all patients. All patients have had excellent airway healing, with no evidence of granulation tissue, necrosis, or dehiscence. No patients have developed late bronchial strictures or malacia, either at the anastomosis or in the distal airways.

Conclusions

In conclusion, BAR is a fairly simple technique that can be performed at the time of SLT with minimal increase in the organ ischemic time and recipient operative time, and there is no interference with other teams at the time of procurement. Special techniques are required at the time of pulmonary allograft procurement to preserve and protect the bronchial arteries. Revascularization at the orifice of the bronchial artery on the donor descending thoracic aorta eliminates the need to dissect the fragile vessels out of the donor mediastinal tissue. The recipient procedure is slightly prolonged by an additional anastomosis and associated hemostasis, but this time is not excessive. The variable bronchial artery anatomy will limit universal application of BAR for SLT, particularly in some cases when both lungs are transplanted (though BAR of both lungs is feasible).

We have attempted BAR using the recipient ITA in 14 consecutive patients undergoing SLT for whom we procured the organs. Excellent bronchial artery perfusion was confirmed in 11 of 13 patients in whom angiography was performed. Bronchial healing was excellent with no short- or long-term airway complications in any patient. We now perform BAR as a routine part of SLT. In addition to improving airway healing, BAR may favorably impact post-transplant implantation response, pneumonia, and late OB.

References

1. Cooper JD: The evolution of techniques and indications for lung transplantation. *Ann Surg* 212:249–256, 1990.
2. Hardy JD, Webb WR, Dalton ML, Walker GR: Lung homotransplantation in man: report of the initial case. *JAMA* 186:1065–1074, 1963.
3. Veith FJ: Lung transplantation. *Surg Clin North Am* 58:357–364, 1978.
4. Toronto Lung Transplant Group: Unilateral lung transplantation for pulmonary fibrosis. *N Engl J Med* 314:1140–1145, 1986.
5. Schafers H-J, Haydock DA, Cooper JD: The prevalence and management of bronchial anastomotic complications in lung transplantation. *J Thorac Cardiovasc Surg* 101:1044–1052, 1991.
6. Egan TM, Westerman JH, Lambert CJ, Detterbeck FC, Thompson JT, Mill MR, et al: Isolated lung transplantation for end-stage lung disease: a viable therapy. *Ann Thorac Surg* 53:590–596, 1992.
7. Shennib H, Massard G: Airway complications after lung transplantation (review). *Ann Thorac Surg* 57:506–511, 1994.
8. Griffith BT, Magee MJ, Gonzalez IF, Houel R, Armitage JM, Hardesty RL, et al: Anastomotic pitfalls in lung transplantation. *J Thorac Cardiovasc Surg* 107:743–754, 1994.
9. Patterson GA, Cooper JD, Goldman B, Weisel RD, Pearson FG, Waters PF, et al: Technique of successful clinical double lung transplantation. *Ann Thorac Surg* 45:626–633, 1988.
10. Loma O, Goldberg M, Peters WJ, Ayabe H, Townsend E, Cooper JD: Bronchial omentopexy in canine lung transplantation. *J Thorac Cardiovasc Surg* 83:418–421, 1982.
11. Morgan E, Lima O, Goldberg M, Ayabe H, Ferdman A, Cooper JD: Improved bronchial healing in canine left lung reimplantation using omental pedicle wrap. *J Thorac Cardiovasc Surg* 85:134–139, 1983.
12. Fell SC, Mollenkopf FP, Montefusco CM, Mitsude S, Kamholz SL, Goldsmith J, et al: Revascularization of ischemic bronchial anastomoses by an intercostal pedicle flap. *J Thorac Cardiovasc Surg* 90:172–178, 1985.
13. Dubois P, Choiniere L, Cooper JD: Bronchial omentopexy in canine lung allotransplantation. *Ann Thorac Surg* 38:211–214, 1984.
14. Morgan E, Lima O, Goldberg M, Ferdman A, Luk SK, Cooper JD: Successful revascularization of totally ischemic bronchial autografts with omental pedicle flaps in dogs. *J Thorac Cardiovasc Surg* 84:204–210, 1982.
15. Khaghani A, Tadjkarimi S, Daly RC, Theodropoulos S, Madden B, Banner N, et al: Influence of different types of wraps versus no wrap in single-lung transplantation: a prospective randomized trial (abstr). *J Heart Lung Transplant* 11:213, 1992.
16. Metras H: Note préliminaire sur la greffe totale du poumon chez le chien. *Proc Acad Sci* 231:1176–1177, 1950.
17. Metras D, Henri Metras: A pioneer in lung transplantation. J *Heart Lung Transplant* 11:1213–1216, 1992.
18. Mills NL, Boyd AD, Gheranpong C: The significance of bronchial circulation in lung transplantation. *J Thorac Cardiovasc Surg* 60:866–874, 1970.
19. Haglin JJ, Ruiz E, Baker RC, Anderson WR: Histologic studies of human lung allotransplantation. In: Wildevuur C (ed). *Morphology in Lung Transplantation*. Basel, Switzerland: S Karger; 13–22, 1973.

20. Griffith BP, Hardesty RL, Trento A, Paradis IL, Duquesnoy RJ, Zeevi A, et al: Heart-lung transplantation: lessons learned and future hopes. *Ann Thorac Surg* 43:6–16, 1987.
21. Novitzky D, Cooper DKC: Surgical technique of the recipient operation. In: Cooper DKC, Novitzky D (eds). *The Transplantation and Replacement of Thoracic Organs.* Boston: Kluwer Academic Publishers; 293, 1990.
22. Raju S, Heath BJ, Warren ET, Hardy JD: Single and double lung transplantation. *Ann Surg* 211:681–693, 1990.
23. Patterson GA, Todd TR, Cooper JD, Pearson FG, Winton TL, Maurer J—The Toronto Lung Transplant Group: Airway complications after double lung transplantation. *J Thorac Cardiovasc Surg* 99:14–21, 1990.
24. Daly RC, Tadjkarimi S, Khaghani A, Banner NR, Yacoub MH: Successful double-lung transplantation with direct bronchial artery revascularization. *Ann Thorac Surg* 56:885–892, 1993.
25. Aeba R, Stout JE, Francalancia NA, Keenan RJ, Duncan AJ, Yousem SA, et al: Aspects of lung transplantation that contribute to increased severity of pneumonia: an experimental study. *J Thorac Cardiovasc Surg* 106:449–457, 1993.
26. Paul A, Marelli D, Shennib H, King M, Wang N-S, Wilson JAS, et al: Mucociliary function in autotransplanted, allotransplanted, and sleeve resected lungs. *J Thorac Cardiovasc Surg* 98:523–528, 1989.
27. Pearson FG, Goldberg M, Stone RM, Colapinto RF: Bronchial arterial circulation restored after reimplantation of canine lung. *Can J Surg* 13:243–250, 1970.
28. Ventemiglia RA, Braverman B, DiMauro J, Castro R, Blair W, Spigos D, et al: The ischemic lung: role of the bronchial arteries in lung function. *Cardiovasc Dis Bull Tex Heart Inst* 8:480–498, 1981.
29. Bando K, Paradis IL, Similo S, Konishi H, Komatsu K, Zullo TG, et al: Obliterative bronchiolitis after lung and heart-lung transplantation: an analysis of risk factors and management. *J Thorac Cardiovasc Surg* 110:4–14, 1995.
30. LoCicero J III, Robinson PG, Fisher M: Chronic rejection in single-lung transplantation manifested by obliterative bronchiolitis. *J Thorac Cardiovasc Surg* 99:1059–1062, 1990.
31. Scott JP, Higenbottam TW, Clelland CA, Stewart S, Smyth RL, McGoldrick JP, et al: Natural history of chronic rejection in heart-lung transplantation. *J Heart Transplant* 9:510–515, 1990.
32. Takao M, Katayama Y, Onoda K, Tanabe H, Hiraiwa T, Mizutani T, et al: Significance of bronchial mucosal blood flow for the monitoring of acute rejection in lung transplantation. *J Heart Lung Transplant* 10:956–967, 1991.
33. Tanabe H, Takao M, Hiraiwa T, Mizutani T, Yada I, Namikawa S, et al: New diagnostic method for pulmonary allograft rejection by measurement of bronchial mucosal blood flow. *J Heart Lung Transplant* 10:968–974, 1991.
34. Takao M, Katayama Y, Tanabe H, Hiraiwa T, Mizutani T, Yada I, et al: Histologic changes in donor bronchi may explain the reduced mucosal blood flow seen during acute lung allograft rejection. *J Heart Lung Transplant* 11:994–1000, 1992.
35. Couraud L, Baudet E, Martigne C, Roques X, Velly J-F, Laborde N, et al: Bronchial revascularization in double-lung transplantation: a series of 8 patients. *Ann Thorac Surg* 53:88–94, 1992.
36. Daly RC, McGregor CGA: Routine, immediate, direct bronchial artery revascularization for single lung transplantation. *Ann Thorac Surg* 57:1446–1452, 1994.
37. Schreinemakers HHJ, Weder W, Miyoshi S, Harper BD, Shimokawa S, Egan TM, et al: Direct revascularization of bronchial arteries for lung transplantation: an anatomical study. *Ann Thorac Surg* 49:44–54, 1990.
38. Laks H, Louie HW, Haas GS, Drinkwater DC, Lewis W, Permut LC, et al: New technique of vascularization of the trachea and bronchus for lung transplantation. *J Heart Lung Transplant* 10:280–287, 1991.
39. McGregor CGA, Daly RC, Peters SG, Midthun DE, Scott JP, Allen MS, et al: Evolving strategies in lung transplantation for emphysema. *Ann Thorac Surg* 57:1513–1521, 1994.
40. Raju S, Heath BJ, Warren ET, Hardy JD: Single and double lung transplantation. *Ann Surg* 211:681–693, 1990.

Chapter 13

Single Lung Transplantion in Children

Sara J. Shumway, MD; R. Morton Bolman, III, MD

Introduction

Single lung transplantation was first successfully performed for an adult recipient in 1983.[1] Its application in the pediatric population was delayed until the technical aspects were further developed for adult recipients. End-stage pulmonary disease involves different diseases in children than in adults, and it is necessary to allow for the potential growth of young recipients. At a conference in Philadelphia in 1991, physicians shared their results with pediatric lung and heart-lung procedures.[2] The numbers were small, but have continued to steadily increase.

Indications and Contraindications

Pediatric patients with end-stage lung disease (of the restrictive or obstructive type) or pulmonary vascular disease (either primary or secondary) require a lung transplant. Eisenmenger's syndrome associated with a correctable congenital heart defect is an indication for a single lung transplant if the defect can be repaired and the transplant done at the same time. Such patients have a life expectancy of less than a year to 18 months without the transplant.

Emphysema is a common indication for a single lung transplant in adults, but not in children. Two major groups of pediatric pulmonary pathology can require a single lung transplant: pulmonary fibrosis and pulmonary vascular disease.[3] Indications under pulmonary fibrosis include: usual interstitial fibrosis; desquamative interstitial fibrosis; pulmonary alveolar proteinosis; idiopathic pulmonary alveolar microlithiasis; cystic fibrosis; radiation-induced pulmonary fibrosis; obliterative bronchiolitis (OB); and bronchopulmonary dysplasia. Indications under pulmonary vascular disease include: primary pulmonary hypertension; pulmonary hypertension, after corrected congenital

From: Franco KL (ed). *Pediatric Cardiopulmonary Transplantation*. Armonk, NY: Futura Publishing Company, Inc.; © 1997.

heart disease; pulmonary hypertension, with a correctable congenital heart defect; and pulmonary atresia or hypoplasia of the lung.

Some suggest that patients with a congenital diaphragmatic hernia could undergo a single lung transplant. Then, once the patient could survive on native lung tissue, the transplanted lung could be removed when it was outgrown.[4] Children with cystic fibrosis would require removal of both lungs because of septic lung disease, so they would undergo a bilateral sequential lung transplant.

Contraindications to a pediatric lung transplant include chest wall deformities such as severe scoliosis, poorly controlled diabetes mellitus, or poor heart function. Previous thoracic surgery can complicate a lung transplant because of difficulties with adhesions and bleeding. High steroid doses pretransplant are associated with increased risk of poor bronchial healing, and even sepsis, post-transplant. Absolute contraindications include active infection, active malignancy, or any permanent end-organ dysfunction. A strong family support system is crucial for any child undergoing any transplant.

If children have been intubated for long periods, they are poor candidates for a single-lung transplant because of problems related to tracheo- or bronchomalacia. Generally, up to 2 weeks of intubation would not be a problem; however, the waiting time on the transplant list is usually longer than that. If patients cannot be extubated within 1 month, tracheostomy is indicated. At the University of Minnesota, we have not done a single lung transplant in any pediatric patient with an indwelling tracheostomy.

Recipient Selection

All pediatric lung transplant candidates are evaluated by a pediatric pulmonologist, a thoracic transplant surgeon, a social worker, a pediatric cardiologist (when appropriate), and of course their own pediatrician (when possible).[5] Candidates should have normal nutritional status; any coexisting congenital heart disease should be well defined. Changes in steroid doses, as well as treatment of antibiotic resistant organisms must be well documented and very carefully followed. Echocardiography is routinely done to rule out the presence of a patent foramen ovale. If present, it would need to be repaired at the time of the transplant and would require cardiopulmonary bypass.

Lung Preservation and Procurement

Lung preservation is the same for pediatric and adult patients. The main pulmonary artery is cannulated using an appropriate-sized pulmonary artery catheter, then secured in place. Modified Euro-Collins solution is administered at about 60 mL/kg as the lungs are gently ventilated. Both lungs are examined to ensure adequate blanching (flushing) of each. The left atrial appendage is amputated at its widest level, so that the heart does not distend and the preservation fluid can freely egress. At the time of procurement and dissection, care is taken to provide adequate left atrial cuffs bilaterally.

The dissection begins once the heart arrests and the lungs receive the necessary amount of pulmonary flush solution. Topical cold is administered over the heart and both lungs. The heart is elevated and the left atrium is opened about midway between the pulmonary veins and the coronary sinus. The incision begins at the left inferior pulmonary vein and is extended superiorly toward the main pulmonary artery. The main pulmonary artery is amputated at its bifurcation. The aorta is amputated at the level of the innominate takeoff. The dissection continues, moving to the right. Care is taken not to injure the right pulmonary artery as the dissection continues on the right side. Again, attempts are made to leave an adequate cuff around the pulmonary veins. The dissection continues as the incision is extended inferiorly. The heart is positioned to the left. Under tension, the left atriotomy is completed in a circumferential fashion.

The lung block is then excised along the posterior surface of the mediastinum. Each lung is reflected upward and away from the dissection, as it continues superiorly. The dissection continues away from the airways. The descending thoracic aorta is divided, as is the thymus along with associated superior mediastinal fat. The trachea is divided, using a stapler, inferiorly (with the lungs partially expanded). The ex vivo lung block is then divided on a back table.

Once the heart is excised, the left atrium is bifurcated. The pulmonary arteries are separated, and the dissection continues posteriorly to reveal the carina. Since the trachea has usually been divided more superiorly, the bronchi are divided at the proximal left mainstem bronchus in order to preserve the otherwise shorter right mainstem bronchus.

Recipient Operation

In single lung transplants, most of the operative techniques for adults can be used successfully for children—with one exception. Telescoping the bronchial anastomosis for children tends to cause stenosis at the anastomosis, due in large part to progressive granulation tissue or bronchomalacia. So, instead, for children, an end-to-end bronchial anastomosis with absorbable suture material is done to promote the growth potential at the anastomotic site and reduce the opportunity for granulation formation.[6] For children, pericardial or omental wraps have not been popular, and any kind of revascularization procedure is not mandatory.

Pediatric lung transplant recipients—particularly those with pulmonary vascular disease—require cardiopulmonary bypass, which is done through a bilateral submammary anterior thoracotomy incision that divides the sternum. This approach obviates the need for double lumen endotracheal tubes or bronchial blockers, which are not easy to use in small children. At the University of Minnesota, we do not use bronchial blockers or double lumen tubes until patients weigh at least 45 kg. Occasionally, a pediatric patient with cystic fibrosis who is larger than a small child can undergo a bilateral sequential lung transplant without cardiopulmonary bypass.

In pediatric single lung transplants, donor and recipient size matching is very important. The chest dimensions of the donor and recipient are compared to minimize difficulties created by space problems and to allow the usual excursion of the diaphragm. It is not known what best predicts a good match: the chest measurements, or the height and weight.[8]

Extracorporeal membrane oxygenation (ECMO) has been used in children as a bridge to transplantation, as well as early post-transplant to support both lung and heart function.[9] Pediatric lung recipients sometimes require protracted vascular access for ganciclovir infusion, blood drawing, and intravenous nutritional support. For that reason, many will have indwelling catheters (e.g., Hickman) for the first 3 months post-transplant.

We used ECMO perioperatively to support a patient who underwent a single right lower lobar lung transplant with a living related donor. This patient had also undergone a right thoracotomy with extension across the sternum. Through this same incision, the patient was cannulated via the aorta and right atrium. For our patients under age 2 who have not undergone a transsternal incision or a bilateral submammary anterior thoracotomy incision, cannulation is done via the carotid artery and jugular vein. The carotid artery is repaired, whenever possible, when the cannula is removed. To date, we have not used ECMO as a bridge to lung transplantation, except when a previous lung transplant has failed.

Immunosuppression

Our current immunosuppressive protocol for pediatric single lung recipients involves triple drug therapy. Preoperatively, azathioprine (2.5 mg/kg orally) and cyclosporine (CsA) (4 to 6 mg/kg orally) are given. Intraoperatively, methylprednisolone (10 mg/kg intravenously) is given before the pulmonary artery clamp is released; if the patient weighs more than 50 kg, then 500 mg of methylprednisolone is given.

Postoperatively, CsA (3 to 5 mg/kg orally b.i.d.) is given; an intravenous drip is started at 1.5 to 2.5 mg/hr to maintain a CsA level of about 300 ng/mL by radioimmunoassay (RIA). For patients with poor absorption via the gastrointestinal tract, CSA may be given three times a day in divided doses. Azathioprine is continued at 2.5 mg/kg/d orally or, if necessary, intravenously. Prednisone is started at 1 mg/kg/d orally in divided doses on post-transplant day 2, or when the patient is extubated; if intravenous administration is indicated, the equivalent dosage is given using methylprednisolone. Prednisone is tapered, depending on the incidence of rejection, over the next 6 months. Antilymphocyte globulin (ATG) has not been used for single lung recipients at our institution since August 1992. Antiviral agents are given for 3 months post-transplant if cytomegalovirus (CMV)-positive status was documented in either the donor or recipient.

Rejection episodes are diagnosed by infiltrates on chest x-ray, fever, leukocytosis, a decrease in peripheral arterial oxygen saturation and ventilatory function, or the development of new pleural effusions.[10] Transbronchial lung biopsies are done for larger children.[11] All rejection episodes are treated with bolus steroids.

Case Report

In July 1990, at age 4, W.L. underwent a right single lung transplant for primary pulmonary hypertension. She required cardiopulmonary bypass at that time. Initially, she did well and was removed from the ventilator on post-transplant day 10, but then developed OB related to multiple episodes of rejection, and required a retransplant. In September 1991, she underwent a bilateral sequential lung transplant, again using cardiopulmonary bypass. Post-transplant, she received several courses of photopheresis when some form of OB syndrome was suspected. She has done well ever since. As of 1996, 5 years after her bilateral sequential lung transplants, she attends school and participates in the usual activities of daily life.

Rejection

As stated earlier, we treat all documented rejection episodes with bolus steroids. Bronchoscopy is done frequently in the early postoperative period to assess the quality of the bronchial anastomosis. Transbronchial biopsies have been done even in infants, using a modified cardiac bioptome and fluoroscopic guidance.[12] In older children, biopsies have been obtained through the fiberoptic bronchoscope, with sampling of at least two areas in a transplanted lung. Ideally, three to six specimens are taken from the transplanted lung. Biopsies are more frequent if the clinical status of the patient changes; usually, they are done about 1 week post-transplant, then one to three times in the first 3 months, then every 6 months after that. Occasionally, if a child's clinical status deteriorates and no diagnosis has been made on the basis of transbronchial biopsies, an open-lung biopsy is necessary. Serial pulmonary function studies are helpful in older children, but are of little use in children under age 6.[13]

Infection

Pulmonary infections are a common cause of morbidity and mortality after single lung transplants. Pneumonia may be secondary to bacteria such as Enterococcus and Staphylococcus.[14] Viral infections are primarily caused by CMV, the respiratory syncytial virus (RSV), or parainfluenza.[15] The adenovirus is especially lethal. All recipients with a CMV-positive donor receive a 12-week course of prophylactic ganciclovir. Fungal infections secondary to Aspergillus or Candida are treated with intravenous amphotericin. Postoperative exposure to varicella in previously unexposed recipients is treated with varicella zoster immunoglobulin (VZIG), within 48 hours if possible.

Obliterative Bronchiolitis

OB is the main problem preventing good long-term results for pediatric single lung recipients.[16] It appears to be slightly more common in children than in adults. To some degree, it responds to increased immunosuppression. Photopheresis may have some role in its treatment, especially when the diagnosis is made early in the disease process. Treatment success, however, remains primarily anecdotal. A retransplant may be the only real option. Note that for single lung recipients with OB, a bilateral sequential lung transplant may be more appropriate for their second transplant; the native lung in immunosuppressed patients may harbor infection.

Living Related Lung Transplants

Lobar transplants may be an effective method to increase the availability of donors.[17] They have primarily been done in small female recipients with cystic fibrosis.

An adult right lower lobe and an adult left lower lobe are used to replace the child's right and left lungs.

Single lung transplants using only a single lobe have also been done at a few centers. They should not be done for patients with acute respiratory distress or pneumonia. No large series has been published.

Results

As of September 1994, the St. Louis International Lung Transplant Registry had data for 133 lung recipients under age 16.[18] Of these, 29 had undergone a single lung transplant; 86, a bilateral single lung transplant; and 16, an en-bloc double lung transplant. The precise operation was unknown for two recipients. The primary indication was cystic fibrosis in 64 recipients, primary pulmonary hypertension in 20, and idiopathic pulmonary fibrosis in 10. The overall reported survival for 127 recipients was 66% at 1 year and 54% at 2 years. More data are being collected annually by the United Network for Organ Sharing (UNOS).

Survival

The main obstacle to significant long-term survival for pediatric single lung recipients is OB. This problem should be the focus of any clinical research in this field. Survival often reflects the patient's condition at the time of the transplant. Transplant candidates must be followed regularly while they are on the waiting list, to make sure their nutritional status and degree of infection are clearly understood. Most children undergoing a single lung transplant for pulmonary vascular disease require cardiopulmonary bypass. It is still a matter of debate whether patients with pulmonary vascular disease, either primary or secondary, would benefit more from bilateral or single lung transplantation.[19] Our knowledge of pulmonary vascular disease in children should improve as more lungs are removed and replaced.

Summary

Controversy remains as to whether a child should undergo a single lung or a bilateral single lung transplant. Another question is whether waiting list time and donor availability should be considered important variables in recipient selection and transplant timing.

A pediatric single lung transplant requires perfect surgical technique. The bronchial anastomosis should be done end-to-end. The omentum is not appropriate for use as a wrap for children. Care must be taken not to kink or twist the pulmonary artery at its anastomotic site. The left atrial anastomosis must be widely patent. Otherwise graft failure will ensue. As with adults, endocardial-to-endocardial anastomosis is mandatory at the left atrial level.

OB requires the immediate attention of researchers to improve long-term results of single lung transplants in children. Anecdotal experience with photopheresis is encouraging. New immunosuppressants may be the answer. In any case, a child who suddenly deteriorates after a single lung transplant needs to be assessed for OB.

The future may see an increase in the application of lobar transplants in children. A few centers are pioneering this work.[20]

References

1. The Toronto Lung Transplant Group: Unilateral lung transplantation for pulmonary fibrosis. *N Engl J Med* 314:1140–1145, 1986.
2. Organ Transplants in Children; Symposium. Philadelphia: April 7–9, 1991.
3. Spray TL, Huddleston CB: Pediatric lung transplantation. In: Patterson GA, Cooper JD (eds). *Lung Transplantation.* Philadelphia: WB Saunders, Co.; 123–143, 1993.
4. Spray TL: Projections for pediatric heart-lung and lung transplantation. *J Heart Lung Transplant* 12:S337–S343, 1993.
5. Mackay B, Lucore P: Pediatric lung transplantation: an emerging program. *Crit Care Nurs Clinics North Am* 4:223–233, 1992.
6. Hislop AA, Odom NJ, McGregor CGA, et al: Growth potential of the immature transplanted lung: an experimental study. *J Thorac Cardiovasc Surg* 100:360–370, 1990.
7. Spray TL, Mallory GB, Canter CE, et al: Pediatric lung transplantation for pulmonary hypertension and congenital heart disease. *Ann Thorac Surg* 54:216–225, 1992.
8. Cohen RG, Barr ML, Starnes VA: Pediatric lung transplantation. *Semin Pediatr Surg* 2:279–288, 1993.
9. Armitage JM, Fricker FJ, Kurland G, et al: Pediatric lung transplantation: the years 1985 to 1992 and the clinical trial of FK506. *J Thorac Cardiovasc Surg* 105:337–346, 1993.
10. Starnes VA, Marshall SE, Lewiston NJ, et al: Heart-lung transplantation in infants, children, and adolescents. *J Pediatr Surg* 26:434–438, 1991.
11. Starnes VA, Lewiston NJ, Theodore J, et al: Cystic fibrosis: target population for lung transplantation in North America in the 1990s. *J Thorac Cardiovasc Surg* 103:1008–1014, 1992.
12. Whitehead B, Scott JP, Helms P, et al: Technique and use of transbronchial biopsy in children and adolescents. *Pediatr Pulmonol* 12:240–246, 1992.
13. Egan T, Kaiser L, Cooper J: Lung transplantation. *Curr Probl Surg* 26:675–751, 1989.
14. Zenati M, Dowling RD, Dummer JS, et al: Influence of the donor lung on development of early infections in lung transplant recipients. *J Heart Transplant* 9:502–509, 1990.
15. Keenan RJ, Lega MA, Dummer JS, et al: Cytomegalovirus serologic status and postoperative infection correlated with risk of developing chronic rejection after pulmonary transplantation. *Transplantation* 51:433–438, 1991.
16. Whitehead B, Rees P, Sorensen K, et al: Incidence of obliterative bronchiolitis after heart-lung transplantation in children. *J Heart Lung Transplant* 12:903–908, 1993.
17. Evans RW: The actual and potential supply of organ donors in the United States. In: Terasaki P (ed). *Clinical Transplants 1990.* Los Angeles: UCLA Tissue Typing Laboratory; 329–341, 1990.
18. International Lung Transplant Registry. Suite 3107, Queeny Tower, One Barnes Hospital Plaza, St. Louis, MO 63110.
19. Miyoshi S, Trulock EP, Schaefers H-J, et al: Cardiopulmonary exercise testing after single- and double-lung transplantation. *Chest* 97:1130–1136, 1990.
20. Cohen RG, Barr ML, Starnes VA: Lobar pulmonary transplantation. In: Shumway SJ, Shumway NE (eds). *Thoracic Transplantation.* Cambridge: Blackwell Science, Inc.; 406–414, 1995.

Chapter 14

Lung Transplantation for Cystic Fibrosis in Children

George B. Mallory, Jr, MD; Thomas L. Spray, MD

Cystic fibrosis (CF) is a genetic disorder of chloride conductance across the apical membrane of epithelial cells within the exocrine glands of the body.[1] The major clinical manifestations of CF appear to be caused by inspissated secretions within the lower respiratory tract, the pancreas, and intestine. The median survival of CF patients is over 27 years and 30% of patients die before the age of 20 years.[2] The cause of death in greater than 95% of CF patients is respiratory failure, due to severe bronchiectasis.[3] Although aggressive therapy including intravenous antibiotics, nutritional supplementation, chest physiotherapy, and oxygen supplementation have been employed successfully to attain longer survival in patients with CF, the progression of lung disease in most patients is relentless. Heart-lung transplantation (HLT) and, more recently, lung transplantation have been utilized to treat selected children, adolescents, and adults with end-stage CF lung disease.[4–10] According to the St. Louis Lung Transplant Registry, as of July 1995, out of a total of 4134 lung transplant operations in the world, 625 (15.1%) have been performed in CF patients.[11] One hundred forty-one (22.6%) of the 625 lung transplants for CF have been performed in patients under 20 years of age. Due largely to the English experience with HLT,[4–6,8] it is likely that a similar number of CF patients have undergone HLT.

In this chapter, we discuss the approach to patients under 20 years of age with CF who are candidates for lung transplantation. Our own experience covers the period of July 1990 through July 1995, during which 86 patients had undergone lung transplantation or HLT at St. Louis Children's Hospital. Of the 86, 33 children and adolescents (18 years of age or younger) had CF. At the Washington University Medical Center, patients over 17 years of age at the time of initial evaluation are referred to the Barnes Hospital Lung Transplant Program. To date, over 40 patients with CF have undergone lung transplantation in the adult program. This chapter provides an overview of the problem of severe pulmonary disease and respiratory failure associated with CF in the pediatric years, and also reviews donor selection criteria, pretransplant

From: Franco KL (ed). *Pediatric Cardiopulmonary Transplantation.* Armonk, NY: Futura Publishing Company, Inc.; © 1997.

care, technical and surgical aspects of lung transplantation and in children, postoperative complications, and outcome.

Pathophysiology

Although all patients with CF have abnormal salt and water secretion within the exocrine glands, the variation in secondary manifestations of disease among affected individuals has been appreciated for decades. Although genotypic variations in CF are now well documented and are an attractive explanation for phenotypic differences between individuals, no correlation between specific mutations and clinical severity of pulmonary disease have been demonstrated in recent studies.[12,13] Nonetheless, the pathophysiology of lower respiratory tract disease in CF has become clearer because of insights into the molecular defect in the CF transmembrane conductance regulator (CFTR) protein.[14] Defective regulation of chloride conductance[15,16] and an accelerated rate of sodium reabsorption[17] lead to dehydration of the airway secretions. The dehydration of mucous secretions within the small airways would account for mechanical obstruction to airflow, but the full clinical picture includes the colonization and infection of the airways with typical organisms, most notably *Staphylococcus aureus* and *Pseudomonas aeruginosa*. It appears that CF respiratory epithelial cells have a higher density of specific membrane receptors for *P. aeruginosa*.[18] Within the dehydrated microenvironment of the CF lung, *P. aeruginosa* also appears to have an enhanced ability to produce mucoid exopolysaccharide which inhibits the ability of host phagocytes to kill the organism.[19] Although an intense host immune response is characteristic of CF patients within the pulmonary compartment, the efficacy of the response is compromised by a number of factors. The immunopathology of CF-associated lung disease has been recently reviewed.[20] The chronic suppurative bronchiectasis of CF is due in part to the dehydrated environment of the small airways, the ineffective and injurious host immune response, and the evasive activities permitting long-term residence of the typical pathogens, especially *Pseudomonas* species.

In the vast majority of patients, mechanical obstruction of the small airways leads to bronchiolitis and then bronchiolectasis. The onset of clinical disease may be in the first weeks of life, or it may be delayed until early or mid-adulthood. Eventually, the intense, chronic inflammatory process and the resultant destruction of airway walls span the entire length of the conducting airways. Chronic infection with increasingly antibiotic resistant organisms, exuberant host response with immune complexes, and huge numbers of neutrophils within the airways, defective mucociliary clearance, and chronic hyperinflation of the lungs leads to failure of gas exchange.[21] At the terminal stage, there is combined hypoxic-hypercapnic respiratory failure, cor pulmonale, severe malnutrition, and failure of the respiratory pump muscles. Death ensues, usually with progressive hypercapnia, but occasionally with an acute event such as massive hemoptysis.

Epidemiology

From recently published data of the Cystic Fibrosis Foundation (Figure 1), significant numbers of children and adolescents with CF die annually. In fact, more pe-

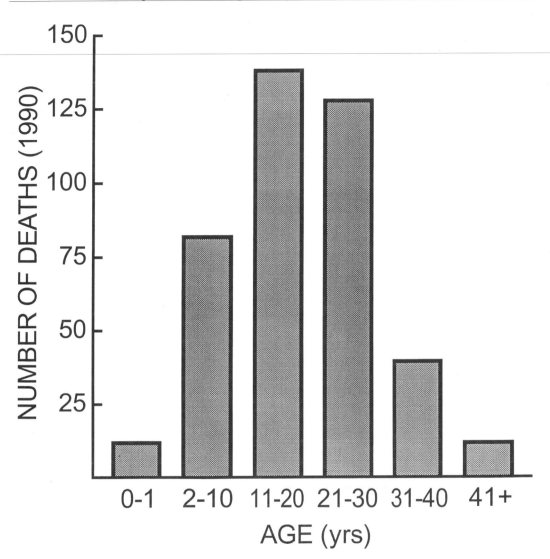

Figure 1. The incidence of death in cystic fibrosis patients by age in 1990. (Reproduced with permission from Reference 2.)

diatric CF patients died than adult CF patients in 1990 because of the skew of the population toward the younger ages.[2] Possible explanations for CF patients progressing to respiratory failure at an earlier stage than others include genetic factors (including coinheritance of another familial factor predisposing to lung disease or respiratory infection), more severe malnutrition, frequent or severe viral respiratory infections early in childhood, early acquisition of virulent or antibiotic resistant bacterial organisms within the lower respiratory tract, environmental factors, or inadequate medical interventions due to delay in diagnosis, parental noncompliance, or nonaggressive physician care.

Recipient Selection Criteria

When a child or adolescent with CF is being evaluated as a candidate for lung transplant, a number of factors must be considered. As with other patients, the primary criterion is that the child is likely to die within 1 to 2 years. Predicting mortality with a disease as protean as CF is obviously both difficult and important. The report of Kerem from the large CF Center at the Hospital for Sick Children in Toronto is helpful in this regard.[22] The best predictor of 50% mortality at 2 years in all groups was forced expiratory volume (FEV$_1$)expressed as percent predicted. For adult males, an FEV$_1$ of 20% or less, and for adult females and younger patients of either gender, an FEV$_1$ of 30% or less was associated with a 50% chance of death within 2 years. We regard this standard as a reasonable guideline. There are, however, limitations to a single index of function at one point in time in patients with dynamic function. It is not clear from the Toronto study whether there was any attempt to utilize a representative or average figure for FEV$_1$ as opposed to a value just prior to or after hospitalization, which might make an enormous difference. Several issues which we consider to be potential mitigating factors in pediatric candidates whose FEV$_1$ is higher than 30% predicted at the time of referral are listed in Table 1. In terms of cardiopulmonary function, patients who have a history of instability indicated by the requirement for frequent or prolonged hospitalizations, patients with increasingly resistant organisms, patients with hypoxia and/or hypercapnia out of proportion to spirometric values, patients with documented exercise intolerance, or patients with cor pulmonale would be considered even if FEV$_1$ were above the 30% predicted guideline. The microbiology and antibiotic sensitivity of *Pseudomonas* organisms can vary significantly over time and may not always correlate with clinical severity. Nonetheless, we utilize sputum cultures and antibiotic sensitivity testing in evaluating patients, treating them during the waiting period, and in the selection of postoperative antibiotic regimens.

Contraindications to lung transplantation in general are listed in Table 2. Severe scoliosis results in an immobile and distorted thorax which would make the selection of donor lungs difficult and limit the adaptability of the recipient. Poorly controlled diabetes mellitus with evidence of irreversible vascular complications is considered a contraindication. A recipient with inadequately controlled diabetes mellitus whose glycemic control measured by glycosylated hemoglobin improves during the pretransplant period will be considered if there is no vasculopathy, especially diabetic nephropathy with albuminuria. It is hoped that islet cell transplants may be available to CF lung transplant recipients with diabetes mellitus in the future. We consider *Burk-*

Table 1.

Factors Contributing to Early Consideration of Cystic Fibrosis Patients for Lung Transplantation With FEV$_1$ >30% Predicted Value

Malnutrition refractory to aggressive intervention
Cor pulmonale
Frequent hospitalizations, despite aggressive antibiotic therapy
Gas exchange abnormalities out of proportion to spirometry
Increasing antibiotic resistance of pulmonary pathogens

Table 2.

Contraindications to Lung Transplantation

Severe scoliosis
Surgical pleurectomy
Organ dysfunction: hepatic or renal insufficiency
                                 left ventricular dysfunction
                                 poorly controlled diabetes mellitus
Neoplasia
Serious psychiatric disorder
Active systemic infection
Antibiotic resistant pulmonary pathogens
Absent financial/insurance resources
Refractory noncompliance

holderia cepacia resistant to all antibiotics a contraindication, and we are reluctant to consider other patients with *B. cepacia* who have experienced rapid deterioration. Our concern is based on our own limited experience and the published experience of others.[23] *P. aeruginosa,* resistant to all antibiotics, is a relative contraindication. Previous thoracic procedures, particularly surgical pleurectomy, are also considered a relative contraindication. In patients with a previous lobectomy or chemical pleurodesis, we have encountered excessive, but manageable bleeding at the time of transplantation. Last, significant irreversible dysfunction of organs other than the lung are considered contraindications except for cor pulmonale which is reversible as long as left ventricular contractility is well preserved. Renal insufficiency defined as less than 50% of predicted glomerular filtration rate (GFR) and biliary cirrhosis with portal hypertension disqualify potential recipients in our program, although combination (liver-lung) transplants may be considered in the future in selected individuals.

Psychosocial and fiscal issues deserve a separate discussion. The rigors of therapy and expected complications after lung transplantation require a functioning, reasoned, and competent family. Because the supply of organs for transplantation is limited, we strongly believe that we have an obligation to our patients and society to exercise wise judgment with regard to patient and family capacity to handle the responsibilities of immunosuppression, daily assessment of respiratory status after discharge, and timely communication with the transplant team. To that end, we require a social work evaluation of the child and family at the time of referral. We do further psychosocial evaluation of the child and family during the initial evaluation. Formal psychologic testing is extensive. We contact the child's teacher and other significant adults in his/her life, if necessary, to judge his/her maturity and character. A history of noncompliance does not necessarily disqualify a child from consideration. However, if concerns arise from the evaluation, the child may be listed for transplant on a probationary status, with the understanding that we will provide a clear list of reasonable expectations with regard to nutrition, physical rehabilitation, chest physiotherapy, and regular clinic visits—first at the home CF Center and then at the transplant center as the patient's name rises higher on the transplant list. Our experience has been that most patients and families who are committed to transplantation are willing to focus on reasonable goals and form a therapeutic partnership with us during this period.

Transplantation is an expensive therapy. Our estimates of the costs for a lung transplant patient with CF are presented in Table 3. Although hospitals have traditionally been willing to provide standard care for members of the community independent of their ability to pay, the expenses of lung transplantation and the current realities of shrinking reimbursement for all health care services require families to have the means of paying most of their transplant-related bills. Most third party payers, including many state Medicaid programs, will consider lung transplantation. Others exclude organ transplantation in their contracts. Some families have no insurance. Community fund raising is an option which has been highly successful for some families. Transplant centers must have administrative personnel with transplant expertise who can work closely with families and third party payers. Thus, the absence of any means of payment for lung transplant is, at present, a contraindication.

PreTransplant Care

The waiting times for both children and adults for lung transplantation have increased steadily since the initiation of lung transplantation as a therapy for CF. Therefore, it is of importance to list the child or adolescent for lung transplantation as promptly as possible once the child reaches the stage of clinical disease which makes transplantation imperative. Waiting times of over 1 year are now common in many centers, especially for children over 10 years of age who are competing with adults for organs. The mortality of patients on waiting lists for pulmonary transplantation has gradually increased, such that now as many as 20% to 25% of children will die while waiting for the availability of a donor. Twelve potential candidates for lung transplantation, including two with CF, have died while waiting for transplantation in our program. In order to maximize the survival of children to the transplant procedure, close attention to the health status of prospective candidates who are waiting for transplantation is required. Such pretransplant chronic care includes weaning of steroids to the lowest possible dose consistent with adequate pulmonary function, the encouragement and maintenance of adequate nutrition by nutritional counseling, monitoring and maintenance of optimal pulmonary function by monitored physical therapy, and the prompt treatment of any pulmonary exacerbations or infections. CF candidates are asked to move to St. Louis

Table 3.

Expenses Excluding Outpatient Drug Therapy and Home Care Services for Cystic Fibrosis Patients at St. Louis Children's Hospital, 1993–1995

	Median	*Minimum*	*Maximum*
Evaluation	$13000	$2600	$38600
Pretransplant center care	$50000	$7200	$190000
Transplant hospitalization	$154000	$107000	$503250
First-year care	$57500	$2300	$376000
Second-year care	$12500	$3171	$100000

when transplantation within 6 months is likely. After coming to St. Louis, we recommend elective endoscopic maxillary sinus surgery with ethmoidectomies[24] in those patients with extensive sinus disease. The surgery and general anesthesia have been well tolerated as a general rule in our patients, even those with hypercapnia. We believe that removing nasal polyps and permitting short-term debulking of the pansinusitis, which is almost universally present in CF patients, may decrease the risk of contaminating the donor lungs after transplantation. The Stanford approach involves initial sinus surgery with repeated, usually monthly maxillary sinus lavage.[25] Intravenous antibiotics are utilized to treat even mild pulmonary exacerbations, either at home or in the hospital at the discretion of the pulmonologist in consultation with the child's family, who are seen by a pediatric pulmonologist every week while waiting for transplantation. Aerobic exercise with continuous oximetry supervised by an experienced pediatric physical therapist 3 to 5 days per week is performed by the child waiting for transplant.

Donor Issues

Matching of donor and recipient size is extremely important in pediatric lung transplantation.[26] The transverse chest dimensions and vertical measurements of the chest cavities from the diaphragm to the apex on chest radiograph are compared in order to minimize the occurrence of potential space problems and to optimize tension on the diaphragm so as to permit good pulmonary function in patients who have had chronically hyperinflated lungs prior to transplant. Excessive size of the donor lungs in comparison to the recipient's chest cavity can result in pulmonary tamponade of the heart when the chest is closed. In this circumstance, it may be necessary to trim the transplanted lungs to allow adequate room for chest closure. For this reason, it is desirable to have donor lungs slightly smaller or the same size than the recipient's chest cavity for bilateral single lung transplantation (BSLT). Often the hyperinflated and expanded chest cavity of the recipient will remodel nicely to accommodate the smaller transplanted lungs and the slight downsizing of the lungs has not been associated with significant space problems in our experience.

The predicted vital capacity of the recipient of double lung transplantation has been correlated with ultimate post-transplant lung volumes in previous studies.[27] Whether weight, chest measurements, age, or height comparison of donor and recipient, or some other factor will prove to be the best predictor of donor and recipient size match has not yet been determined; however, in our experience, age and height have correlated well with the critical variable of bronchial size in pediatric patients. Nevertheless, in pulmonary transplantation in children with CF, significant size discrepancies between donor and recipient have been tolerated with good functional results.

Because CF is a septic lung process and implantation of a single lung would result in chronic contamination of the transplanted lung by secretions from the remaining contaminated lung, BSLT is the preferred technique in children and adults with CF. Assessment of the potential donor for possible significant lung injury which may predispose to pulmonary infectious complications is important; however, use of two lungs in the CF patient makes it possible to utilize donor lungs when there is some evidence for contusion or trauma to one of the potential donor lungs by history and chest radiography. We have utilized flexible fiberoptic bronchoscopy to detect purulent secretions or significant contamination by aspiration into the donor lungs. Additionally, visual assessment of the lungs prior to harvesting at the time of thoracotomy is important in order to evaluate the presence of any significant traumatic injury or infiltrates. Adequate oxygenation, as assessed by a PaO_2 of greater than 300 mm Hg on an FIO_2 of 1.0 with a positive end-expiratory pressure (PEEP) of 5 mm Hg is mandatory for consideration of the donor for lung transplantation. With adequate gas exchange by this criterion, ischemic times of up to 8 hours have been tolerated with good functional results in the transplanted lungs.

The technique of donor harvest has been described elsewhere.[28] The lungs are removed en bloc and transported to the transplanting center prior to separation of the lungs for bilateral sequential lung transplantation. With cooperation between the heart and lung transplant harvesting teams, adequate atrial cuffs can be created for both the lung transplant pulmonary venous anastomoses and the left atrial anastomosis of the donor heart.

Technique of Operation

Although lung transplantation for CF initially was done by the en bloc double lung technique, the majority of transplant surgeons now use the bilateral sequential technique to improve bronchial revascularization and, in some cases, to avoid the need for

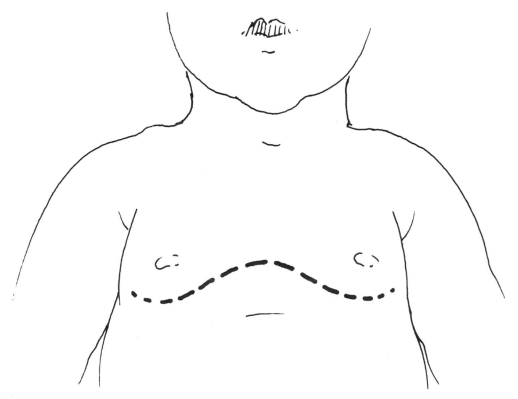

Figure 2A. Chest incision utilized for lung transplantation in children.

cardiopulmonary bypass. Tracheal anastomotic complications with the en bloc double lung transplant technique have been significant.[29] Although BSLT can be performed through a median sternotomy incision, the use of a bilateral thoracotomy incision crossing the sternum transversely has made exposure of the pleural spaces much easier and has allowed takedown of often significant adhesions between the lungs and the chest wall in patients with CF who may have had previous pleurodesis or lobectomy.[30] In addition, this incision permits easy exposure of the heart for use of cardiopulmonary bypass if necessary. For these reasons, the bilateral thoracosternotomy technique has become our incision of choice for lung transplantation (Figure 2).

The majority of children who undergo pediatric lung transplantation require the use of cardiopulmonary bypass for the procedure. The use of cardiopulmonary bypass eliminates the need for double lumen endotracheal tubes or bronchial blockers which

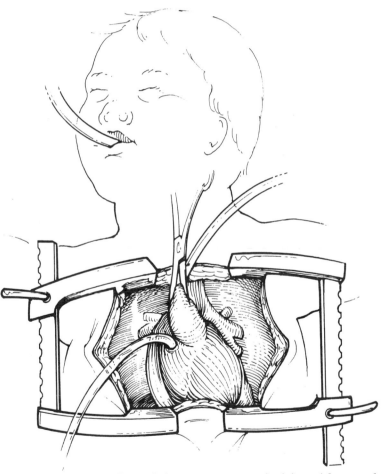

Figure 2B. Exposure through the bilateral thoracosternotomy incision with cannulation for bypass, aortic cross-clamping if necessary, and excision of both recipient lungs prior to implantation of each donor lung sequentially. (Reproduced with permission from Spray TL: Heart-lung and lung transplantation in children. In: *Glenn's Thoracic and Cardiovascular Surgery*. Appleton & Lange; 1491–1507, 1996.)

are cumbersome and often not suitable for use in very small children or small adolescents. The copious secretions in CF patients make single lung ventilation difficult, and can result in contamination of the newly transplanted lung when the bilateral sequential technique is performed. In addition, the hyperinflation and stiffness of the lungs have made it difficult to dissect the hilum in many children with CF at the time of transplant.

Although cardiopulmonary bypass has not been routinely used in adult lung transplant programs for CF patients, it has been utilized in virtually all children who undergo BSLT at St. Louis Children's Hospital. The bilateral transverse thoracotomy incision has permitted cannulation for bypass in the chest, avoiding the need to cannulate small femoral vessels in children. In addition, it has been possible to remove both lungs, cleanse and irrigate the blind trachea with antibiotic solution before implantation of the donor lungs, thus preventing spill-over contamination of the transplanted lung in patients who have copious secretions. This avoidance of contamination is particularly important in patients whose respiratory tracts are infected with multiple antibiotic resistant *Pseudomonas* species. Although significant periods of cardiopulmonary bypass have been necessary in many of our patients, there have been no complications of bypass noted in these children to date. We have found it useful to utilize aprotinin (Trasylol®) to aid in decreasing the amount of postoperative hemorrhage in CF patients during transplantation. The use of this drug has decreased bleeding both in adult patients who have not required the use of cardiopulmonary bypass and in our pediatric patients in whom cardiopulmonary bypass is routinely utilized.[31]

The technical aspects of pulmonary transplantation in children are similar to those in adult patients. After making a bilateral transverse thoracotomy incision crossing the sternum in the midline and ligation of the internal mammary pedicles, the chest is entered through the fourth or fifth intercostal space bilaterally. Any indwelling central venous catheter is removed if it crosses the area for the chest incision. The pericardium is opened and the heart suspended in a pericardial cradle, and sutures placed in the aorta and right atrium for cannulation for bypass. Dissection of pleural adhesions is completed as much as possible before heparin is given in order to decrease the magnitude of hemorrhage on bypass. Nevertheless, the hyperinflated nature of the lungs in CF patients often makes dissection in the hilum of the lung difficult and, therefore, once pleural adhesions are taken down as completely as possible, bypass is initiated. Single aortic and right atrial cannulation is generally used. With the patient on cardiopulmonary bypass at a systemic temperature of 34°C, the hilum of the lung is dissected bilaterally. The branches of the pulmonary artery are ligated and divided, as are the branches of the pulmonary veins. The pulmonary veins are divided as far into the parenchyma of the lung as possible to maximize the length of the pulmonary veins in order to accomplish the widest possible anastomosis to the recipient pulmonary venous confluence. Bronchial arterial supply to the lung is carefully controlled with ligaclips and cautery, and the bronchi mobilized bilaterally back to within 1 cm of the carina. The bronchi are then stapled, divided, and both lungs are removed. While the donor lungs are prepared for anastomosis, the anesthesiologist suctions the trachea well and instills antibiotic solution tailored to the sensitivities of the organisms cultured from the patient preoperatively in order to cleanse the trachea and decrease the bacterial contamination of the newly transplanted lungs. The donor bronchi are then trimmed approximately two cartilaginous rings from the takeoff of the upper lobe orifices bilaterally, and the lungs are then implanted sequentially using absorbable suture for the anastomoses in children in hopes of encouraging maximum growth. We utilize a running suture for the membranous bronchus and then interrupted sutures for the cartilaginous portion of the bronchus. In addition, the pulmonary arterial and pulmonary venous anastomoses are created using running absorbable suture. Just prior to completion of the pulmonary venous anastomosis, the pulmonary arterial clamp is briefly released in order to evacuate air prior to completion of the venous anastomosis and full release of the clamps.

Although early in the lung transplantation experience omental pedicles were used to wrap the bronchial anastomosis in order to maximize revascularization and to prevent disruption or erosion into the pulmonary artery, several centers have now shown that omental wraps are not necessary.[32] In addition, the thin and tenuous nature of omentum in many malnourished pediatric patients has led to abandonment of its use for bronchial wrapping. Many children with CF have had a gastrostomy for feeding purposes, and entering the abdomen and taking down adhesions for mobilization of the omentum is more complicated in these children. We have utilized pericardial pedicles taken down at the time of opening the pericardium as a means of wrapping the bronchial anastomoses, although in our more recent experience no bronchial wrap has been used. Peribronchial tissue of donor and recipient is tacked around the bronchial anastomosis with absorbable sutures to cover the suture line. We have not identified any increase in the incidence of anastomotic complications with the use of this technique.

Bronchial anastomoses in children have been performed in an end-to-end fashion. In our experience, the utilization of absorbable suture prevents residual foreign body in the airway and may maximize growth potential. If donor and recipient size discrepancy is severe, a telescoping bronchial anastomosis of the smaller bronchus into the larger bronchus is performed.

After completion of implantation of both lungs, the trachea is again suctioned extensively and irrigated, and then ventilation begun and the patient weaned off cardiopulmonary bypass. With the use of cardiopulmonary bypass and removal of both lungs prior to implantation of the donor lungs, ischemic times can be minimized, since it is not necessary to dissect the recipient lung and remove it prior to implantation of the second lung as is required in a sequential bilateral lung transplant technique without the use of cardiopulmonary bypass.

Living-Related Donors and Downsizing of Adult Lungs

Because of the smaller sizes of children waiting for transplantation, it was hoped that the waiting times for lungs would be significantly shorter in this group than for adult patients. In spite of this theoretical advantage, however, it is clear that the average waiting time for pediatric donor lungs is now 6 months to 1 year in our center. Significant mortality may occur in children waiting for pulmonary transplantation. Because some adult lung transplant recipients are small due to chronic illness and smaller lungs can be utilized in significantly larger adults due to the capacity of the lung to expand and of the thorax to remodel, the number of organs available for pediatric patients is quite limited. In addition, there are relatively few pediatric donors available nationwide, and large lungs from adult patients may not be suitable for use in pediatric recipients due to problems with pulmonary tamponade of the heart. Thus, a potential source of organs for lung transplantation in children are downsized adult lungs or living-related donor lobes.

While it may be possible to utilize a single lung from an adult as two lobes implanted into separate chest cavities for a bilateral sequential transplant in a child, the range of volumes of lobes in adult patients would limit this technique to children between 8 to 10 years of age in most cases. In addition, the much larger number and longer waiting times for lung transplants by adult patients in the United States make the chance of obtaining a suitable large adult lung relatively unlikely for a pediatric recipient waiting for lung transplantation. Thus, although there may be rare instances where downsizing of adult lungs can be performed for pediatric CF recipients, it is unlikely that a significant number of these procedures will occur.

Another potential ready source for donor lungs are the parents or other family members of the CF patient. Several BSLT have been performed from living-related donors to date.[33] While there may be some hope that living-related lungs may be less subject to rejection, at present there is no evidence to support such a contention. In addition, the growth potential of adult pulmonary lobes in pediatric recipients has not been demonstrated, although there has been some experimental evidence to suggest that growth will occur in the immature lung after it is used for transplant.[34,35] Lobar tissue from adults may offer adequate lung volume. In the experimental animal after transplantation of a mature lobe, alveolar number does not increase along with alveolar volume.[36,37] Reduced potential for lung growth is less likely to be a major concern in the child with CF needing lung transplantation, since very few children with CF will require transplantation before the age of 8 to 10 years. Use of living-related adult lobes for transplantation into children with CF is likely to be a particular benefit in severely ill patients with acute exacerbations of their pulmonary disease who would otherwise die before a suitable cadaveric donor was available.

At St. Louis Children's Hospital, we have reserved consideration of living-related lobar transplantation to those children with CF who require intubation, and have already been evaluated and placed on the waiting list for a cadaveric donor. In these patients, once intubation is required for progressive respiratory insufficiency, survival is unlikely if a donor is not available within 1 to 4 weeks. In addition, our own experience with these children has been that even when donor lungs become available within days after intubation, the postoperative course may be prolonged. Thus, it may be reasonable to consider living-related lobar transplantation from the parent to a CF patient once intubation is required, but before septic complications intervene. To date, we have performed three living donor transplants in CF patients: one involving parents; the second a father and an uncle; and the third, unrelated family friends for an adopted child. All patients were on mechanical ventilatory support. Short-term follow-up has been good with all three patients discharged from the hospital on room air. Because donation of pulmonary lobes subjects both parents to a real, albeit small, risk and removes them from participation in the immediate post-transplant care of the recipient, we do not believe that routine use of living-related donors is warranted at the present time in children who are otherwise stable and can wait for a cadaveric donor. Careful evaluation of living-related donors and recipients within the few centers most active in this procedure will provide valuable guidance for all physicians involved in lung transplantation, especially for children and adolescents.

Postoperative Care

Immunosuppression is critical to the survival of organ transplant patients. Most lung transplant centers utilize the same triple immunosuppressant protocol as used in other solid organ transplantation (Table 4). Experience has led current practice to higher dosing for most of the immunosuppressants in the context of lung transplantation compared to kidney, liver, and heart transplantation. The presumed reasons for the higher propensity for graft rejection when the target is the lung are: 1) the enormous endothelial surface area within the lung, which may express the antigens of the major histocompatibility complex; and 2) the large number and type of immune effector cells, which reside in the lung under normal circumstances to dispose of the infectious and particulate debris inhaled on a constant basis. In most centers, cyclosporine (CsA) is the mainstay of immunosuppression. CsA is begun either intraoperatively or immediately postoperatively as an IV infusion. We prefer a loading dose (0.5 mg/kg over 2 hours) followed by a constant infusion of 0.1 mg/kg/hr up to 4.0 mg/hr. Transition to oral dosing occurs after extubation and the commencement of oral feedings. We give pancreatic enzyme supplementation with oral CsA because its solvent is corn oil, glycerol, and other lipophilic agents in capsule form and olive oil in the oral solution. The initial dose for CF patients with pancreatic insufficiency is 7.5 to 10 mg/kg twice daily. Trough blood levels are followed daily for the first 2 weeks and then less frequently with

---

Table 4.

Immunosuppresant Regimen After Lung Transplantation for Cystic Fibrosis Patients

Preoperative: Azathioprine 2–3 mg/kg IV

Immediate postoperative:

        Azathioprine 2–3 mg/kg IV daily
        Cyclosporine 0.5 mg/kg IV over 2 hours, then 0.1 mg/kg/hr (maximum
           dose: 4.5 mg/hr) titrated to a steady state serum level of 300–400 ng/mL
           (whole blood)
        Methylprednisolone 0.5 mg/kg IV on arrival in intensive care unit and
           then each AM
        Antithymocyte globulin 10–15 mg/kg IV for 7 days in selected patients

After resumption of enteral feedings:

        Azathioprine 2–3 mg/kg orally, daily
        Cyclosporine 6–8 mg/kg P.O. every 12 hours with pancreatic enzyme
           supplement titrated to trough level of 300–350 ng/mL
        Prednisone 0.5 mg/kg orally each AM

AT 12 months post-transplant:

        Azathioprine 2–3 mg/kg orally, daily
        Cyclosporine titrated to trough level of 250 ng/mL
        Prednisone 0.2 mg/kg orally each AM (maximum dose 10 mg)

stability in the patient's condition and blood levels.[38,39] The target for CsA trough level in the early post-transplant period is 300 to 400 ng/mL. Azathioprine is given intravenously on a daily basis at a dose of 2 to 3 mg/kg and then changed to oral administration at the same time as the CsA. Complete blood cell counts and transaminases are utilized to monitor for azathioprine toxicity. Except for transient neutropenia, our patients have tolerated this drug extremely well. Our use of corticosteroids has evolved over the past 3 years. We originally withheld steroids for the first week after transplantation to enhance wound healing, but over the last 2 years, we have initiated intravenous methylprednisolone on arrival in the intensive care unit (ICU) after surgery at a dose of 0.5 mg/kg/d. It is our impression that we have seen fewer and milder episodes of organ rejection since introducing steroids immediately in the postoperative period. Last, we have utilized antilymphocyte preparations, primarily Minnesota antilymphocyte globulin and, more recently, antithymocyte globulin, selectively in those patients in the first week after surgery if the patient is hypergammaglobulinemic and there have been no resistant bacteria on recent sputum culture.

Antimicrobial therapy after transplantation is critically important in CF patients.[40,41] Our surgical technique permits cleansing and irrigation of the trachea and proximal mainstem bronchi, which decreases the likelihood of contaminating the transplanted lungs with a high density load of *Pseudomonas* organisms. We utilize an antibiotic regimen based on the most recent pretransplant sputum culture and sensitivity testing. Generally, tobramycin and a beta lactam or fluoroquinolone antibiotics are utilized both preoperatively and postoperatively. Vancomycin is added to prevent methicillin resistant *Staphylococcus* and other gram positive organisms which may be transmitted to the patient via the donor lungs or the operative procedure itself. Aminoglycoside and vancomycin serum drug levels are monitored carefully because of the frequency of mild renal insufficiency and associated decreased renal drug clearance occurring in the first days after transplantation. Intravenous antibiotics are usually given for 7 to 10 days after transplantation or until thoracostomy tubes have been removed. If there is no indication of ongoing lower respiratory infection, aerosolized tobramycin 80 to 160 mg tid or colistin 150 mg tid is substituted for 4 to 6 weeks at the time that intravenous antibiotics are discontinued. Although the lower airways of the transplanted lungs no longer demonstrate the electrophysiologic properties of CF, the trachea does. During the critical period of anastomotic healing, we prefer this aggressive antibiotic approach.

If the CF recipient has had either *C. albicans* or *Aspergillus* species consistently in the sputum cultures monitored pretransplant, or if there is a history of allergic bronchopulmonary aspergillosis (ABPA), we have used a prophylactic program of intravenous amphotericin B 0.25 mg/kg/d for 7 to 10 days followed by a 2-week course of aerosolized amphotericin B 10 mg bid or tid. All patients are given nystatin 500,000 units by mouth, "swish and swallow" from extubation onward. For those who find nystatin particularly distasteful, we substitute clotrimazole troches bid. If *Aspergillus* is cultured from bronchoalveolar lavage (BAL) cultures beyond the first month, oral itraconazole is usually prescribed for a minimum of 1 month with careful attention to impact on CsA clearance.[42]

If the recipient or donor is positive for cytomegalovirus (CMV) IgG antibody before transplant, we utilize a prophylactic course of ganciclovir 5 mg/kg IV daily for 6 to 8 weeks. We screen for CMV infections via blood buffy coat cultures every 2 weeks during the first 3 months post-transplant and CMV IgM antibody conversion if the recipient is seronegative at the time of transplant.

P. carinii pneumonia is a preventable pulmonary infection after organ transplantation. We begin trimethoprim-sulfamethoxazole within the first 2 weeks at a dose of 20 mg/kg of trimethoprim once daily. At the time of discharge from the hospital, the schedule is changed to the same dose 3 mornings per week. In patients who are allergic to sulfa antibiotics, aerosolized pentamidine at a dose of 300 mg once a month can be given instead.

As might be expected in children with a chronically infected airway, a significant incidence of bronchial anastomotic complications (disruption or stenosis of bronchial suture lines and bronchomalacia) has been noted in our patients. Localized airway complications have been managed with placement of silastic stents (Hood Labs, Pembroke, MA, USA) which have generally been successful in preventing progressive stenosis of the anastomoses in our pediatric patients. In our limited experience with pediatric lung transplantation, it is unclear that the technique of bronchial anastomosis or the age of the patient significantly affects the incidence or severity of bronchial complications. One CF patient in our series developed early *Aspergillus* infection of the bronchial anastomosis and after disruption had occurred on two separate occasions in the first 10 days after transplant, she required pneumonectomy of the transplanted right lung. An additional patient developed bronchial dehiscence with mediastinal cavity formation which eventually healed without further intervention. Other children have had bronchomalacia or localized anastomotic disruption resulting in stenosis which has required dilatation and implantation of stents (Figure 3).

A mainstay in the care of the lung transplant recipient is careful monitoring. We utilize pulse oximetry both during the transplant hospitalization and after discharge. Oxyhemoglobin saturation is a physiologic parameter sensitive to subtle changes in lung health. Spirometry requires relative freedom from thoracic discomfort, and is not very practical in children until they have been transferred to the floor and the thoracostomy tubes have been removed. The use of serial spirometry after discharge is almost universally used in adult lung transplant programs. We procure a portable spirometer with printer (Puritan-Bennett model PB110, Wilmington, MA, USA) and ask our patients to measure spirometry twice daily after discharge. A drop in FEV_1 of more than 10% for 2 consecutive days is considered significant enough to merit a call to the transplant nurse, pulmonologist, or primary physician.

Flexible fiberoptic bronchoscopy (FFB) is utilized to monitor bronchial anastomotic healing and to test the transplanted lungs for infection and rejection.[43,44] Our general protocol for surveillance FFB is shown in Figure 4. The initial bronchoscopy occurs approximately 24 hours after admission to the ICU. The goal of the procedure is to inspect the anastomosis for configuration and integrity, assess the bronchial mucosa of the transplanted lungs for color indicating adequacy of blood flow, and to perform the first BAL for culture for bacteria, fungi, and viruses. Subsequent procedures almost always include transbronchial biopsies. We use a 4.9 mm flexible fiberoptic bronchoscope (Olympus PD30, Tokyo, Japan) with video attachment to record anatomic findings for future review and comparisons. Standard cup forceps (small or large depending on patient size) are used for transbronchial biopsy; we generally choose a single lower lobe based on auscultation and recent radiograph, and perform a minimum of six separate biopsies under fluoroscopy. Unless otherwise indicated, we

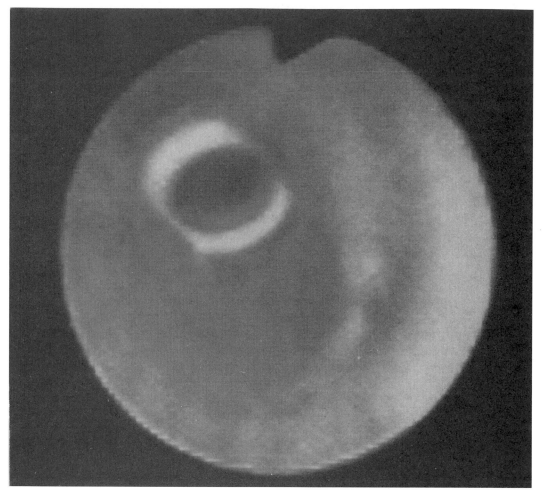

Figure 3. Endoscopic view of silastic stent placed across bronchial anastomosis in a child following bilateral sequential lung transplantation. The flange on the stent seats the stent across the anastomosis preventing stenosis or malacia.

alternate lungs on consecutive procedures. In our experience, it is more difficult to obtain satisfactory specimens from the upper lobes, yet we do not hesitate to use the upper lobe if radiographically indicated, or if there have been several recent biopsies involving both lower lobes. The frequency of procedure depends on the patient's clinical course. In addition to the surveillance times for biopsy listed in Figure 4, patients are rebiopsied 2 weeks after methylprednisolone bolus for acute vascular rejection or 3 to 4 weeks after completing cytolytic therapy to assess response to augmented immunosuppression. BAL and transbronchial biopsy with immunohistochemistry are required to identify CMV pneumonitis in a definitive manner. In other instances of suspected acute lower respiratory infection, bronchoscopy with BAL with or without transbronchial biopsy is usually performed if practical. The greater the time since transplant and the greater the distance from the transplant center, the less likely is bronchoscopy to be performed and empiric treatment chosen instead.

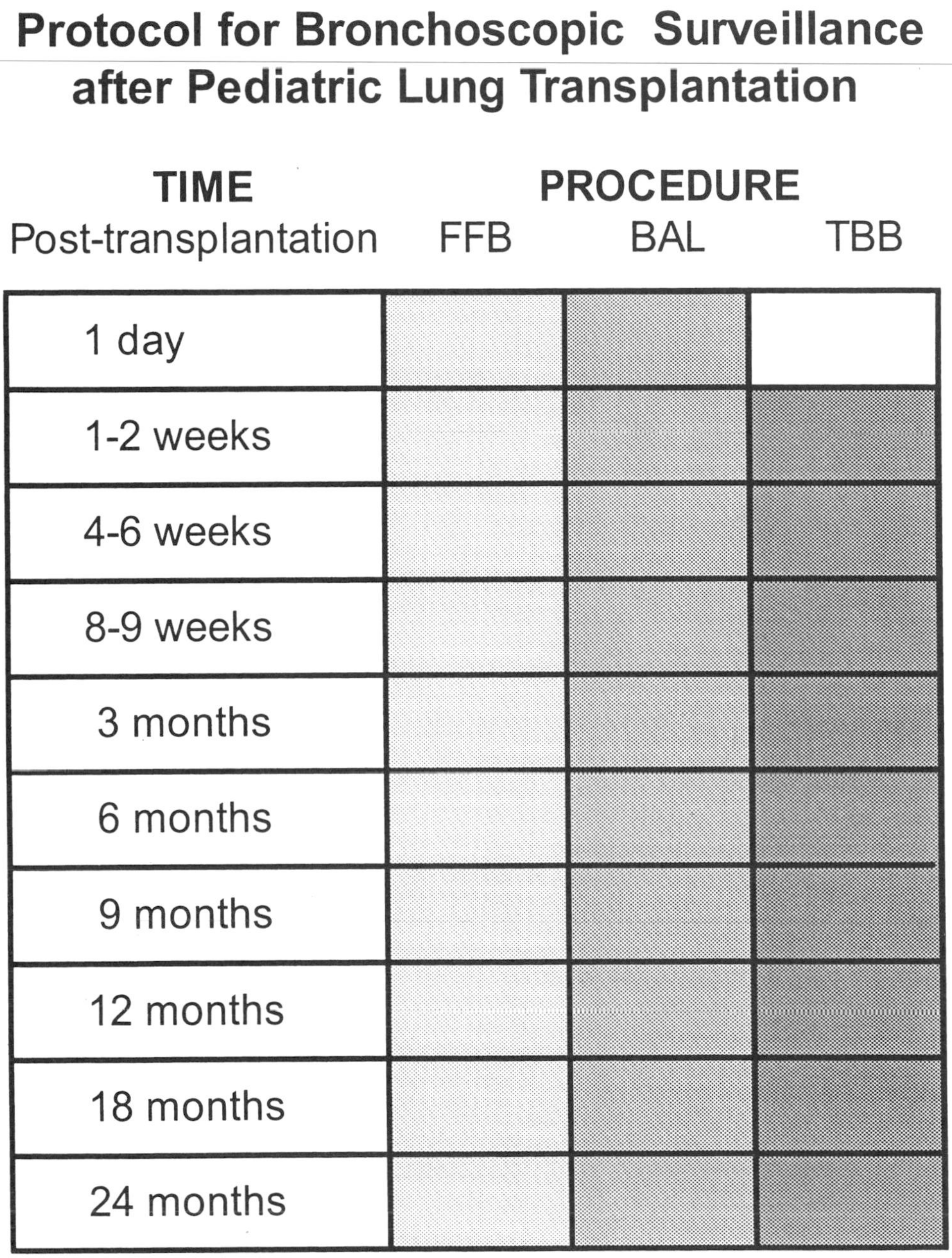

Protocol for Bronchoscopic Surveillance
after Pediatric Lung Transplantation

TIME	PROCEDURE		
Post-transplantation	FFB	BAL	TBB
1 day			
1-2 weeks			
4-6 weeks			
8-9 weeks			
3 months			
6 months			
9 months			
12 months			
18 months			
24 months			

Figure 4. Schedule of surveillance bronchoscopies.

The infections which affect lung transplant patients after the initial hospitalization can be divided into categories (Table 5). Reactivation of latent viruses may involve any of the herpes family viruses. Herpes simplex virsus (HSV) rarely causes a severe systemic infection; more commonly, it causes a typical focal vesicular eruption. Although clinical diagnosis is straightforward, our practice is to scrape and culture all

Table 5.

Infections Which Affect Lung Transplant Recipients

Viruses
    Herpes simplex
    Varicella zoster
    Ebstein Barr virus
    Cyctomegalovirus
    Adenovirus
    Respiratory syncytial virus
    Parainfluenza
    Influenza
Bacteria
    Pseudomonas aeruginosa
    Other gram negative organisms
    Staphylococcus aureus
    Staphylococcus epidermis
Fungi
    Candida albicans
    Torulopsis glabrata
    Aspergillus fumigatus
    other aspergillus species

suspicious vesicular eruptions. Treatment of focal herpetic dermatitis is a 2-week course of oral acyclovir; a longer course of treatment may be necessary if the patient has recently had an episode of rejection or is undergoing augmentation of immuno-suppression. Primary varicella infection is more common in children than adults because of exposure. Patients who have absent IgG antibody to varicella are identified prior to transplant and then followed carefully after any exposure to an infectious vector. We have avoided the expense and difficulty of procuring varicella-zoster immune globulin and have chosen early and aggressive treatment of clinical varicella in the post-transplant patient with intravenous acyclovir with good results to date. In this way, effective long-term immunity, hopefully, will follow. Reactivation of varicella as shingles does occur in transplant patients with serologic protection from natural infection. Since the dose of oral acyclovir is higher for the treatment of herpes zoster than for HSV, culture of the scraped vesicles is recommended. Epstein-Barr virus (EBV) is a greater danger to the child without previous infection than is reactivation of the virus in a child who has been serology-positive prior to immunosuppression. EBV appears to be the primary risk factor for post-transplant lymproliferative disorder (PTLD).[45] Seven of our patients (five with CF) have developed PTLD, four of which were associated with primary EBV infection and two with reactivation of EBV. Three of the patients succumbed to this complication. We survey all of our EBV-negative recipients with EBV serologies monthly after transplantation. In the event of primary infection, immunosuppression is reduced as follows: CsA decreased to give whole blood trough levels of 200 to 250 ng/mL; azathioprine dose halved; and prednisone dose halved. Oral acyclovir is added in a dose of 20 mg/kg/d. We believe the keys to treating PTLD are a high degree of suspicion and early diagnosis and treatment.[46] In terms of prevention, we now have all blood products used during and after surgery irradiated and passed through a leukocyte-trapping filter to lessen the chance of passing live virus, active or latent, to our patients.

CMV has been the most feared pathogen for transplant physicians in previous decades.[47,48] Now that therapy is available in different forms, CMV has lost some of its ignominious reputation. We believe that a well-informed, systematic approach can prevent most of the morbidity and virtually all the mortality associated with CMV in the preganciclovir era.[49] We use ganciclovir prophylaxis in the first 6 weeks post-transplant as indicated earlier in situations where either the donor or the recipient is serology-positive for CMV. In the less common situation when both the recipient and the donor are CMV serology-negative, we ask for all blood products to be from CMV-negative donors. We screen these patients weekly with buffy coat cultures with shell vial assay during the first weeks after transplantation. The hallmark for diagnosing CMV pneumonitis is a patient with positive BAL and transbronchial biopsy. Biopsies which demonstrate histopathology typical of CMV pneumonitis are confirmed with immuno-histochemistry. Treatment of symptomatic CMV pneumonitis includes 2 to 3 weeks of intravenous ganciclovir 5 mg/kg bid. If the symptoms are associated with significant impairment of lung function and/or oxygenation, CMV hyperimmune globulin is also given daily for 1 week, then weekly for an additional 2 to 4 weeks depending on response to therapy. Ganciclovir is also given in patients during and for 1 week after cytolytic therapy to prevent reactivation of disease. Asymptomatic patients with positive buffy coat or BAL cultures in whom transbronchial biopsies are negative for interstitial pneumonitis and CMV antigen are observed, not treated.

Other viral infections are common. Most school-aged children return to school within 3 to 6 months after transplantation and are thus exposed to community pathogens. Most respiratory viral infections are minor and have minimal effect on SaO_2 or FEV_1. Others are more potentially serious. Influenza A and B, parainfluenza, adenovirus, and respiratory syncytial virus (RSV) are well-known respiratory pathogens with a predilection to more severe infection in immunocompromised patients. Influenza vaccine should be given each autumn. Because antibody response to vaccine may be suboptimal, both a second dose in early winter and the use of amantadine or rimantidine with symptomatic illnesses during a known influenza A epidemic is recommended. The only available specific treatment for influenza B, adenovirus, parainfluenza, and RSV is ribavirin, which is available only in the inhaled form.[50] This treatment should be considered in severe infections, but must be given early in the course of the infection to be effective.

Bacterial infections may be more common in CF patients than other transplant recipients, presumably because of the persistence of pathogenic organisms in the sinuses. Surveillance culturing by BAL of the transplanted lungs in CF patients is of particular importance, especially if the patient's pretransplant organisms are relatively or absolutely resistant to antibiotics. Most of our patients have a central venous catheter to facilitate the delivery of intravenous medications and to permit frequent blood sampling in the first 6 months after transplant. Bacteremia from central lines has occurred in almost 10% of our patients. Early diagnosis and treatment with vancomycin and a third generation cephalosporin (ceftazidime is preferred in CF patients) until culture and sensitivity testing is completed has been associated with prompt resolution of symptoms in almost all of our patients. Otitis media and symptomatic sinusitis requires aggressive oral antibiotic treatment in lung transplant patients. Refractory infections of the upper respiratory tract are an indication for surgical treatments. We choose ofloxacin as the oral drug of choice in CF patients with symptomatic sinusitis since it does not impact CsA hepatic clearance as significantly as ciprofloxacin. If the patient's upper respiratory tract organisms are known to be resistant to oral antibiotics, intravenous antibiotics may be required.

Fungal infections of the lower respiratory tract are of great concern after lung transplantation because they may be difficult to diagnose and very serious. *A. fumigatus* has been associated with both a tracheobronchitis[51] and pneumonia with invasion of the bloodstream[48,52] after transplantation. Candidal infections are less commonly serious. Differentiating a true lower respiratory tract infection from colonization especially in the context of a bronchial stent or abnormal bronchial anastomosis impairing efficient bronchial clearance is particularly difficult with candidal organisms. The false-negative rate for any diagnostic procedure, whether BAL, transbronchial biopsy, protected specimen brush, or open-lung biopsy is high. Therefore, the suspicion must be high and the threshold for treatment low. The treatment of serious lower respiratory infections is intravenous amphotericin B. When tracheobronchitis or airway colonization is suspected, aerosolized amphotericin B[53] or oral intraconazole may be used. The mortality rate for invasive *Aspergillosis* despite aggressive treatment is high. In areas where *Aspergillosis* may be common, prophylactic intraconazole may be the best approach through the first months after transplant.

Graft rejection has two major manifestations in the lung. Acute vascular rejection most commonly occurs in the first 6 months after transplant and is graded by histologic classification.[54] Although a clinical syndrome of low-grade fever, bibasilar crackles, interstitial infiltrates on chest radiograph, and hypoxemia is well described, we have found this syndrome to be nonspecific and often absent with histologically proven mild and moderate grade rejection. Thus, we try to document any suspected rejection episode with transbronchial biopsy. Mild, moderate, and severe grades of rejection are treated with intravenous methylprednisolone 10 mg/kg for 3 consecutive days. Persistent acute rejection is an indication for antithymocyte globulin (15 mg/kg/d for 10 days). The second form of rejection is obliterative bronchiolitis (OB), which is also called chronic rejection. We believe that OB may be more common in children than in infants or adults, although currently available data is insufficient to make a definitive conclusion. We do know that it is more difficult to maintain a therapeutic level of CsA in CF patients than others, which, we presume, is due to the pancreatic insufficiency and attendant inefficient fat absorption from the small intestine. Greater variability in blood levels of CsA put CF patients at greater risk of both toxic effects and inadequate immunosuppression. OB rarely occurs before 3 months after transplant. It usually presents insidiously with a gradual drop in FEV_1 without fever. There may be a semiproductive cough in some cases and a variable amount of dyspnea with exercise. Chest radiograph and chest computed tomography (CT) scan are usually normal or minimally abnormal. Ventilation perfusion nuclear medicine scans will often show heterogeneity of perfusion and focal areas of delayed wash-out of xenon. We attempt to diagnose OB via transbronchial biopsy, but the false-negative rate is high.[55] On occasion, we move to open-lung biopsy if therapeutic options depend on the diagnosis. If there is histologic evidence of active lymphocytic inflammation, cytolytic therapy and a short course of intravenous methylprednisolone is administered. Response to therapy is highly variable. Some children have had an unrelenting, rapid course; the health and pulmonary function of others have stabilized for many months at a time. Because of augmented immunosuppression and abnormalities in small airway function, these patients are at high risk of serious infection. Death from pneumonia or systemic infection is more common than uncomplicated respiratory failure in patients with severe obstructive lung disease due to OB. Retransplantation is an option about which we are more positive if the patient has not been overly immunosuppressed prior to retransplant, and there is a therapeutic strategy available which has a higher chance of success than the initial therapy.

Outcome

After successful lung transplantation, patients must take immunosuppressant medication daily and monitor their health closely for the rest of their lives. Fortunately, patients with CF are well acquainted with complex medical regimens and the imposition on their lifestyle is far less than those with pulmonary hypertension who often have a short-term relationship with chronic illness and daily medication.

By 3 months after transplantation, most patients with CF have achieved a remarkable improvement in lung function, nutrition, and general well-being. Most patients can return to school or work 3 months after surgery. In adolescents, we recommend delaying contact sports for the first 6 months after surgery to permit healing of the sternal incision. The FEV_1 of the CF patients in our program who survived the first 6 months post-transplant compared to their preoperative values are demonstrated in Figure 5.

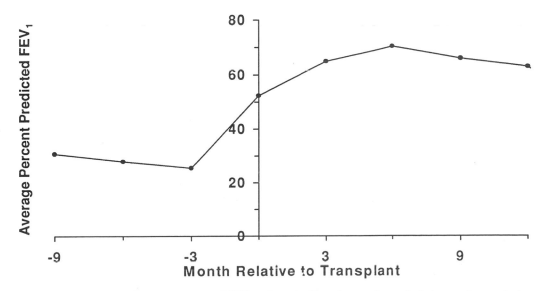

Figure 5. Lung function, measure as FEV_1, of cystic fibrosis survivors (minimum 6 months) at St. Louis Children's Hospital.

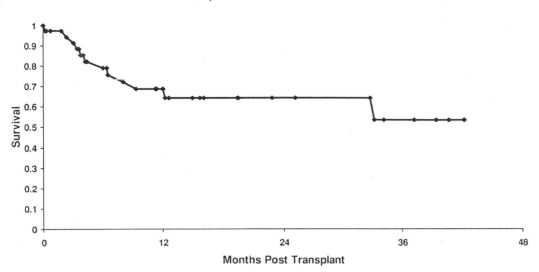

Figure 6. Kaplan-Meier survival curve for the 33 patients with cystic fibrosis who have undergone bilateral single lung transplantation at St. Louis Children's Hospital from 1990 to 1995.

Long-term survival is the goal of every transplant patient. Given that the first successful lung transplant in the post-CsA era was performed in 1983, we obviously must be cautious in projecting survival beyond 5 years. The Kaplan-Meier survival curve for our first 33 CF patients is shown in Figure 6. It should be noted that four of the nine deaths occurred in our first four patients. Causes of death have included PTLD in two, invasive *Aspergillosis* in one after retransplant for OB, primary graft failure in one, three from respiratory failure due to OB, one from unrelenting *B. cepacia* lower respiratory infection, and one from progressive pulmonary fibrosis of uncertain etiology. Of the remaining 24 patients, five have proven OB, two have suspected OB, and one has chronic PTLD in the central nervous system.

Conclusion

Our early experience with lung transplantation in children and adolescents with CF demonstrates the feasibility of the procedure and acceptable short-term survival. There are technical considerations unique to children because of variation in size between donor and recipient and the advent of living-related lung transplantation. The CF patient provides a challenge because of the severity of infection and the nature of the *Pseudomonas* organisms which are universally present in end-stage CF lungs, often with a variable antibiotic resistance. On the other hand, the long experience of CF patients and their families with chronic illness and their remarkable courage have made them a particularly attractive group of patients for lung transplantation. The major challenge of the future for all lung transplant recipients is understanding and preventing OB.

References

1. Collins FS: Cystic fibrosis: molecular biology and therapeutic implications. *Science* 256: 774–779, 1992.
2. FitzSimmons SC: The changing epidemiology of cystic fibrosis. *J Pediatr* 122:1–9, 1993.
3. Wheeler WB, Colten HR: Cystic fibrosis: correct approach to diagnosis and management. *Pediatr Rev* 9:241–248, 1988.
4. Whitehead B, Helms P, Goodwin M, et al: Heart-lung transplantation for cystic fibrosis. I: assessment. *Arch Dis Child* 66:1018–1022, 1991.
5. Whitehead B, Helms P, Goodwin M, et al: Heart-lung transplantation for terminal cystic fibrosis. II: outcome. *Arch Dis Child* 66:1018–1022, 1991.
6. DeLeval MR, Smyth R, Whitehead B, et al: Heart and lung transplantation for terminal cystic fibrosis. *J Thorac Cardiovasc Surg* 101:633–642, 1991.
7. Ramirez JC, Patterson GA, Winton TL, de Hoyos AL, Miller JD, Maurer JR: Bilateral lung transplantation for CF. *J Thorac Cardiovasc Surg* 103:287–294, 1992.
8. Tsang V, Hodson ME, Yacoub MH: Lung transplantation for cystic fibrosis. *Br Med Bull* 48:949–971, 1992.
9. Starnes VA, Lewiston N, Theodore J, et al: Cystic fibrosis: target population for lung transplantation in North America in the 1990s. *J Thorac Cardiovasc Surg* 103:1008–1014, 1992.
10. Egan M: Lung transplantation in cystic fibrosis. *Semin Respir Inf* 7:227–239, 1992.
11. Pohl M: St. Louis International Lung Transplant Registry (personal communication).
12. Santis G, Osborne L, Knight RA, Hodson ME: Independent genetic determinants of pancreatic and pulmonary status in cystic fibrosis. *Lancet* 336:1081–1084, 1990.
13. The Cystic Fibrosis Genotype-Phenotype Consortium: Correlation between genotype and phenotype in patients with cystic fibrosis. *N Engl J Med* 329:1308–1313, 1993.
14. Welsh MJ, Anderson MP, Rich DP, et al: Cystic fibrosis transmembrane conductance regulator: a chloride channel with novel regulation. *Neuron* 8:821–829, 1992.
15. Knowles M, Gratzy J, Boucher R: Increased bioelectric potential differences across respiratory epithelia in cystic fibrosis. *N Engl J Med* 305:1489–1495, 1981.
16. Quinton PM, Byman J: Higher bioelectric potentials due to decreased chloride absorption in the sweat glands of patients with cystic fibrosis. *N Engl J Med* 308:1185–1189, 1983.
17. Boucher RC, Stutts MJ, Knowles MR, Cantley L, Gratzy JJ: Sodium transport in cystic fibrosis respiratory epithelia: abnormal basal rate and response to adenylate cyclase activation. *J Clin Invest* 78:1245–1252, 1986.
18. Saiman L, Prince A: *Pseudomonas aeruginosa Pili* bind to asialo GM1 which is increased on the surface of cystic fibrosis epitheial cells. *J Clin Invest* 92:1875–1880, 1993.
19. Cabral DA, Loh BA, Speert DP: Mucoid *Pseudomonas aeruginosa* resists nonopsonic phagocytosis by human neutrophilis and macrophages. *Pediatr Res* 22:429–431, 1987.
20. Buret A, Cripps AW: The immunoevasive activities of *Pseudomonas aeruginosa:* relevance for cystic fibrosis. *Am Rev Respir Dis* 148:793–805, 1993.
21. Davis PB: Pathophysiology of pulmonary disease in cystic fibrosis. *Semin Respir Med* 6:261–270, 1985.
22. Kerem E, Reisman J, Corey M, Canny GJ, Levison H: Prediction of mortality in patients with cystic fibrosis. *N Engl J Med* 326:1187–1191, 1992.
23. Snell GI, de Hoyos A, Krajden M, Winton T, Maurer JR: *Pseudomonas cepacia* in lung transplant recipients with cystic fibrosis. *Chest* 103:466–471, 1993.
24. Lusk RP: Endoscopis approach to sinus disease. *J All Clin Immunol* 90:496–505, 1992.
25. Lewiston N, King V, Umetsu D, et al: Cystic fibrosis patients who have undergone heart-lung transplantation benefit from maxillary sinus antrostomy and repeated sinus lavage. *Transplant Proc* 23:1207–1208, 1991.
26. Noirclerc M, Shennib H, Gindicelli R: Size matching in lung transplantation. *J Heart Lung Transplant* 11:S203–S208, 1992.
27. Miyoshi S, Schaefer HJ, Trulock EP, et al: Donor selection for single and double lung transplantation: chest size matching and other factors influencing post-transplantation vital capacity. *Chest* 98:308–313, 1990.

28. Sundaresan S, Trachiotis GD, Aoe M, Patterson CA, Cooper JD: Donor lung procurement: assessment and operative technique. *Ann Thorac Surg* 56:1409–1413, 1993.
29. Patterson GA, Todd TR, Cooper JD, et al: Airway complications after double lung transplantation. *J Thorac Cardiovasc Surg* 99:14–21,1990.
30. Pasque MK, Cooper JD, Kaiser LR, et al: Improved technique for bilateral lung transplantation: rationale and initial clinical experience. *Ann Thorac Surg* 49:785–791, 1990.
31. Jacquiss RD, Huddleston CB, Spray TL: Use of aprotinin in pediatric lung transplantation. *J Heart Lung Transplant* 14:302–307, 1995.
32. LoCicero J III, Massad M, Oba J, Bresticker M, Greene R: Short-term and long-term results of experimental wrapping techniques for bronchial anastomosis. *J Thorac Cardiovasc Surg* 103:763–766, 1992.
33. Theodore PR, Starnes VA: Reduced-size lung transplantation: clinical experience. In: Kern JA, Kron IL (eds). *Reduced-Size Lung Transplantation.* Georgetown, TX: RG Landes Co.; 76–87, 1993.
34. Haverich A, Dammenhayn L, Demertzis J, Kemnitz J, Reimers P: Lung growth after experimental pulmonary transplantation. *J Heart Lung Transplant* 10:288–295, 1991.
35. Kern JA, Tribble CG, Chan BB, Flanagan TL, Kron IL: Reduced-size porcine lung transplantation: long-term studies of pulmonary vascular resistance. *Ann Thorac Surg* 53:583–589, 1992.
36. Kern JA: Function and growth potential of experimental reduced-size lung transplants. In: Kern JA, Kron IL (eds). *Reduced-Size Lung Transplantation.* Georgetown, TX: RG Landes, Co.; 54–65, 1993.
37. Kern JA: The ideal pediatric lung allograft: mature lobe versus immature whole lung. In: Kern JA, Kron IL (eds). *Reduced-Size Lung Transplantation.* Georgetown, TX: RG Landes, Co.; 54–65, 1993.
38. Mancel-Grosso V, Bertault-Peres P, Barthelemy A, Chazalette JP, Durand A, Nonclerc M: Pharmacokinetic of cyclosporine A in bilateral lung transplantation candidates with cystic fibrosis. *Transplant Proc* 22:1706–1707, 1990.
39. Tan KKC, Trull AK, Hue KL, Best NG, Wallwork J, Higgenbottan TW: Pharmacokinetics of cyclosporine in heart and lung transplant candidates and recipients with cystic fibrosis and Eisenmenger's syndrome. *Clin Pharmacol* 53:544–554, 1993.
40. Flume PA, Egan TM, Paradowski LJ, Detterbeck FC, Thompson JT, Yankaskas JR: Infectious complications of lung transplantation: impact of cystic fibrosis. *Am J Respir Crit Care Med* 149:1601–1607, 1994.
41. Kurland G, Orenstein DM: Complications of pediatric lung and heart-lung transplantation. *Curr Opin Pediatr* 6:262–271, 1994.
42. Back DJ, Tjia JF: Comparative effects of the antimycotic drugs ketoconazole, fluconazole, itraconazole, and terbinafine on the metabolism of cyclosporine by human liver metabolism. *Br J Clin Pharmacol* 32:624–626, 1991.
43. Scott JP, Higgenbotam TW, Smyth RL, et al: Transbronchial biopsies in children after heart-lung transplantation. *Pediatr* 86:698–702, 1990.
44. Kurland G, Noyes BE, Jaffe R, Atlas AB, Armitage J, Orenstein DM: Bronchoalveolar lavage and transbronchial biopsy in children following heart-lung and lung transplantation. *Chest* 104:1043–1048, 1993.
45. Randhawa PS, Yousem SA, Paradis IL, Dauber JA, Griffith BP, Locker J: The clinical spectrum, pathology, and clonal analysis of Epstein-Barr virus-associated lymphoproliferative disorders in heart-lung transplant recipients. *Am J Clin Pathol* 92:177–185, 1989.
46. Armitage JM, Kormos RL, Stuart RS, et al: Post-transplant lymphoproliferative disease in thoracic organ tranplant patients: ten years of cyclosporine-based immunosuppression. *J Heart Lung Transplant* 10:877–887, 1991.
47. Brooks RG, Hofflin JM, Jamieson SW, Stinson EB, Remington JS: Infectious complications in heart-lung transplant recipients. *Am J Med* 79:412–422, 1985.
48. Dauber JH, Paradis IL, Dummer JS: Infectious complications in pulmonary allograft recipients. *Clin Chest Med* 11:291–308, 1990.
49. Ettinger NA, Bailey TC, Trulock EP, et al: Cytomegalovirus infection and pneumonitis: impact after isolated lung transplantation. *Am Rev Respir Dis* 147:1017–1023, 1993.

50. Smith RA, Kirkpatrick W (eds): *Ribavirin: A Broad Spectrum Antiviral Agent.* New York: Academic Press; 100–120, 1980.
51. Kramer MR, Denning DW, Marshall SE, et al: Ulcerative tracheobronchitis after lung transplantation: a new form of invasive *Aspergillosis. Am Rev Respir Dis* 144:552–556, 1991.
52. Maurer JR, Tullis E, Grossman RF, Vellend H, Winton TL, Patterson GA: Infectious complications following isolated lung transplantation. *Chest* 101:1056–1059, 1992.
53. Schmitt HJ: New methods of delivery of amphotericin B. *Clin Inf Dis* 17(2):S501–S506, 1993.
54. Berry GJ, Brunt EM, Chamberlain D, et al: A working formulation for the standardization of numenclature in the diagnosis of heart and lung rejection:Lung Rejection Studt Group. *J Heart Lung Transplant* 9:593–601, 1990.
55. Kramer MR, Stoehr C, Whang JL, et al: The diagnosis of obliterative bronchiolitis after heart-lung and lung transplantion: low yield of transbronchial lung biopsy. *J Heart Lung Transplant* 12:675–681, 1993.

Chapter 15

Lung Transplantation for Pulmonary Hypertension

Kenneth L. Franco, MD

Lung and heart-lung transplantation (HLT) is offered to any patient with end-stage pulmonary or cardiopulmonary disease for which is there is no effective medical treatment. There are approximately 2000 patients waiting for transplantation in the United States; about 10% of these patients are children. The first human lung transplant was performed by Hardy et al in 1963 and the recipient survived only 18 days.[1] Over the next 20 years, approximately 40 lung transplants were performed by a number of centers with only one patient surviving a total of 10 months. The surgical procedure was technically successful, but the outcome was poor because of pulmonary sepsis, rejection, and anastomotic airway complications, a sequela of the unsophisticated immunosuppression that existed at that time. HLT was introduced clinically by Cooley and associates in 1968.[2] This report and others showed that an individual could function satisfactorily with a transplanted heart and lungs even though all patients died in the early perioperative period. In 1979, the immunosuppressive agent cyclosporine (CsA) became available and reduced the requirements for high-dose steroids in the early perioperative period. After an extensive laboratory investigation at Stanford, Reitz et al performed the first long-term successful HLT in 1981.[3] This patient, a 45-year-old woman with end-stage primary pulmonary hypertension (PH), survived more than 5 years, dying from causes unrelated to her allograft. Similarly, Cooper et al, in 1983, performed the first long-term successful isolated lung transplant on a 58-year-old man with pulmonary fibrosis.[4] This patient survived for 6 years, dying ultimately of chronic renal failure. Over the last 10 years, the field of lung transplantation has grown significantly as the results have continued to improve, due to better patient selection, surgical techniques, immunosuppression, and postoperative care. The improved results of lung transplantation in adults made it easier to extend this procedurce to children.

PH is a condition resulting from altered mechanical properties of the pulmonary vascular bed leading to increased pulmonary vascular resistance and impedance to blood flow through the lungs (Figure 1). The major consequence of this condition is

From: Franco KL (ed). *Pediatric Cardiopulmonary Transplantation.* Armonk, NY: Futura Publishing Company, Inc.; © 1997.

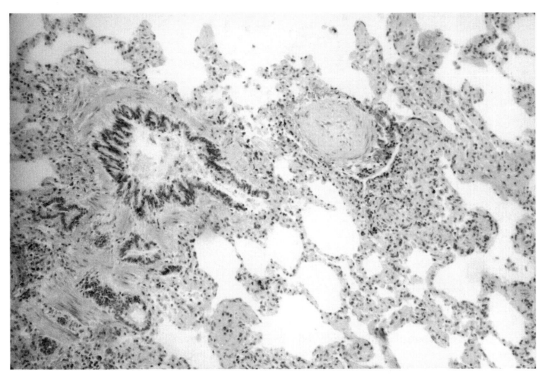

Figure 1. Lung pathology from 13-year-old boy with primary pulmonary hypertension (PH) showing pulmonary arteriopathy.

increased afterload on the right ventricle (RV) leading to structural and functional changes in that chamber of the heart. The causes of PH are listed in Table 1. The incidence of PH among children and young adults is unknown. Primary PH appears to involve young women and those of child-bearing age more than any other group.[5] The prognosis of these patients is poor once they develop symptoms of dyspnea or syncope with survival probably less than 3 years.[6] Survival was poorest in those patients with a right atrial pressure greater than 20 mm Hg, a mean pulmonary artery pressure greater than 80 mm Hg, cardiac index less than 2 L/min/m^2, and a very low mixed ve-

Table 1.

Etiology of Pulmonary Hypertension

1. Primary pulmonary hypertension
2. Eisenmenger's syndrome (PH and congenital heart defect)
3. PH after repaired congenital heart defect
4. Thromboembolic
5. Congenital pulmonary vein stenosis
6. Inadequate pulmonary vascular bed
    a. Pulmonary atresia, ventricular septal defect
    b. Congenital diaphragmatic hernia

PH = pulmonary hypertension

nous oxygen saturation.[7] Since the waiting time for lung donors has increased to several years at many programs, it would seem prudent to list patients with PH as soon as the diagnosis is made.

Recipient Selection

Lung transplantation and HLT is appropriate for any patient with PH who develops disabling end-stage pulmonary disease and whose life expectancy is less than 2 years. Ideally, these patients should be in good condition apart from their lung disease and not desperately ill, infected, or suffering from multisystem organ failure. Patients should have adequate nutrition, be medically compliant, have no contraindications to immunosuppression, and have strong family support. The indications for lung transplantation and HLT are listed in Table 2. Single lung transplantation (SLT) for PH

Table 2.

Recipient Operation for Pulmonary Hypertension

1. Single lung transplantation (SLT)

PH and adequate right heart function

Eisenmenger's syndrome with correctable intracardiac lesion

Advantages:	More organs available for other recipients
	More transplants
	Shorter waiting time
	Technical ease of operation
Disadvantages:	Early hemodynamic instability
	V/Q imbalance and decreased reserve if allograft dysfunction develops

2. Bilateral Single Lung Transplantation (BSLT)

PH and adequate right heart function

Eisenmenger's syndrome with correctable intracardiac lesion

Advantages:	Use of marginal donors
	Use if recipient lives long distance from transplant center
	More reserve if allograft dysfunction develops
Disadvantages:	Less transplants
	Longer waiting time
	Longer operation and cardiopulmonary bypass time

3. Heart-Lung Transplantation (HLT)

PH and biventricular failure

Eisenmenger's syndrome with noncorrectable complex congenital heart disease

Advantages:	More secure airway anastomosis
	More reserve if lung allograft dysfunction develops
Disadvantages:	Less transplants
	Longer waiting time
	More difficult operation

PH = pulmonary hypertension; V/Q = ventilation/perfusion

requires adequate or reversible right heart function. Patients with fixed PH and congenital heart defects, such as atrial septal defect,[8] ventricular septal defect,[9] or patent ductus arteriosus,[10] are candidates for surgical correction at the time of lung transplantation. Bilateral single lung transplantation (BSLT) may be the operation of choice if there is an adequate donor supply, because it avoids the early hemodynamic instability seen with patients after SLT and allows a greater reserve if allograft dysfunction develops postoperatively. HLT should be reserved for those patients with complex congenital heart disease or severe biventricular failure.

Patients referred for transplantation are evaluated by the transplant team and undergo an extensive workup which includes a history, physical exam, and a battery of laboratory tests and procedures. The procedures include two-dimensional or transesophageal echocardiogram (ECHO) of the heart, left ventricle (LV) and RV ejection fractions by nuclear angiocardiography, right heart catheterization with pharmacologic testing, and angiography to define the anatomy and collaterals in patients with congenital heart disease.

Contraindictions to lung transplantation and HLT include an active extra pulmonary systemic infection, severe malnutrition, cirrhosis, renal failure, systemic disease limiting survival, obesity, and prolonged ventilatory dependence. Prolonged ventilatory dependence makes these patients more prone to airway sepsis, multisystem organ failure; in addition, they have poor stamina and will have a difficult time being weaned from the ventilator early postoperatively which places them at high risk for airway complications. Tracheostomy is a contraindication for HLT, but not lung transplantation. Previous cardiothoracic surgery or pleurodesis used to be a contraindication to HLT and BSLT, but is no longer the case as many programs have adopted the clamshell incision (Figure 2). This incision involves bilateral anterolateral thoracotomies with transection of the sternum, and allows excellent exposure of the mediastinum and both pleural cavities. Pleurodesis and previous thoracic surgery are not contraindications to SLT because most surgeons will transplant the other side. Diabetes mellitus is not a contraindiction to transplantation, unless it is poorly controlled or there is end-organ involvement such as renal failure, myocardial dysfunction, or severe peripheral vascular disease. Patients who need chronic vascular access either for hyperalimentation or antibiotic therapy should have lines placed on the left side if they are being considered for HLT to protect the right internal jugular vein which is used for postoperative endomyocardial biopsy procedures.

Patients with PH who deteriorate while awaiting transplantation may respond to selective pulmonary vasodilators like prostacyclin or nitric oxide (NO) (Figure 3) with a lowering of pulmonary artery pressures and improvement in RV function. Patients can be maintained on continuous intravenous infusions of prostacyclin until a suitable donor is found.[11] There have been isolated reports of patients being rescued by an atrial septostomy.[12] This procedure can be performed percutaneously and unloads the RV with improvement in overall cardiac function, but at the expense of arterial desaturation. In addition, extracorporeal membrane oxygenation (ECMO) can be used as a bridge to lung transplantation to support both cardiac and pulmonary function.[13] Venoarterial ECMO can be accomplished with cannulation of the carotid or axillary artery and the right internal jugular vein. Venovenous ECMO can be used in patients who need only respiratory support and cannulation involves the right internal jugular vein and return of arterialized blood to the common femoral vein.

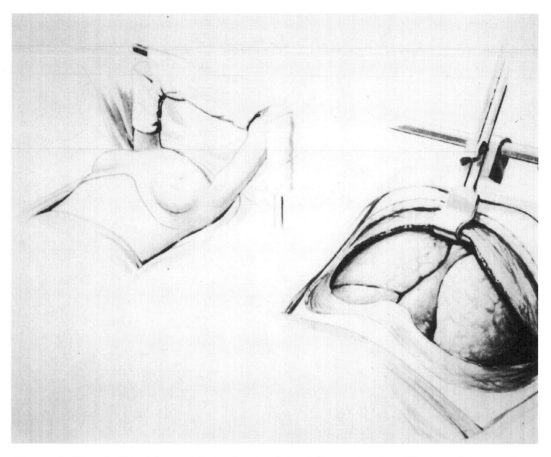

Figure 2. Clamshell incision or bilateral anterolateral thoracotomies with sternal transection. (Reproduced with permission from Patterson GA: Bilateral lung transplant: indications and technique. *Sem Thorac Cardiovas Surg* 4:95–100, 1992.)

Donor Selection and Management

Criteria for the selection of donors for lung transplantation and HLT are more stringent than for isolated cardiac transplantation. Most donors are victims of traumatic deaths involving severe head injuries from motor vehicle accidents, rupture of an intercerebral aneurysm, cerebral vascular accident, or a gunshot wound to the head. Protection of the airway is often impossible and aspiration may occur. This becomes evident on chest x-rays during the first 12 to 24 hours following traumatic injury. In addition, neurogenic pulmonary edema is often an accompaniment to brain death. Many of these donors are placed on mechanical ventilation with no positive end-expiratory pressure (PEEP) or suctioning which causes progressive atelectasis and leads to bacterial colonization and pneumonitis. Because of these problems, there continues to be a shortage of lung and heart-lung donors.

Many donor operations involve multiorgan harvesting by surgeons from different institutions and require close cooperation. There should be judicious fluid management

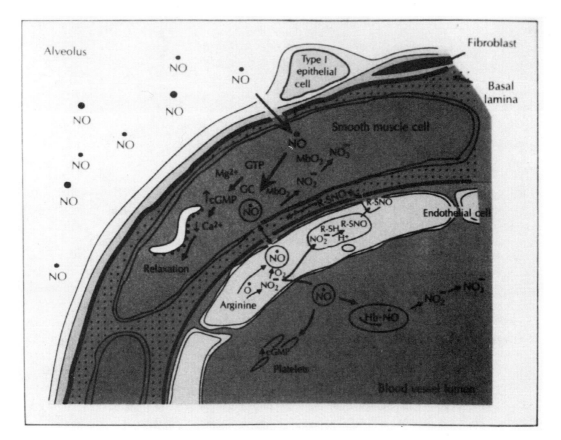

Figure 3. The proposed routes of nitric oxide (NO) uptake and mechanism for pulmonary vasodilatation. (Reproduced with permission from Soifer SJ: Pharmacologic and surgical treatment of the pulmonary circulation in the fetus, newborn, infant, and child. *Curr Opin Cardiol* 8:138, 1993)

with losses replaced with either albumin or blood. Patients should be placed on inotropes if they have a drop in blood pressure, instead of receiving more volume. All lung and heart-lung donors should be ABO identical and have an adequate size match between donor and recipient. Overall, large lungs are avoided because of the possibility of cardiac tamponade and compressive atelectasis with subsequent risk of infection. Occasionally, a lobectomy of the donor lung may be required to allow an adequate fit.

A suitable heart-lung donor has no history of major chest trauma, a normal electrocardiogram (EKG), an ECHO with absence of any regional wall abnormalities, and is on inotropic support of less than 10 mcg/kg/min of dopamine. A suitable lung donor for both lung transplantation and HLT has no history of pulmonary disease, a clear chest x-ray, and absence of infected sputum by bronchoscopy, a short period of mechanical ventilation, excellent gas exchange (a $PO_2 > 300$ on FIO2 of 100% and PEEP of 5, or a $PO_2 > 100$ on FIO_2 of 40% and a PEEP of 5) normal lung compliance, and a central venous pressure (CVP) of between 5 and 10.

All lung donors should undergo fiberoptic bronchoscopy to define endobronchial anatomy, look for gross contamination or foreign bodies of the endobronchial tree, and have specimens sent for gram stain and sputum culture. Any gram stain which reveals fungus or heavy contamination of gram negative bacteria precludes lung transplantation. Occasionally, a lung donor will present with borderline oxygenation and unilateral pathology. This dilemma has been addressed by intraoperative unilateral ventilation of the normal lung by x-ray with documentation of excellent single lung function.[14] This lung can then be used for transplantation. Serologic tests including hepatitis, HIV, cytomegalovirus (CMV), and Epstein-Barr virus (EBV) are performed on all potential lung donors.

Donor Operation

The donor operation is performed via a median sternotomy. The heart is carefully examined, the pleural spaces are entered, and the lungs inspected for areas of contusion or atelectasis. Our current lung donor preservation technique involves pretreatment with prostaglandin (PGE_1) 15 minutes before aortic cross-clamping and flush perfusion cooling using 60 mL/kg of a modified Euro Collins solutions at 4°C. The solution is administered at a rate of 15 mL/kg/min via a pulmonary artery catheter placed in the main pulmonary artery by the surgeon. After pretreatment with PGE_1, the cross-clamp is applied, and the heart is arrested in the usual fashion with cold potassium cardioplegia. The inferior vena cava and left atrial appendage are transected to prevent any distention of the heart. The lungs are perfused as previously described. If there has been excellent lung preservation, the lungs will appear white at the end of the pulmonoplegic solution. The heart-lung bloc is removed in an inflated state and may be separated on the back table if the heart and lungs are to go to separate institutions (Figure 4). The heart and lungs are separated so that each has an adequate left atrial cuff (Figure 5). When the lungs are divided, a short donor bronchus should be used for the anastomosis because the distal main bronchus is better vascularized than either the carina or the proximal main bronchus (Figure 6).

Recipient Operation

The technique used to perform lung transplantation and HLT has evolved at our institution over the last 5 years. Monitoring of older children includes placement of a pulmonary artery catheter, a pulse oximeter, a peripheral arterial catheter, and a transesophageal echocardiographic probe to follow RV function and also assess gradients across atrial or pulmonary arterial anastomoses. Intubation is usually performed as sterilely as possible, with a single lumen endotracheal tube for bronchoscopy at the end of the case. All operations are performed with the use of cardiopulmonary bypass and aprotinin.

Successful SLT for PH requires an ideal graft because the entire cardiac output must go through the newly transplanted lung. If the recipient requires repair of a congenital cardiac defect, it can be accomplished easily through a right thoracotomy with cannulation of the right atrium, ascending aorta, and replacement of the right lung. After a congenital heart defect is repaired, the recipient pneumonectomy is carried out. Central dissection around the recipient bronchus is kept to a minimum to avoid

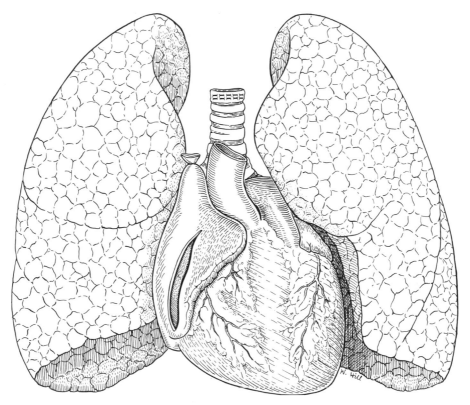

Figure 4. Heart-lung graft.

damage to the blood supply. Implantation of the donor lung involves three anastomoses including the bronchial, left atrial, and pulmonary artery. Bronchial anastomoses is performed end-to-end with continuous prolene or polydioxanone suture (PDS). After completion of the procedure, air is vented, the clamps are removed, and the lung is reexpanded, and all anastomoses are inspected for bleeding. BSLT is performed via a clamshell incision and the conduct of the operation is as for the SLT procedure.

Important aspects of the recipient operation for HLT include removing the heart and lungs without injury to the phrenic, vagus, or recurrent laryngeal nerves, and to ensure hemostasis. The operation is performed through a median sternotomy or clamshell incision. If possible, any adhesions are taken down with the electrocautery prior to heparinization. After the patient is placed on cardiopulmonary bypass, the recipient heart is excised, and the phrenic nerve pedicles are fashioned. The pulmonary hilum is mobilized, bronchial arteries are secured, which may be enlarged in patients with Eisenmenger's syndrome, and using a TA 30 stapling device, the bronchus is divided. The left lung is removed first and then the right in a similar fashion. The remnants of the pulmonary artery are now removed, leaving a 3-cm ribbon around the ductus ligament so as to preserve the left recurrent laryngeal nerve. After removal of the diseased heart and lungs, the posterior mediastinum is irrigated and inspected for hemostasis as the perfusion pressure is increased by the heart-lung machine (Figure 7).

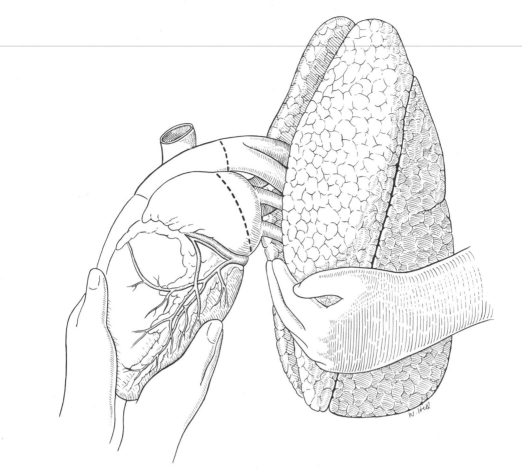

Figure 5. Heart-lung graft removed from the chest. Incision marked to allow separation of heart from the lungs leaving adequate atrial cuffs for both grafts.

The trachea is now dissected by grasping the stumps of the left and right bronchi. Care should be taken to leave the surrounding blood supply to the trachea as intact as possible. The trachea is divided immediately above the carina. The donor heart and lungs are passed onto the field, the donor trachea is trimmed immediately above the carina, the right lung is passed beneath the right atrium and the phrenic nerve pedicle and the left lung beneath the left phrenic nerve pedicle. The tracheal anastomosis is performed with continuous prolene suture. After completion of the tracheal anastomosis, ventilation is commenced avoiding high oxygen concentrations. The atrial and aortic anastomosis are completed as the patient is rewarmed. Once all anastomoses are completed, the chest cavities are emptied of fluid, air is evacuated from the heart, and the aortic cross-clamp is removed (Figure 7). Vigorous diuresis is begun in the operating room with the administration of lassix and mannitol. Lung allograft dysfunction in the operating room can be treated with inhaled NO, independent lung ventilation in those patients who have undergone SLT or ECMO. All patients undergo fiberoptic bronchoscopy, prior to leaving the operating room, to inspect the airway anastomosis and to remove any secretions or blood clots.

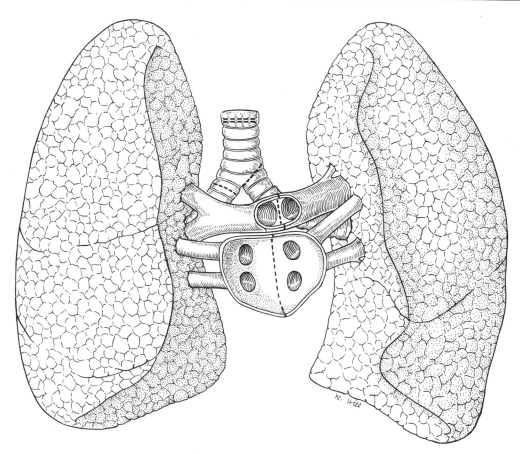

Figure 6. Double-lung graft.

Postoperative Care and Immunosuppression

Patients with PH who undergo SLT may develop severe hemodynamic instability postoperatively, probably related to persistent ventilation of the native lung and perfusion of the entire cardiac output through the newly transplanted lung.[15] Techniques to stabilize these patients include PEEP, sedation and paralysis, elevation of the transplanted side, and delay of extubation for several days. Patients who have undergone HLT or BSLT can usually be extubated within 24 to 48 hours. Antibiotics are continued for 7 days or are modified if positive donor cultures are identified from intraoperative specimens. Antifungal prophylaxis consists of fluconazole and bactrim is used for prophylaxis against pneumocystis. All lung transplant patients receive ganciclovir and cytogam for 4 to 8 weeks postoperatively if a significant serologic mismatch exists (recipient is CMV negative and the donor is CMV positive, or the recipient is CMV positive and the donor is CMV negative).

Our immunosuppression protocol consists of preoperative CsA and azathioprine. Intraoperatively, the patient is given methylprednisolone just prior to removal of the vascular clamp. Immediate postoperative immunosuppression consists of CsA twice a day

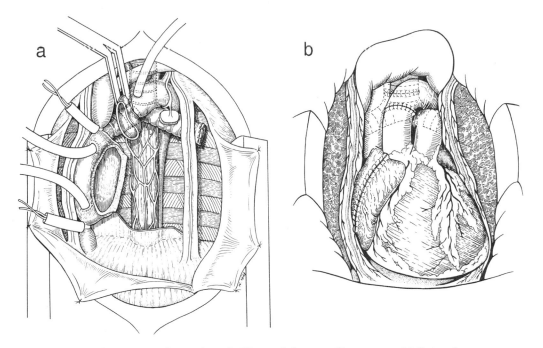

Figure 7. Heart-lung transplantation. **A.** The recipient cardiectomy and bilateral pneumonectomies have been performed with the patient on cardiopulmonary bypass. Phrenic nerve pedicles are fashioned and present in each pleural cavity. Dissection around the trachea is limited. **B.** The completed procedure shows anastomoses of the trachea, right atrium, and aorta.

(three times a day in the pediatric patient) and azathioprine once a day. CsA levels are obtained and the dosage adjusted based on the level and renal function. Azathioprine is held if the white count is less than 4000. Intravenous steroids are given for 24 hours and then discontinued. Prednisone is begun at 0.5 mg/kg/qd on day 2 for lung transplant recipients and on day 7 for HLT recipients. At 2 weeks, the immunosuppression protocol consists of triple drug therapy: CsA, azathioprine, and prednisone.

Lung rejection occurs more frequently during the first 3 months post-transplantation.[16] Patients present with a febrile illness, have decreased oxygen saturations, and may develop an infiltrate on chest x-ray. This should prompt immediate bronchoscopy with specimens sent for gram stain, bacterial, fungal and viral cultures, and a transbronchial lung biopsy obtained. Lung rejection is treated with IV pulse steroids for 3 days. Recurrent lung rejection can be treated with a second pulse of steroids, OKT3, or photochemotherapy. An accurate diagnosis of acute lung rejection enables the prompt use of augmented immunosuppression and may reduce the risk of bronchiolitis obliterans. Rejection in the HLT patient may involve either organ, the heart or the lungs, and at different times.[17] Isolated lung rejection is more common in these patients. Isolated heart rejection is rarely seen, and many programs are not performing routine endomyocardial biopsies.

Airway complications after lung transplantation have decreased due to limiting dissection around the anastomosis, a primary end-to-end anastomosis, and the routine early use of perioperative steroids.[18] Anastomotic airway problems after HLT are uncommon because of the extensive tracheobronchial coronary collateral flow that is present to the supracarinal trachea and main bronchi postoperatively.[19] Significant bronchial stenosis, if they do develop, can be treated by dilatation and placement of a stent. Many Silastic stents can be removed and need not remain in the tracheobronchial tree indefinitely.

Follow-Up and Results

Follow-up of patients after lung transplantation for PH includes chest x-ray, pulmonary function tests, nuclear angiocardiograms and right heart catheterizations. After lung transplantation, pulmonary vascular resistance and pulmonary pressures dramatically decrease and these changes are stable over a follow-up period beyond 3 years.[20] These decreases in pulmonary vascular resistance are associated with significant improvement in RV function (Figures 8 and 9). HLT recipients also receive endomyocardial biopsies and coronary arteriography. Cardiac allograft vasculopathy appears to be less common in the heart-lung recipient than the heart recipient.[21]

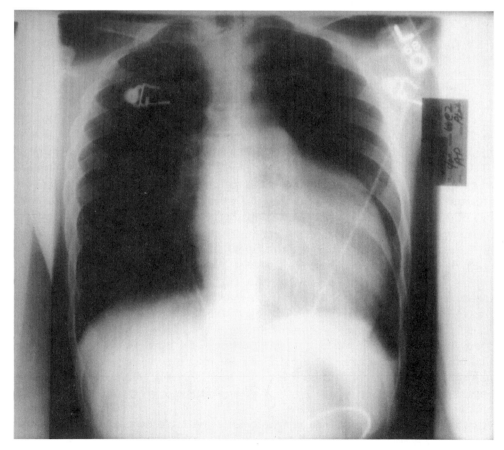

Figure 8. Preoperative chest x-ray from 13-year-old boy with primary pulmonary hypertension (PH).

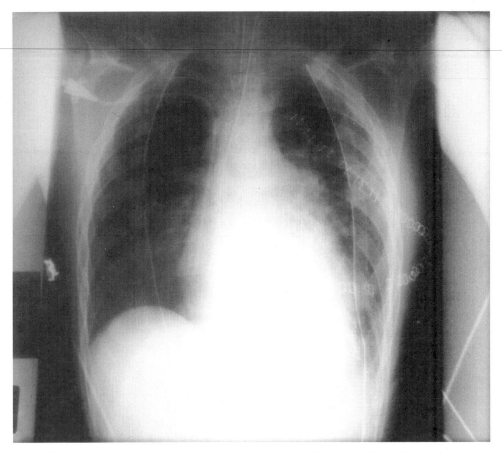

Figure 9. Postoperative chest x-ray from same patient in Figure 8 after left single lung transplant (SLT) showing decrease in size of right ventricle.

Bronchiolitis obliterans limits long-term survival in lung and HLT patients. Bronchiolitis obliterans develops in 15% to 40% of lung recipients[22] and in about 30% to 40% of heart-lung recipients[23] (Figure 10). One must have a high index of suspicion to make the diagnosis because it has been shown that bronchiolitis obliterans may be reversed and airway function stabilized by early detection and aggressive high-dose steroid therapy. Patients who do not respond to augmented immunosuppression or total lymphoid irradiation and continue to have a downhill course may be candidates for retransplantation, but the results are not as good as the original transplant.[24]

Two-year survival for lung transplant recipients is 65% and 55% for heart-lung recipients (Figure 11). Controversy exists with regards to the best operation for PH. Lung transplantation (single or bilateral) and HLT appear to give equal results, but the debate concerns donor issues, and the potential ventilation/perfusion (V/Q) mismatch and decreased reserve that can occur in patients after SLT. Most patients have substantial improvement in the quality of life and improved exercise tolerance. Lung transplantation and HLT remain effective therapeutic options for patients with end-stage pulmonary and cardiopulmonary disease. With increasing experience and improved results, more transplants will need to be performed, but the limiting factor will be the donor supply.

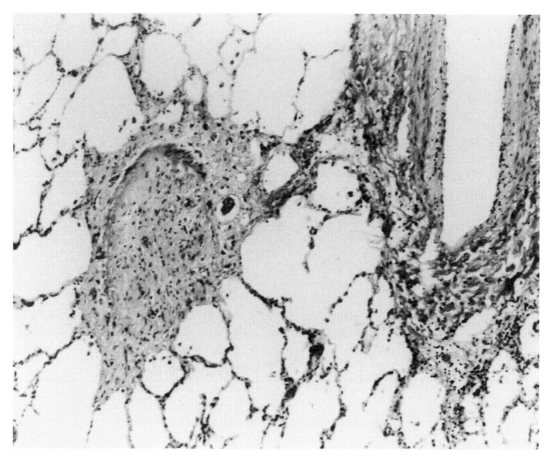

Figure 10. Transbronchial lung biopsy showing bronchiolitis obliterans from a young female with primary pulmonary hypertension after heart-lung transplantation (HLT).

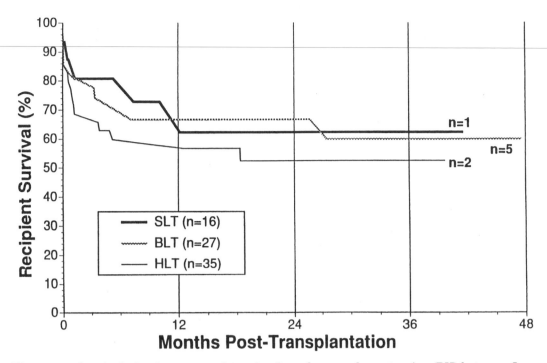

Figure 11. Survival after lung transplantation for pulmonary hypertension (PH) between January 1, 1990 and January 1, 1995 at the University of Pittsburgh by type of transplant procedure. (Reproduced with permission from United Network for Organ Sharing.)

References

1. Hardy JD, Webb WR, Dalton ML, Walker GR: Lung homotransplantation in man. *JAMA* 186:1065–1074, 1963.
2. Cooley DA, Bloodwell RD, Hallman GL, Nora JJ, Harrison GM, Leachman RD: Organ transplantation for advanced cardiopulmonary disease. *Ann Thorac Surg* 8:30–46, 1969.
3. Reitz BA, Wallwork J, Hunt SA, Pennock JL, Billingham ME, Oyer PE: Heart-lung transplantation: successful therapy for patients with pulmonary vascular disease. *N Engl J Med* 306:557–564, 1982.
4. Cooper JD, Pearson FG, Patterson GA, Todd TR, Ginsburg RJ, Goldberg M: Technique of successful lung transplantation in humans. *J Thorac Cardiovasc Surg* 93:173–181, 1987.
5. Rich S, Dantzker DR, Ayres SM, Brundage BH: Primary pulmonary hypertension: a national prospective study. *Ann Intern Med* 107:216–220, 1987.
6. Rubin LJ: Primary pulmonary hypertension. *Chest* 104:236–250, 1993.
7. D'Alonzo G, Barst RJ, Ayers SM, Bergofsky EH: Survival in patients with primary pulmonary hypertension. *Ann Intern Med* 115:343–349, 1991.
8. McCarthy PM, Rosenkranz ER, White RD, Rice TW, Stevba R, Mehta AC: Single-lung transplantation with atrial septal defect repair for Eisenmenger's syndrome. *Ann Thorac Surg* 52:298–303, 1991.
9. Spray TL, Mallory GB, Canter CE, Huddleston CB, Kaiser LR: Pediatric lung transplantation for pulmonary hypertension and congenital heart disease. *Ann Thorac Surg* 54:240–248, 1992.
10. Fremes SE, Patterson GA, Williams WA, Goldman BS, Todd RT, Maurer J: Single lung transplantation and closure of patent ductus arteriosus for Eisenmenger's syndrome. *J Thorac Cardiovasc Surg* 100:1–5, 1990.

11. Rubin LJ, Mendoza J, Hood M, McGoon M, Barst R, Williams WB: Treatment of primary pulmonary hypertension with continuous intravenous prostacyclin (epoprostenol). *Ann Intern Med* 112:485–491, 1990.
12. Kerstein D, Hsu DT, Hardof AJ, Barst RJ: Efficacy of blade balloon atrial septostomy in advanced pulmonary vascular disease. *Am Rev Resp Dis* 145:717, 1992.
13. Spray TL: Pediatric lung transplantation. *Sem Thorac Cardiovasc Surg* 4:113–121, 1992.
14. Puskas JD, Winton TL, Miller JD, Patterson GA: Unilateral donor lung dysfunction does not preclude successful contralateral single lung transplantation. *J Thorac Cardiovasc Surg* 103:1015–1018, 1992.
15. Pasque MK, Kaiser LR, Dresler CM, Trulock E, Triantafillou AN, Cooper JD: Single lung transplantation for pulmonary hypertension: technical aspects and immediate hemodynamic results. *J Thorac Cardiovasc Surg* 103:475–482, 1992.
16. Trulock EP, Ettinger NA, Brunt EM, Pasque MK, Kaiser LR, Cooper JD: The role of transbronchial lung biopsy in the treatment of lung transplant recipients. *Chest* 102:1049–1054, 1992.
17. Griffith BP, Hardesty RL, Trento A, Bahnson HT: Asynchronous rejection of the heart and lungs following cardiopulmonary transplantation. *Ann Thorac Surg* 40:488–493, 1985.
18. Ramirez J, Patterson GA: Airway complications after lung transplantation. *Sem Thorac Cardiovasc Surg* 4:147–153, 1992.
19. Dawkins KD, Jamieson SW, Hunt SA, Baldwin JC, Burke CM, Morris A: Long-term results, hemodynamics and complications after combined heart and lung transplantation. *Circulation* 71:919–928, 1985.
20. Dohoyos A, Patterson G, Maurer J: Pulmonary transplantation: early and late results. *J Thorac Cardiovasc Surg* 103:767–772, 1992.
21. Madden BP, Hodson ME, Rodley-Smith R, Khaghani A, Yacoub MY: Intermediate-term results of heart-lung transplantation for cystic fibrosis. *Lancet* 339:1583–1588, 1992.
22. Bolman RM, Shumway SJ, Estrin JA, Hertz MI: Lung and heart-lung transplantation. *Ann Surg* 214:456–470, 1991.
23. McCarthy PM, Starnes VA, Theodore J, Stinson EB, Oyer PE, Shumway NE: Improved survival after heart-lung transplantation. *J Thorac Cardiovasc Surg* 99:54–60, 1990.
24. Miller JD, Patterson GA: Retransplantation following isolated lung transplantation. *Sem Thorac Cardiovasc Surg* 4:107–112, 1992.

Chapter 16

Bilateral Lobar Transplantation With Split Cadaver Lung

Jean-Paul Couetil, MD

Introduction

Pulmonary transplantation for the pediatric population, or for patients of small size, is particularly limited by the now well-described scarcity of organs available for transplantation.[1,2] Limitations of size mismatch and shortage of suitable donors make these groups of recipients especially difficult to accommodate. To circumvent these obstacles, we have developed a technique of lung transplantation inspired from previous experience with liver bipartition.

Bismuth and Houssin[3] have shown that splitting the liver into its constituent lobes allows two children to be transplanted with one liver. Recent studies of transplantation of pulmonary lobes in animals have been successful at medium-term follow-up, with respect to hemodynamics and equitation of volume and conformity of the lobes in the thorax of the recipient.[4-8] Satisfactory results of pulmonary reduction and lobar transplantation and liver bipartition, from either cadaveric[9,10] or living donors,[11-13] have been reported clinically. We postulated that bipartition of one large donor lung into its constituent lobes would allow bilateral pulmonary transplantation into a recipient of smaller thorax size.

We first showed the feasibility of the procedure experimentally.[14] Using adult dogs as donors, single lungs, either right or left, were divided into separate lobes which were subsequently implanted unilaterally and bilaterally into young dogs. Follow-up of up to 21 weeks demonstrated satisfactory bronchial and vascular anastomoses, and perfect adaptation of the transplanted lobes to the morphology of the recipient thorax. Following the success of these animal experiments, the procedure was applied clinically for the first time in 1993.

From: Franco KL (ed). *Pediatric Cardiopulmonary Transplantation*. Armonk, NY: Futura Publishing Company, Inc.; © 1997.

Materials and Methods

Between May 1993 and November 1994, seven bilateral lobar transplantations using a bipartitioned left donor lung were performed at the Broussais Hospital. There were five female and two male recipients. There were three children, aged 13 to 17 years (median 14), and four adults, aged 40 to 53 years (median 45). The etiology of the end-stage lung disease was cystic fibrosis (CF) in the case of the three children; two adults had primary pulmonary hypertension, one had bronchiectasis, and one had idiopathic pulmonary fibrosis. All patients required continuous O_2 therapy, and had grade IV dyspnea. Preoperative lung function tests are shown in the Table. All were judged to have a life expectancy of less than 18 months.

The criteria of suitability for a donor were similar to those of single lung transplantation, except that bilateral lobe transplantation was performed when there was a discrepency of height or weight of more than 20% between donor and recipient. In the present reported cases, the weight discrepency was 44% to 50% and the height discrepency was 12% to 17%. Vertical and transverse chest x-ray measurements were also used in an attempt to assess the suitability of the match.

Surgical Technique

Donor Operation

A median sternotomy is performed and the pericardium and pleural cavities are opened. The lungs are inspected and particular attention paid to the left oblique fissure to ensure that it is well defined. In most young adult donors, the fissure is well defined and, therefore, does not present any difficulty in separating the fissure. If the fissure is ill defined or likely to cause a major difficulty, this information is passed to the recipient hospital at this stage and an alternative recipient is sought. However, this has not occurred to date in our experience.

Table				
Adult Recipients				
	R1:D1	R2:D2	R3:D3	R4:D4
Height (cm)	150:180	158:190	163:180	160:188
TLC:LLC (L) (predicted)	4.10:3.26	5.57:3.06	5.10:3.26	5.40:3.46
Child Recipients				
	R5:D5	R6:D6	R7:D7	
Height (cm)	154:174	140:178	135:170	
TLC:LLC (L) (predicted)	4.01:3.04	3.06:3.26	2.76:2.42	

R = recipient; D = donor; TLC = total lung capacity (Predicted TLC has been calculated using the European Community for Coral and Steel Formula). LLC = estimated left lung capacity of donor (as 45% of calculated TLC of the donor).

The trachea, aorta, pulmonary artery, and both venae cavae are dissected free. Heparin is administered in a central venous line followed by prostacyclin (500 mcg over 10 minutes) into the pulmonary artery. The heart is then excluded from the circulation by cross-clamping the aorta and the venae cavae. Cardioplegia is administered via the ascending aorta, and when the heart is arrested and the lungs still ventilated, pneumoplegia is infused via the pulmonary artery (Papworth solution 60 mL/kg). The heart is decompressed by incising the inferior vena cava and the left atrial appendage. Topical cardiac and lung cooling is applied. The heart is then excised, taking care to leave enough atrial tissue surrounding the left and right pulmonary veins. After aspiration of bronchial secretions, the lungs are inflated, the endobronchial tube removed, and the trachea stapled and transected. The double lung block is then excised, leaving the esophagus and the descending aorta in the donor chest. If the decision is made to transplant one lung in two different recipients (twinning procedure), the pulmonary block is divided on a back table. The pericardium is split vertically midway between the two atrial cuffs, and the pulmonary artery is divided at its bifurcation. The dissection is then completed at the level of the carina, and the proximal left main bronchus is stapled and divided after having inflated the lungs. Each lung and heart are placed in cold containers for transportation.

Recipient Operation

The patients are anesthetized and monitored with standard single lumen tube, radial artery line, two central venous catheters, and Swan-Ganz catheter. Surgical exposure is via a bithoracotomy and transverse sternotomy through the fourth or fifth intercostal space, the "clamshell" incision. The pulmonary ligaments and any pleural adhesions are divided with cautery. The pulmonary artery is dissected intra- and extrapericardially on both sides of the hilum and dissected as distally as possible into the parenchyma of the lung, beyond the upper lobe branch, to have sufficient length for subsequent anastomosis. The pulmonary veins, both inferior and superior, are dissected free and a tape passed around the superior pulmonary vein on the right.

Preparation of the Donor Lung

Bench preparation of the donor left lung involves separation of the upper and lower lobes, and may be completed within 15 minutes. Initial inspection determines the direction and completeness of the fissure and the presence or not of anatomic variants. Pulmonary veins are dissected free to the hilum (Figure 1). The oblique fissure is dissected down to the pulmonary artery. Small vessels crossing the fissure are clipped and divided. Parenchymal bridges are divided after stapling. After completion of dissection of the fssure, the pulmonary artery is divided between the apical branch of the lower lobe and the lingular artery (Figure 2). The two pulmonary veins are exposed on the mediastinal surface of the lung and divided, leaving a small cuff of atrial tissue. The two veins are separated from each other. The upper and lower lobe bronchi are dissected down to the level of the segmental branches with minimal dissection to preserve retrograde vascularization. Both upper and lower lobe bronchi are transected at their origin, just before implantation of the donor lobes (Figure 3). Both upper and lower lobes are separated, aligned, and ready for implantation (Figure 4).

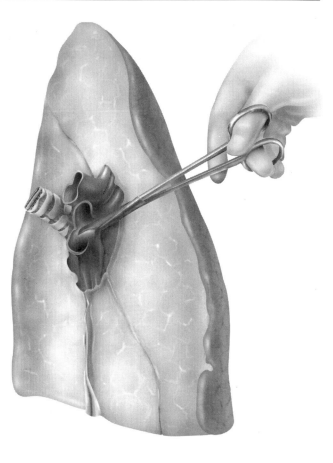

Figure 1. The left lung showing the hilum with the bronchus posteriorly, the pulmonary artery anterosuperior, and the confluence of the veins anteroinferior.

Excision of the Recipient's Right Lung

Full normothermic cardiopulmonary bypass with a beating heart is established between the ascending aorta and the right atrium using a two-stage venous cannula, and ventilation is then stopped. The recipient right lung is then excised in a standard fashion,[15] but ensuring that as long a vascular pedicle as possible remains (Figure 5). The first branch of the pulmonary artery is ligated to achieve greater length. This is also useful to orient the anastomosis. The inferior vein is sutured closed in the adult, but in the pediatric cases, the recipient cuff is fashioned to incorporate both inferior and superior veins.

Implantation of the Left Upper Lobe in the Right Thorax

The donor left upper lobe is then placed in the right thorax, having undergone a 180 degree vertical axis rotation for approximation of donor and recipient hila (Figure 6). Thus, in this situation, the posterior border of the donor left upper lobe becomes anterior, and its anterior border lies posteriorly along the spine. This has the effect of placing the membranous portion of the donor bronchus opposite the cartilaginous portion of the recipient bronchus and vice versa. The donor pulmonary artery is postero-

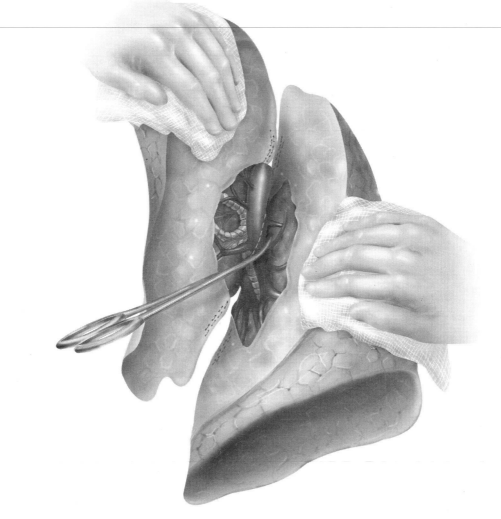

Figure 2. After completion of dissection of the fissure, the pulmonary artery is divided between the apical branch of the lower lobe and the lingular artery (**dotted line**).

superior to the donor bronchus, and the recipient artery is anterior and slightly inferior to the recipient bronchus. The donor and recipient superior veins are well aligned. The bronchial anastomosis is performed with continuous 4/0 prolene (Figure 6). Any size mismatch is overcome by using an end-to-end anastomotic technique, avoiding telescoping as much as possible. They are sutured as they were aligned, cartilaginous portion of donor to membranous portion of recipient and vice versa (Figure 7). Bronchial wrapping is not performed. This is followed by anastomosis of the donor pulmonary vein to the recipient superior pulmonary vein (continuous 5/0 prolene). The proximal pulmonary artery of the donor is posterior to the bronchus, but leads forward to the fissural section which is anterior and in good alignment with the artery of the recipient. Therefore, the proximal portion is trimmed close to the upper segmental branches and

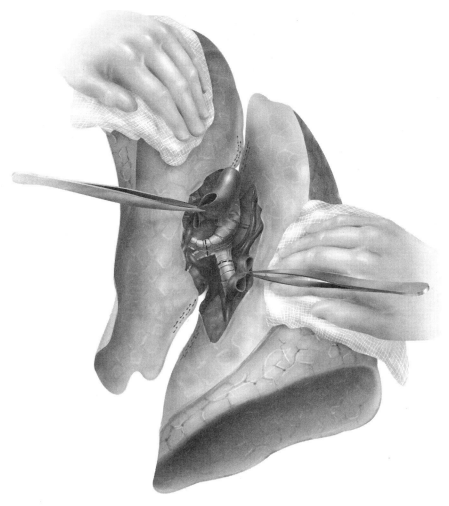

Figure 3. The upper and lower lobe bronchi are dissected down to the level of the segmental branches and are transected at their origin (**dotted lines**).

oversewn, and the anastomosis is fashioned end-to-end with the recipient artery using 6/0 prolene (Figure 8). The pulmonary artery anastomosis is made possible by having dissected sufficient length of recipient artery to allow it to come forward in front of the bronchial anastomosis without tension or twist.

Retrograde deairing is achieved by releasing the venous clamp and evacuating air through the pulmonary artery before securing that anastomosis. The right lung is then ventilated gently with 50% FiO$_2$. Continuous pressure breathing (CPB) is reduced to allow perfusion of the right lung.

Excision of the Left Lung

The recipient left lung is resected in a standard manner, but again leaving a long vascular pedicle.

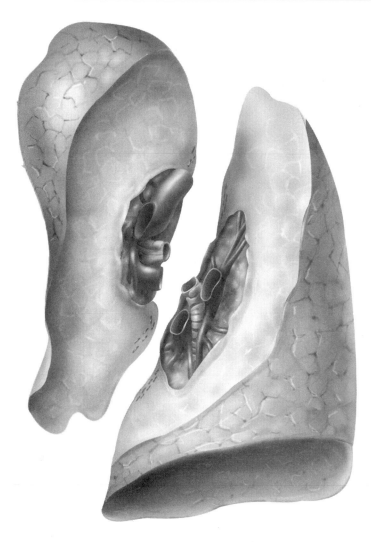

Figure 4. The upper and lower lobes aligned ready for implantation on the right and left sides, respectively. Note the fissural opening of the pulmonary artery anterosuperior to the bronchus.

Implantation of the Left Lower Lobe in the Left Thorax

The donor left lower lobe is placed in the anatomic position in the thorax of the recipient. Alignment of the bronchi and vessels is uncomplicated (Figure 9). Anastomoses are fashioned in the same order, bronchi followed by vein, followed by artery. The bronchial anastomosis involves the main recipient bronchus. Again, any size mismatch is overcome while suturing the bronchi end-to-end. The venous anastomosis differs slightly from the right in that the recipient cuff is fashioned incorporating both superior and inferior veins, as they are more closely aligned than on the right (Figures 10 and 11). Both recipient and donor arteries present anteriorly, and there are no special difficulties forming the anastomosis.

Deairing procedures are repeated before the vascular anastomoses are secured. CPB was gradually discontinued. At this stage, it was apparent, in some cases, that the right graft in its new position was too long for the thorax. In such situations, the lingula may be resected using a linear stapler.

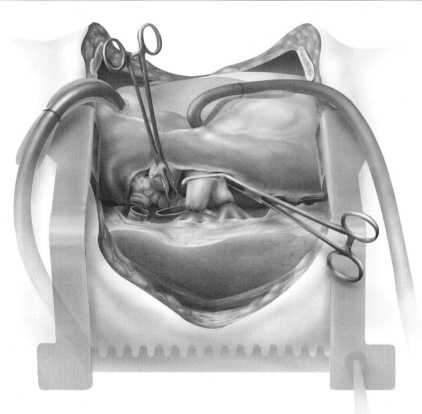

Figure 5. Excision of the recipient right lung showing intra- and extrapericardial dissection of the pulmonary artery to allow as long a pedicle as possible.

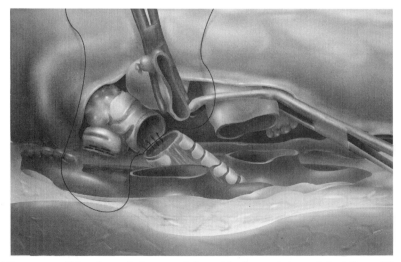

Figure 6. Alignment of the donor left upper lobe with the recipient right hilum. The end-to-end bronchial anastomosis is commenced and is followed by the well-aligned pulmonary venous anastomosis.

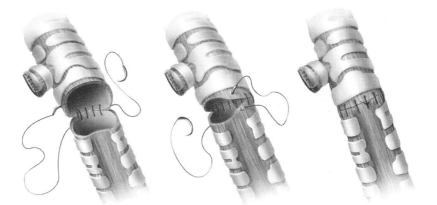

Figure 7. The technique of bronchial anastomosis; a continuous end-to-end stitch sutures cartilaginous portion to membranous portion and vice versa.

Thereafter, bilateral drains were placed and the thoracotomy closed in layers. Postoperatively, patients were extubated as soon as oxygenation was adequate. Transbronchial biopsies were not performed in the initial 2 weeks, and rejection episodes were diagnosed on clinical grounds. Otherwise, bronchoscopy, transbronchial biopsy, and bronchoalveolar lavage were performed on a routine basis and, when clinically indicated, in the investigation of chest x-ray abnormalities, altered gas exchange, or unexplained fever. After discharge from the hospital, patients were enrolled in a physiotherapy and rehabilitative program.

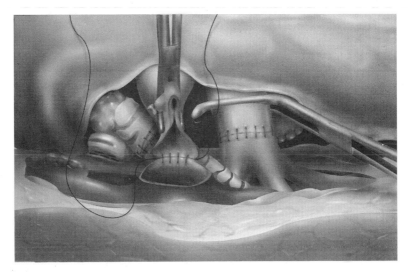

Figure 8. The long pulmonary artery pedicle of the recipient may be aligned with the fissural aspect of the donor pulmonary artery to form the anastomosis in front of the bronchial anastomosis.

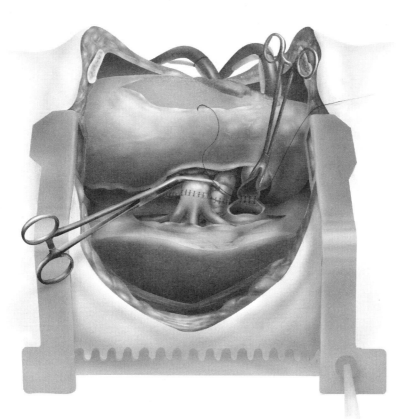

Figure 9. The donor left lower lobe implantation showing the completed bronchial and pulmonary venous anastomosis and the pulmonary artery anastomosis in progress.

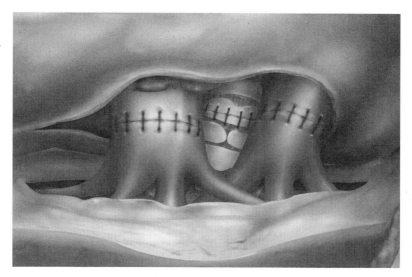

Figure 10. The donor left lower lobe pulmonary vein is fashioned incorporating both superior and inferior veins of the recipient.

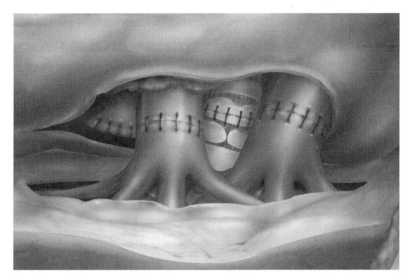

Figure 11. The donor left upper lobe pulmonary vein is anastomosed to the superior recipient pulmonary vein.

Results

Early Results

There were no technical failures at the time of operation and all patients were successfully weaned from bypass. The graft ischemic time was 150 minutes for the first lobe (range 90 to 172), and 210 minutes for the second lobe (range 145 to 305). Additional procedures performed included: patent ductus arteriosus division and ligation; patent foramen ovale closure; and a reduced liver transplantation in a CF patient. The duration of ventilation postoperatively ranged from 12 to 105 hours (median 30). There was one early mortality in a CF patient in whom widespread systemic aspergillosis could not be controlled, and the patient died of a cerebral hemorrhage on day 21, postoperatively. Morbidity was minimal. There were no bleeding complications, and neither bronchial stenosis nor dehiscence became apparent. There was a persistent air leak in two patients, and three others were noted to have partial pneumothoraces. Hospital stays ranged from 21 to 70 days (median 42).

Late Results

Follow-up of the six survivors now ranges from 6 to 23 months (median 11). All patients are subjectively very well, with no major morbidity and minimal problems of rejection or infection. Early and late results were assessed on respiratory function tests, forced vital capacity (FVC), forced expiratory volume (FEV_1), total lung capacity (TLC), and TLCO. Percentage of predicted normal values for the recipients demonstrate an improvement with time after transplantation. There has been no bronchial anastomotic problems, and bronchoscopy has demonstrated patent lumina free of ulceration or stricture. Follow-up computed tomography (CT) scans have demonstrated disappearance of residual pneumothoraces and perfect adaptation of the transplanted lobes to the shape of the recipient thorax.

Conclusion

Following the success of our animal experiments, we have now shown that the technique of lobar separation followed by bilateral transplantation is feasible and easily performed without an increase in mortality or morbidity. Carefully selected patients with a large size discrepency with their donors demonstrate good functional results. Discharged patients have returned to a normal lifestyle with adequate arterial gaseous exchange on exertion. There has been full adaptation of the lobes to the shape of the recipient thorax. Further long-term studies in animals and humans are awaited to assess the full potential of this technique in increasing the number of transplantations in children and adults of short stature.

References

1. Couetil JP, Scott JP, Serrano-Fiz S, Higenbottam TW, Wallwork J: Transplantation cardiopulmonaire: experience de Cambridge. *Coeur* 4:209–213, 1989.
2. Spray TI, Mallory GB, Cantter CB, Huddleston CB: Pediatric lung transplantation: indications, techniques, and early results. *J Thorac Cardiovasc Surg* 107:990–1000, 1994.
3. Bismuth H, Houssin D. Reduced-size orthoptic liver grafts in hepatic transplantation in children. Surgery 95:367–370, 1984.
4. Lillehei CW, Everts E, Shamberger RC: Reduced-size lung transplantation from adult to neonatal sheep. *J Pediatr Surg* 8:1153–1156, 1992.
5. Cromblehome TM, Adzick NS, Longaker MT: Reduced-size lung transplantation in neonatal swine: technique and short-term physiologic response. *Ann Thorac Surg* 49:55–60, 1990.
6. Haverich A, Dammenhayn L, Demertzis S, Kemnitz J, Reimers P: Lung growth after experimental pulmonary transplantation. *J Heart Lung Transplant* 10:288–295, 1991.
7. Hislop AA, Odom NJ, McGregor CG, Haworth SG: Growth potential of the immature transplanted lung: an experimental study. *J Thorac Cardiovasc Surg* 100:360–370, 1990.
8. Huggins E: Reimplantation of lobes of the lung: an experimental technique. *Lancet* 2:1059–1061, 1959.
9. Otte JB, de Ville de Goyet J, Sokal E, et al: Size reduction of the donor liver is a safe way to alleviate the shortage of size-matched organs in paediatric liver transplantation. *Ann Surg* 211:146–157, 1990.
10. Starnes VA, Barr ML, Cohen RG: Lobar implantation: indications, techniques, and outcome. *J Thorac Cardiovasc Surg* 3:403–411, 1994.
11. Strong RW, Lynch SW, Ong TH, Matsunami H, Koidy L, Balderson G: Successful liver transplantation from a living donor to her son. *N Engl J Med* 322:1505–1507, 1990.
12. Backer CL, Ohtake S, Zales VR: Living-related lobar lung transplantation in beagle puppies. *J Pediatr Surg* 4:429–433, 1991.
13. Cohen RG, Barr ML, Schenkel FA, DeMeester TR, Wells WJ, Starnes VA: Living-related donor lobectomy for bilateral lobar transplantation in patients with cystic fibrosis. *Ann Thorac Surg* 57:1423–1428, 1994.
14. Couetil JP, Grousset A, Tolan MJ, Benaim A, Fayolle P, Carpentier A: Experimental bilateral lobar lung transplantation and its application in the human. *Thorax* 1995. (In press.)

15. Pasque MK, Cooper JD, Kaiser LR, Haydock DA, Triantafillou A, Trulock EP: Improved technique for bilateral lung transplantation: rationale and initial clinical experience. *Ann Thorac Surg* 49:785–791, 1990.
16. Otte JB, de Ville de Goet J, de Hemptinne B, et al: The concept and technique of the split liver in clinical transplantation. *Surgery* 107:605–612, 1990.
17. Kern JA, Tribble CG, Zografakis JG, Cassada DC, Chan BB, Kron IL: Analysis of airway function of immature whole lung transplants versus mature lobar translants. *Ann Thorac Surg* 57:1089–1094, 1994.
18. Kern JA, Tribble CG, Flanagan TL, Chan BB, Cassada DC, Kron IL: Growth potential of porcine reduced-size mature pulmonary lobar transplants. *J Thorac Cardiovasc Surg* 104:1329–1332, 1992.
19. Kern JA, Tribble CG, Chan BK, Flanagan TL, Kron IL: Reduced-size porcine lung transplantation: long-term studies of pulmonary vascular resistance. *Ann Thorac Surg* 53:583–589, 1992.

Chapter 17

Living-Related Pediatric Lobar Transplantation

Giovanni B. Luciani, MD; Mark L. Barr, MD
Vaughn A. Starnes, MD

Introduction

The recent improvements in survival and quality of life after pulmonary transplantation have made it a safe therapeutic option for children and adults with end-stage pulmonary parenchymal or vascular disease.[1-3] Thus, an increasing number of patients are considered for transplantation each year, while the availability of organ donors remains insufficient.[1-3] The resulting mismatch of supply and demand has become even more dramatic in the pediatric population, where the size of the donor grafts required also becomes a factor.[4]

In order to meet the increasing need for pediatric pulmonary donors, laboratory and clinical investigation using reduced-size lung grafts (lobes) has been undertaken.[5,6] Moving from this experimental background, we began a clinical program of lobar transplantation in selected children, adolescents, and adults with end-stage pulmonary disease. Our practice has evolved from the use of single lobes from cadaveric donors to the use of lobes from living-related donors for single or double lung transplantation.[7,8]

Indications

The original indications for living-related lobar transplantation in children and adults did not substantially differ from those for conventional cadaveric lung transplantation (Table 1). Because of issues relating to the size of the lobar graft compared to the whole lung, this technique may be more ideally suited for children, adolescents, or adults with a small to medium build. All the recipients of a lobar transplant were previously

From: Franco KL (ed). *Pediatric Cardiopulmonary Transplantation*. Armonk, NY: Futura Publishing Company, Inc.; © 1997.

Table 1.

Indications for Living-Related Lobar Transplantation

	Children	
bilateral	Cystic fibrosis	5
bilateral	Obliterative bronchiolitis	1
unilateral	Bronchopulmonary dysplasia	1
unilateral	Eisenmenger's syndrome	1
	Adults	
bilateral	Cystic fibrosis	18
bilateral	Chemotherapy-induced pulmonary fibrosis	1

listed for cadaveric lung transplantation. Acute clinical deterioration was used initially as a prerequisite for enrollment into the lobar transplantation program. As the experience with this procedure has grown and the clinical results with critically ill patients have proved satisfactory, living-related lobar transplantation has been extended to include patients with end-stage pulmonary disease in noncritical, but deteriorating conditions.[9] Given all these considerations, an ideal recipient population has proven to be the group of children, adolescents, and young adults affected by end-stage cystic fibrosis (CF).[8,9] Because of the coexisting metabolic problems, these patients tend to present with reduced somatic development and cachexia.[9] The majority of the recipients have had a decrease in forced expiratory volume (FEV_1) to 30% or less of predicted, severe hypoxemia, severe hypercapnia, marked weight loss, and increased antibiotic resistance.

Donor Selection Criteria

The selection of donors for living-related donor lobar transplantation involves assessment of both psychosocial and physiologic factors. In each case, the potential donors have been interviewed by a committee of transplant coordinators, social workers, and physicians, including a psychiatrist, to safeguard against coercion and ensure donor comprehension of the surgical procedure.

Selection of the donors is done to minimize the risk that will occur when the lobes are removed. After determination of ABO compatibility, all donors undergo thorough clinical investigation with specific focus on cardiopulmonary anatomy and physiology. It is important that no significant events or recent viral infections be reported on the past medical history. Both the electrocardiogram and echocardiogram must be within limits for age and sex. A negative standard chest roentgenogram is also required. The evaluation continues with room air arterial blood gases, spirometry, ventilation/perfusion scan, and computerized tomography of the chest to exclude pathology and permit volumetric assessment of the lobes considered for donation.

Serologic tests performed include hepatitis A, B, and C virus, human immunodeficiency virus (HIV) and cytomegalovirus (CMV) status. While evidence of hepatitis or HIV infection is considered as absolute contraindication to donation, CMV status is only used to predict which recipients will need prophylactic antiviral therapy. Finally, tissue typing is performed to rule out a positive donor-specific cross-match to the recipient and provide retrospective information. Human leukocyte matches/mismatches are not a contraindication to donation. After a suitable donor pair has been selected, the larger donor, if possible, is used for donation of the right lower lobe. An intraoperative fiberoptic bronchoscopy is performed in each donor immediately before the lobectomy, in order to exclude evidence of inflammatory processes or unexpected variations in bronchial anatomy (Table 2).

Living-Related Donor Lobectomy

While in the early experience with living-related lobar donation only the parents had been considered, we have since extended the selection criteria to include siblings, cousins, aunts, and uncles (Table 3). The selection of the most suitable lobes for donation has evolved with our clinical experience. Unlike lobectomy performed for pulmonary neoplasms or infections, two general rules apply to the donor lobectomy: 1) the volume of the lobe must be adequate to sustain the recipient's respiratory function; and 2) the procedure must be conducted in a way that will avoid any compromise of the remaining donor lobes. A posterolateral thoracotomy is used to facilitate exposure of the pulmonary arteries and intrapericardial pulmonary vein. While manipulation of the lobe is kept to a minimum, dissection in the pulmonary fissures is always carried out on the side of the remaining lung to avoid air leaks in the recipient. Fissures are sealed with both surgical staplers and cautery to reduce the risk of donor or recipient air leaks. In general, bronchial and pulmonary arterial cuffs of only 2 or 3 mm are sufficient for implantation, while it may be important to harvest the intrapericardial pulmonary vein.[8,10] As the right upper lobe has proved to be technically more difficult to remove because of the anatomy of the arterial blood supply, the right middle lobe, although more easily harvested, has inconsistent pulmonary venous drainage and may theoretically have an inadequate microvascular bed. Our preference has, thus, ultimately developed for the right lower lobe to be utilized as the right-sided graft, and the left lower lobe as the left-sided

---

Table 2.

Donor Selection Criteria

ABO compatible
Age ≤ 55 years
No significant past medical history
No recent viral infections
Normal electrocardiogram
Normal chest roentgengram
Normal echocardiogram
$PaO_2 > 80$ mm Hg on room air
FEV_1 and FVC > 85%
No significant pulmonary pathology on computed tomography
No previous thoracic operation on donor side
Negative intraoperative bronchoscopy on donor side

PaO_2 = arterial blood partial oxygen tension; FEV_1 = forced expiratory volume in 1 second; FVC = forced vital capacity.

Table 3.

Donor Demographic Data

		Children	Adults
Kinship			
	parent	10/14	16/38
	sibling	—	10/38
	cousin	2/14	6/38
	uncle/aunt	2/14	6/38
Lobe donated			
	RLL	5/14	16/38
	LLL	5/14	19/38
	RML	1/14	—
	RUL	1/14	—
	RLL + RML	—	3/38

RLL = right lower lobe; LLL = left lower lobe; RML = right middle lobe; RUL = right upper lobe.

graft. Although the right lower lobectomy may sometimes be more challenging because of the variable origin of the bronchus intermedius, requiring removal of both the lower and the middle lobe in our early cases, we have been successful in preserving the integrity of the right middle lobe bronchus at the expense of a shorter length on the donor side (Figure 1). The left lower lobe seems to be the most easily removed with only occasional need for reimplantation of a lingular artery, when its takeoff is distal to the origin of the artery to the superior segment of the left lower lobe (Figure 2).

After dissection of the lobar vasculature to define the arterial and venous anatomy, the fissure is completed with stapling devices. Minimal dissection of peribronchial tissue is then performed to avoid compromise of blood supply to the donor and remaining lobes. Heparin (300 μ/kg) is then administered and the pulmonary artery, the pulmonary vein, and finally the bronchus are divided above clamps. Care is taken to respect this sequence in order to avoid venous congestion of the graft.[8]

Preservation of Lobes

An intravenous infusion of prostaglandin is started at the beginning of the donor operation to dilate the pulmonary vasculature. After excision of the donor lobe, it is moved to a sterile back table where selective intubation of the bronchus and cannulation of the lobar artery are performed. While being gently hand-ventilated using a sterile Ambu bag, the lobe is flushed with approximately 1 liter of cold (4°C) modified Euro-Collins solution. Care is taken to avoid spillage of the crystalloid bath or pneumoplegic solution into the bronchus. The lobe is then placed in cold storage and transferred to the recipient's operating room for implantation.[10]

Recipient Operation

Given the overall condition of the recipient, cardiopulmonary bypass is used routinely to perform the single or bilateral lobar transplant. While the single lobe transplantations have been done through standard posterolateral thoracotomies, all double

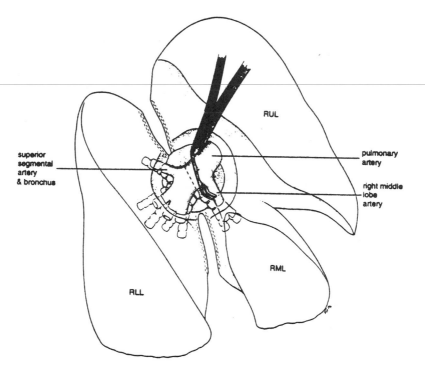

Figure 1. Dissection and division of the pulmonary artery for donor right lower lobectomy. (Reproduced with permission from Reference 10.)

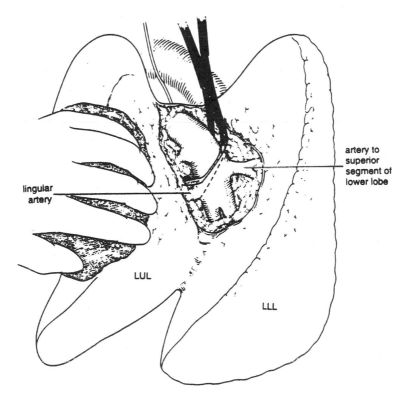

Figure 2. Dissection of the right inferior pulmonary vein so that a vascular clamp can be placed on the intrapericardial left atrium. (Reproduced with permission from Reference 10.)

lobar implants have been performed through a bilateral thoracosternotomy (clamshell) incision as sequential single lung transplants. This approach provides excellent exposure for both cannulation purposes and dissection of the pleural space, apex, and hilum of the lung. Preliminary dissection of the hilar areas and lysis of adhesions are completed before institution of cardiopulmonary bypass to minimize bleeding. The recipient pneumonectomy is now begun with care to divide the pulmonary artery and vein as distally in the parenchyma of the lung as possible. This technique provides the additional vascular tissue often needed to perform the allograft implantation. The bronchus is then divided at the level of the takeoff of the upper lobe bronchus (Figure 3). The sequence of the recipient anastomoses starts with a running 4–0 monofilament polypropylene suture for the bronchus, followed by a running 6–0 suture of the donor lobar vein to the recipient *superior* pulmonary vein, and ending with a running 5–0 suture for the lobar artery to the recipient pulmonary artery (Figures 4, 5, and 6). By limiting the amount of peribronchial dissection and mild telescoping of the donor into the recipient bronchus, we have obtained excellent healing of the airways without the need for an omental wrap.[8] The recipients undergo intraoperative bronchoscopy and transesophageal echocardiography to exclude technical complications with the bronchial and pulmonary venous anastomoses. The postoperative management thereafter is similar to that of our patients undergoing cadaveric lung transplantation.

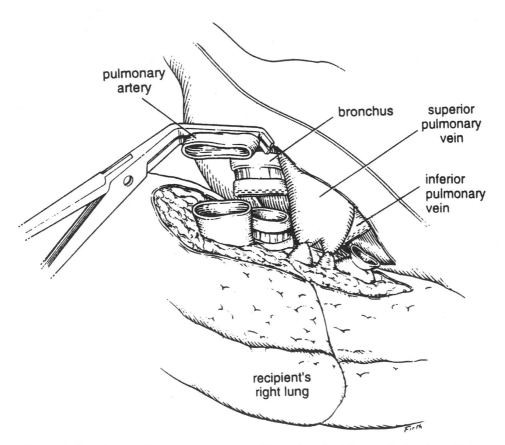

Figure 3. Recipient right pneumonectomy. (Reproduced with permission from Reference 8.)

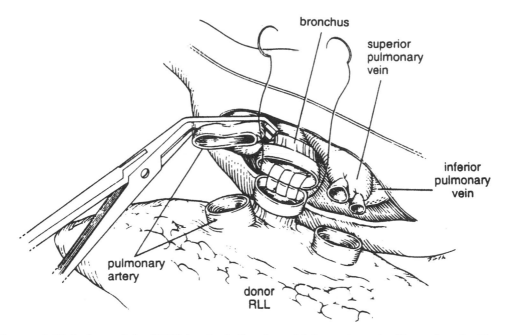

Figure 4. Right lower lobe (RLL) implantation: bronchial anastomosis. (Reproduced with permission from Reference 8.)

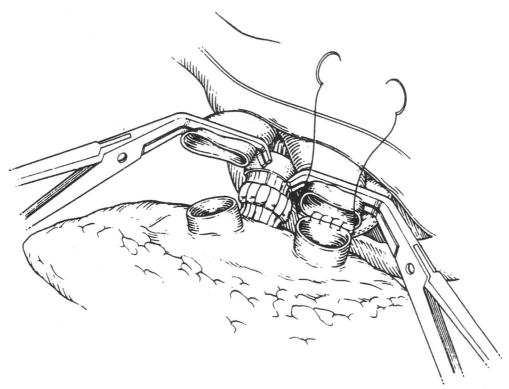

Figure 5. Right lower lobe implantation: pulmonary venous anastomosis. (Reproduced with permission from Reference 8.)

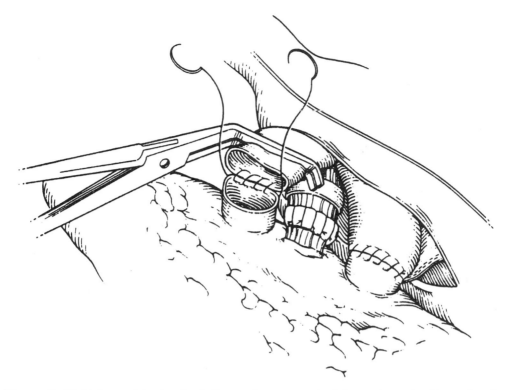

Figure 6. Right lower lobe implantation: pulmonary arterial anastomosis. (Reproduced with permission from Reference 8.)

Postoperative Care and Immunosuppression

The postoperative management of the living-related donors undergoing lobectomy does not significantly differ from that of patients undergoing lobectomy for more common indications. All patients are extubated in the operating room. Their chest tubes are usually removed once the drainage has subsided and no evidence of air leak is noticed. The average hospital stay of the donors ranges 6 to 10 days. All of them are discharged within 24 hours of removal of the chest tubes.

All recipients receive the standard triple drug regimen consisting of cyclosporine, azathioprine, and prednisone. An initial dose of cyclosporine (2 mg/kg intravenous) and azathioprine (4 mg/kg intravenous) are administered shortly before the operation. In addition, a single dose of methylprednisolone (10 mg/kg) is given on discontinuance of cardiopulmonary bypass. Postoperative immunosuppression is maintained with cyclosporine (2 mg/kg/d) to maintain a whole blood level of 250 to 350 ng/mL, azathioprine (2 to 4 mg/kg/d) to leukocyte tolerance (approximately 6000 cells/mL) and methylprednisolone (15 mk/kg for the first 24 hours and 1 mg/kg/d thereafter). We do not currently use cytolytic therapy as part of our induction immunosuppression. The immunosuppressive agents are then converted to oral administration as soon as oral medications are again tolerated. Steroids are generally slowly weaned to a maintenance dose of 0.2 mg/kg/d of prednisone by the end of the first 6 months.

Prophylaxis for CMV infection has been utilized if either donor is positive, regardless of the recipient's CMV status. Two weeks after the day of transplantation, intravenous ganciclovir (5 mg/kg/d) is begun for 4 weeks. Thereafter, chronic treatment with oral acyclovir (10 mg/kg/dose tid) is administered for the following 6 months. All children have received chronic *Pneumocystis carinii* pneumonia prophylaxis with oral sulfamethoxazole/trimethoprim (10 mg/kg/d 3 days per week).

Monitoring of allograft rejection and infection has included clinical parameters of hypoxemia, tachypnea, and decreasing pulmonary function tests. The roentgenographic findings typical of lung rejection with hilar distribution of infiltrates have been observed in recipients of lobar transplants, as well. Bronchoalveolar lavages (BALs) and transbronchial biopsies have been liberally performed, especially in children with CF, who continue to be more prone to opportunistic infections. In patients with CF, preoperative and postoperative irrigation of the sinuses have been aggressively used both to treat recurrent purulent sinusitis and to obtain cultures for specific antimicrobial therapy. Acute rejection episodes have been treated with pulse steroids (oral or intravenous), provided the diagnosis of infection had been excluded on BAL.

Results and Follow-Up

Between January 1992 and March 1995, a total of 28 patients underwent living-related lobar transplantation. Nine patients (32%) were children and represent the cohort discussed for the remainder of this chapter. The mean age at transplantation was 12 years (range 4 to 17 years), while the mean weight was 29 kg (range 15 to 42 kg). The most common indication for lobar transplantation was CF (5/9 patients). Additional indications included primary pulmonary hypertension, viral obliterative bronchiolitis (OB), bronchopulmonary dysplasia, and Eisenmenger's syndrome secondary to a ventricular septal defect (Table 1). Clinical deterioration in the patients with CF, OB, and bronchopulmonary dysplasia manifested with decrease in body weight (greater than 20% of normal weight), worsening pulmonary function (FEV_1 15% to 27% of predicted), and increasing antibiotic resistance. The patient with primary pulmonary hypertension and the one with bronchopulmonary dysplasia manifested progressive dyspnea, fatigue and home O_2 requirements. The patient with Eisenmenger's syndrome developed increasing cyanosis and dyspnea.

Seven patients (five with CF, one with primary pulmonary hypertension, and one with OB) underwent bilateral lobar transplantation, and two patients (one with bronchopulmonary dysplasia and one with Eisenmeger's syndrome) underwent single lobar transplantation. The patient with Eisenmenger's syndrome also had simultaneous repair of her ventricular septal defect.

There was one perioperative death, due to persistent post-transplant pulmonary hypertension in the patient with Eisenmenger's syndrome who received a right middle lobe from her father, and one death, 1 month after bilateral lobar transplantation due to necrotizing bonchiolitis in a patient transplanted for viral OB. All the patients with CF survived the operation and are currently doing well 1 to 38 month after transplant (mean follow-up 13 months). The overall survival is 78% at 1 year (84% at 1 year for the pediatric and adult series combined)(Figure 7), which does not significantly differ from previously reported data for pediatric cadaveric lung transplantation.[4,11]

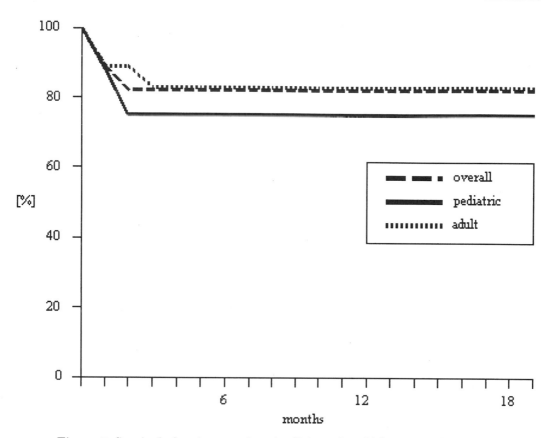

Figure 7. Survival of patients undergoing living-related lobar transplantation.

Considering the critical clinical conditions of the children undergoing lobar transplantation, these results appear quite satisfactory.

Currently, our indications for pediatric and adult living-related lobar transplantation have been most commonly in CF, given the excellent preliminary results in this difficult subset of patients. Indeed, commonly reported survival in both children and adults undergoing cadaveric lung transplantation for CF have often been lower (60% to 76%).[11,12] In addition, it has been estimated that up to 30% of the patients with end-stage CF die while waiting for a donor.[12] Based on these considerations, we believe that this group of patients may represent a target population for living-related bilateral lobar transplantation.

Complications

There have been no serious complications among the 54 donors who underwent lobectomy or bilobectomy for living-related lobar transplantation. A postoperative air leak occurred in one donor who underwent right lower and middle lobectomy. This resulted in prolonged need for chest tube drainage and hospital stay (16 and 18 days, respectively). The finding that donors undergoing right lower and middle lobectomy had prolonged postoperative air leaks, confirmed by our adult series, has led us to strenuously avoid sacrificing the right middle lobe.

Postoperative complications in our recipients included bilateral pulmonary reperfusion injury in two patients, manifesting with severe hypoxemia and pulmonary edema and requiring prolonged ventilatory support, and episodes of generalized seizures, occurring in two patients, within the first postoperative week, which resolved rapidly without the need for chronic anticonvulsant therapy. No airway complications have been observed in any of the recipients of a living-related lobar transplant.

Despite the invariable colonization of the upper airways with gram negative bacilli in the children with CF, no major clinically evident episode of organ or systemic infection was observed in the pediatric recipient group. This may represent an artifact of the small sample size as we have had serious infectious complications in our adult CF population. Two patients experienced unilateral acute allograft rejection, with resolution using pulse steroid treatment in both. In agreement with the preliminary data in the adults receiving living-related lobar transplants, the overall incidence of rejection does not appear significantly different to conventional cadaveric lung transplantation and is unrelated to the number of human leukocyte antigen (HLA) mismatches. However, both the occurrence of unilateral rejection and the complete response to steroid pulses without the need for adjuvant immunosuppression have been commonly observed in our series.

No occurrence of post-transplantation OB has been observed in the pediatric population. Longer follow-up will be needed to establish the relevance of this very preliminary finding. Preliminary data relative to follow-up pulmonary function tests have shown significant improvement in all patients assessed.

Conclusion

Living-related lobar transplantation has been steadily evolving. This technique has proved to be a safe and realistic therapeutic alternative for children and adults with end-stage pulmonary disease, who are in critical or rapidly deteriorating clinical conditions.[8–10] Despite isolated reports of successful cadaveric or living-related lobar transplantation,[13] our experience has been responsible for the development of bilateral living-related lobar transplantation, definition of the clinical indications, technical aspects of the surgical procedure, and outcome after this form of organ replacement.

The interest in living-related lobar transplantation has largely developed because of the chronic donor shortage, even more critical for children waiting for lung transplantation.[12] As laboratory investigations demonstrated reduced-size lung transplantation to be feasible, we have embarked on a program of living-related lobar transplantation.[5–8] Additional experimental evidence is needed to establish the growth potential of pediatric pulmonary lobes. The majority of our lobar transplants have, however, been performed in older children and adolescents, in whom two adult-size lobes may offer sufficient parenchyma to support future pulmonary functional needs. Because the rationale for living-related lobar transplantation is to overcome the problem of donor shortage in the face of a clinically deteriorating recipient, the subset of patients afflicted by CF has represented a target population for this innovative therapy. The high attrition rate of these patients on the transplant list and the natural history of the disease have convinced us that children and adults with CF may be the primary beneficiary of bilateral lung transplantation in general.[12] The good early clinical results with living-related lobar transplantation in terms of survival and prevalence of complications have allowed expansion of this treatment modality also to patients in noncritical, but deteriorating conditions, as well as those with other underlying disease processes. Comparison of the clinical results offered by cadaveric lung transplantation demonstrates at least equivalent survival for both the pediatric and adult recipients of lobes from living donors.[4,11] However, taking into consideration the number of transplant candidates who die while waiting for a donor, we believe living-related lobar transplantation offers a realistic and safe therapeutic opportunity for selected patients with end-stage pulmonary disease.

References

1. Toronto Lung Transplant Group: Experience with single transplantation for pulmonary fibrosis. *JAMA* 29:2258–2262, 1988.
2. Egan TM, Kaiser LR, Cooper JD: Lung transplantation. *Curr Probl Surg* 26:673–752, 1989.
3. Starnes VA, Theodore J, Oyer PE, et al: Evaluation of heart-lung transplant recipients with prospective, serial transbronchial biopsies and pulmonary function studies. *J Thorac Cardiovasc Surg* 98:683–690, 1989.
4. Kaye MP: Pediatric thoracic transplantation: the world experience. *J Heart Lung Transplant* 12:344–350, 1993.
5. Kern JA, Tribble CG, Chan BBK, Flanagan TL, Kron IL: Reduced-size porcine lung transplantation: long-term study of pulmonary vascular resistance. *Ann Thorac Surg* 53:583–589, 1992.
6. Goldsmith MF: Mother to child: first living donor lung transplant. *JAMA* 264:2724, 1990.
7. Starnes VA, Lewiston NJ, Luikart A, Theodore J, Stinson EB, Shumway NE: Current trends in lung transplantation: lobar transplantation and expanded use of single donors. *J Thorac Cardiovasc Surg* 104:1060–1066, 1992.
8. Starnes VA, Barr ML, Cohen RG: Lobar transplantation, indications, technique, and outcome. *J Thorac Cardiovasc Surg* 108:403–411, 1994.
9. Barr ML, Schenkel FA, Cohen RG, et al: Living-related lobar transplantation: recipient outcome and early rejection patterns. *Transplant Proc* 27:1995–1996, 1995.
10. Cohen RG, Barr ML, Schenkel FA, DeMeester TR, Wells WJ, Starnes VA: Living-related donor lobectomy for bilateral lobar transplantation in patients with cystic fibrosis. *Ann Thorac Surg* 57:1423–1428, 1994.
11. Armitage JM, Furland G, Michaels M, Cipriani LA, Griffith BP, Fricker FJ: Critical issues in pediatric lung transplantation. *J Thorac Cardiovasc Surg* 109:60–65, 1995.
12. Starnes VA, Lewiston N, Theodore J, et al: Cystic fibrosis: target population for lung transplantation in North America in the 1990s. *J Thorac Cardiovasc Surg* 103:1008–1014, 1992.
13. Bisson A, Bonnette P, Ben El, Kadi N, Leroy M, Colchen A: Bilateral pulmonary lobe transplantation: left lower and right middle and lower lobes. *Ann Thorac Surg* 57:219–221, 1994.

Chapter 18

Obliterative Bronchiolitis

Bruce F. Whitehead, MB, BS, FRCP

Introduction

Since the "new age" of thoracic transplantation began in the early 1980s following the clinical introduction of cyclosporin A (CsA), long-term success of lung transplantation has been thwarted by the prominence of the complication, obliterative bronchiolitis (OB).[1] This condition involves a progressive fibroproliferative process within the smaller airways which produces an obstructive lung defect often associated with bronchiectasis. Clinically, it is represented by increasing dyspnea, falling lung flows, and recurrent lower respiratory tract infections. Ultimately, it leads to hypoxic respiratory failure and death.

It has been particularly evident in the pediatric lung transplant population which appears to have an increased propensity to its development. In addition, this younger age group may exhibit a more severe form of the disease, often developing within months of transplantation.[2]

The etiology of OB remains obscure and, as a consequence, attempts to prevent its occurrence or treat it once it has become established have been frustrated. At present, the only "cure" for OB is retransplantation, which has been associated with poor results.

This chapter reviews the current knowledge regarding OB and details definitions, pathology, etiologic factors, incidence, clinical characteristics, and treatment, in particular, as they pertain to children. Also included is a review of contemporary research strategies utilized in an attempt to unravel the mysteries of this devastating disease.

Definitions and Pathology

The term *chronic rejection* is often used synonymously with OB in the context of pulmonary transplantation. However, this is somewhat erroneous as chronic rejection implies a pathophysiologic process which may or may not exist (see under etiology), rather than a specific disease entity. OB defines a distinct histopathology: "it is a term

From: Franco KL (ed). *Pediatric Cardiopulmonary Transplantation*. Armonk, NY: Futura Publishing Company, Inc.; © 1997.

restricted to membranous and respiratory bronchioles having evidence of submucosal scarring that may be ecentric, concentric, or associated with total obliteration of the bronchiolar lumens; it may be associated with foam cells in distal air spaces" (Figure 1).[3,4] It is a condition which may also be found in the nontransplant setting,[5] but has been most evident within the transplant patient group.

A histologic diagnosis may not always be possible by using transbronchial biopsy,[6] and histology alone does not encompass the associated functional abnormalities. In an attempt to resolve these issues, an ad hoc working group under the auspices of the International Society for Heart and Lung Transplantation (ISHLT) was commissioned to prepare a clinically applicable formulation for the assessment of chronic dysfunction of lung allografts. This incorporated a staging scheme which included a measure of pulmonary function (forced expiratory volume at 1 second [FEV_1]) as a percentage decline from the greatest baseline value obtained, associated with or without histologic evidence of OB (Table 1). Accordingly, the term *bronchiolitis obliterans syndrome* (BOS) was introduced to describe lung allograft dysfunction, reserving the term *obliterative bronchiolitis* for histologic diagnosis only.[7]

Obviously, this grading system may not be applicable in young children who are unable to satisfactorily or reliably perform spirometry. Nor does it adequately identify those patients who do not achieve a reasonable level of pulmonary function following transplantation. However, in older children and adolescents, this scheme may be a useful tool for assessing the level of graft dysfunction, as well as enabling comparison between both different treatment groups and transplant centers.

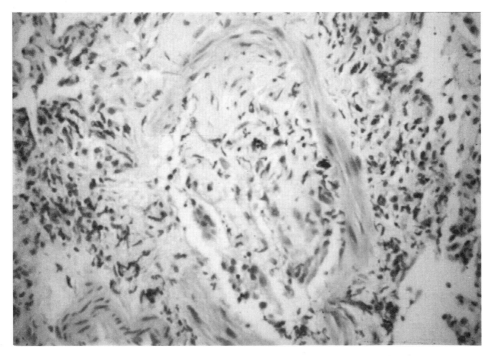

Figure 1. Photomicrograph of lung biopsy from a patient with obliterative bronchiolitis. Note the complete obliteration of the airway in the **center** of the picture by fibroproliferative tissue.

Table 1.

Bronchiolitis Obliterans Syndrome Staging System

Stage 0	No significant abnormality: FEV_1 80% or more of baseline value
Stage 1	Mild bronchiolitis obliterans syndrome: FEV_1 66% to 80% of baseline value
Stage 2	Moderate bronchiolitis obliterans syndrome: FEV_1 51% to 65% of baseline value
Stage 3	Severe bronchiolitis obliterans syndrome: FEV_1 50% or less of baseline value.

Each of the above stages can be subclassified as (a) without pathologic evidence of obliterative bronchiolitis, or (b) with pathologic evidence of obliterative bronchiolitis. (Reproduced with permission from Reference 7.)

Etiology

Factors leading to the development of OB are poorly understood, and no clear etiologic process to explain the pathophysiology has been identified. Suggested mechanisms include rejection, infection, ischemia, interruption of lymphatic drainage, and lung denervation.[4,8-10] As mentioned above, the term chronic rejection is often used (incorrectly) to denote OB. Chronic rejection has been proposed as a major etiologic factor contributing to OB, however investigations have failed to define the immunologic mechanisms of chronic rejection in a comprehensive fashion. The topic has been well reviewed by Tilney et al.[11] They described chronic rejection as an "undefined conundrum" and as an "ill-understood process leading to the bulk of late graft failures. . . . it is inexorable, undefined and, as yet, uncontrollable." In addition, they noted that the common denominator in chronic rejection occurring in all solid organ allografts entailed the development of an obliterative fibrosis of hollow structures within the graft whether they be vessels, bronchioles, or bile ducts, etc. The pathophysiology has not been defined, and it is unknown as to whether this process results from a persistent host immunologic attack or from progressive graft ischemia, secondary to arterial insufficiency.

Most reports of chronic rejection of pulmonary allografts are descriptive. There may be a peribronchial inflammatory infiltrate associated with bronchiolar epithelial ulceration, but this subsides with progressive fibrosis of the bronchiole.[4] Arteriosclerotic changes are also noted in small arteries and veins. Immunoglobulin or complement deposits have not been identified, although an increase in class II major histocompatibility complex (MHC) has been found in biopsies of pulmonary vasculature and bronchiolar epithelium.[12]

Scott et al[8] identified a relationship between histologically confirmed severe, frequent, and persistent acute lung rejection and the development of OB in adult heart-lung transplantation (HLT) recipients, as did Yousem et al.[9] Acute rejection was also identified as a contributory factor in the development of OB in children.[2] In this latter series, pediatric HLT recipients who developed OB within the first year experienced more episodes of acute rejection in the first 6 months (5.7 episodes per patient), than did those who did not develop early OB (mean 3.2 episodes per patient)(Table 2).

Conflicting reports on what role infection plays in the development of OB exist. In the adult transplant literature, postoperative cytomegalovirus (CMV) infection has been implicated in increasing the risk of OB,[10] although this has not been consistently proven.[8] In children, the number of episodes of pulmonary infection was weakly associated with the development of OB.[2] However, in the same report, two children were

Table 2.

Pulmonary Rejection and Infection in Heart-Lung Transplant Recipients*

	OB within 1 Year	No OB at 1 year	
	(n = 6)	(n = 15)	P Value +
Rejection episodes	5.7	3.2	<0.05
Infection episodes	2.8	1.6	NS

* Mean number of pulmonary rejection and infection episodes during the first 6 postoperative months in patients in whom obliterative bronchiolitis (OB) had developed within 1 year and those in whom OB had not developed. (No OB).
+ Fisher's exact test; NS = Not significant.
(Reproduced with permission from Reference 2.)

diagnosed with rapid onset OB after contracting adenovirus pneumonitis. It is established that adenovirus pneumonia can lead to OB de novo in nontransplant, nonimmunosuppressed patients,[13] and, therefore, it is reasonable to suggest that infection does play a major role in the development of OB in certain situations. An increased incidence of organizing pneumonia has also been observed in adult lung transplant recipients who developed OB.[14] The diagnosis of organizing pneumonia preceded that of OB, suggesting that it may be an etiologic factor rather than simply a coincidental finding.

Apart from those already mentioned, other more unusual etiologic factors may play a role. One such factor is chronic aspiration associated with delayed gastric emptying and/or esophageal dysmotility, presumably secondary to vagus nerve injury during surgery. This has been observed in one series of five patients.[15] Despite specific antireflux therapy which effected an improvement in the symptoms of chronic cough, three of those affected developed OB and bronchiectasis.

In children and adolescents, another major contributing factor to the development of OB is noncompliance (or nonadherence) to the immunosuppression treatment regimen. Side effects, including hypertrichosis, gingival hypertrophy, and tremor secondary to CsA therapy, and obesity, and Cushingoid features secondary to glucocorticoid administration, may precipitate poor adherence to treatment. Nonadherence has been observed in children following renal transplantation[16] and has been identified as a major cause of renal graft loss beyond 2 years.[17] There are limited data on nonadherence in pediatric cardiothoracic transplant recipients,[18] although an incidence of 20% was reported in one pediatric HLT series.[2] It is imperative that this problem be further investigated in an attempt to identify and treat those patients who are potentially nonadherent, thus minimizing graft (and life) loss. In conclusion, OB appears to be the product of a final common pathway of lung injury which may be of uni- or multifactorial origins.[19]

Incidence

It is difficult to derive accurate data on the incidence of OB due to discrepancies in definition. With the increasing use of the BOS criteria, as outlined above, the incidence may be more accurately defined. Reports of adult lung transplant series have yielded an overall incidence ranging from 24%[8] to 50%.[20] As OB is a time-related phenomenon, a more appropriate method of determining incidence may be defining actuarial freedom from the disease over time. This method was applied in a pediatric cohort which showed an actuarial freedom from OB (in survivors) of 76%, 59%, and 37% at 1, 2, and 3 years post-transplant, respectively (Figure 2).[2]

Although the incidence of OB was not age-related in this series, a report from Harefield Hospital in the United Kingdom demonstrated a higher incidence in children under the age of 8 years—32% freedom from OB at 5 years compared to 62% freedom from OB in those recipients aged over 8 years.[21] Despite this difference, both these reports indicate an increased incidence of this complication in children, compared to that found in adult lung transplant recipients.

This raised incidence of OB has been confirmed in children who have received isolated lung transplantation,[22] while another series demonstrated no difference in the increased incidence (21% at a mean follow-up of only 12.7 months) between children undergoing HLT or bilateral sequential single lung transplantation.[23]

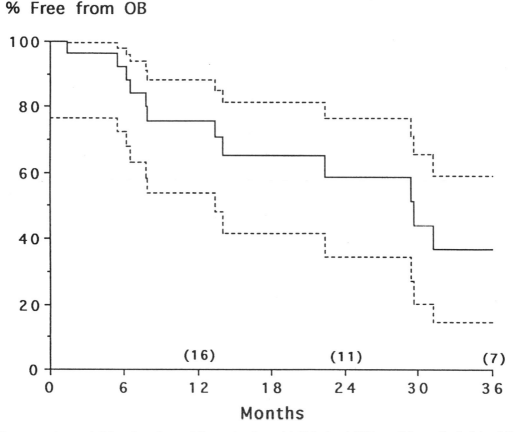

Figure 2. Actuarial freedom from obliterative bronchiolitis (and 95% confidence limits) in children and adolescents surviving after heart-lung transplantation. Number of survivors at each year is indicated in **brackets**. (Reproduced with permission from Reference 2.)

Clinical Characteristics

OB is characterized by progressive pulmonary dysfunction over a variable timescale, eventually leading to hypoxic respiratory failure. There is often an associated central bronchiectasis precipitating recurrent infective exacerbations compounding the pulmonary incapacity.[24] The usual presentation is one of an obstructive lung defect associated with hyperinflation of the chest and falling spirometric values. The usual time of onset is 2 to 3 years post-transplant, but this varies considerably. Disease commencement is often heralded by a decrease in expiratory flow values, particularly FEV_1 and forced expiratory flow at 25% to 75% of vital capacity (FEF 25% to 75%) (Figures 3A and 3B). Dyspnea on exercise ensues, though auscultatory findings may be minimal.

Radiologically, evidence of hyperinflation is observed with attentuation of vascular markings (Figure 4).[25] With disease progression, bronchiectatic changes may become apparent. High-resolution computerized tomography (HRCT) of the chest may elucidate these latter developments (Figure 5A).[26] Other HRCT findings that are observed in OB include: patchy opacification; septal lines; fibrosis; and small pneumothoraces and pneumomediastinum. Another finding which may appear preceding the on-

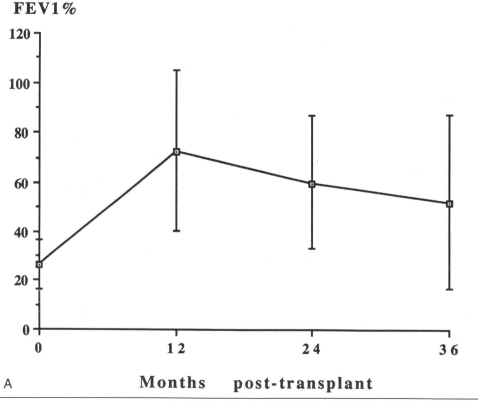

Figure 3. Mean (SD) FEV_1 (A) and FEF 25%

set of OB, (and which may possibly be predictive) is ground glass opacification, usually observed in a patchy symmetrical distribution (Figure 5B).[27]

In the author's experience, pediatric HLT recipients show a bimodal pattern of presentation of OB. The more common form, as described above, has an onset many months or years after transplantation, with an insidious onset of obstructive lung disease complicated by secondary bronchiectasis and chronic infection. This variety tends to follow a more chronic course with patients remaining debilitated, but stable for extended periods of time. The other pattern of presentation is more acute, occurring within months of transplant, demonstrating rapid progression and often early death.[2] This aggressive form of OB often occurred in those patients who experienced more episodes of rejection in their early post-transplant course. In addition, pulmonary infective episodes, particularly when due to adenovirus, influenced the early development of OB in some patients, although overall, pulmonary infections were not significantly associated with this form of premature-onset OB (Table 2).[2]

This unfortunate group of patients who experienced early progressive OB showed accelerated clinical deterioration leading to early incapacity associated with dyspnea on minimal exertion and then at rest, increasing hypoxia, weight loss, often rapidly

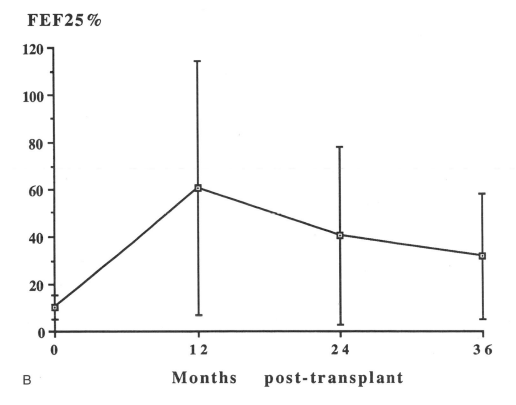

FEF25%

B **Months post-transplant**

Figure 3 (*continued*). (B) in children following heart-lung transplantation expressed as percentage of predicted normal. Note the decline in values at 2 and 3 years post-transplant indicating worsening airway obstruction associated with the development of obliterative bronchiolitis in many of the patients.

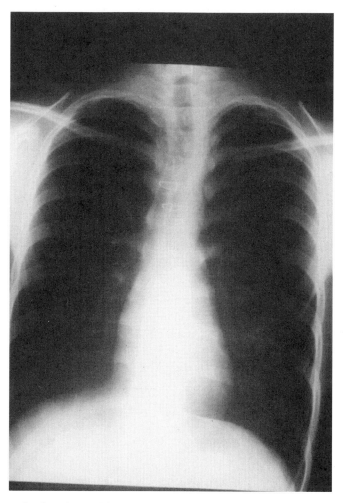

Figure 4. Radiograph of patient with "usual" presentation of obliterative bronchiolitis. This patient presented at 3 years post-heart-lung transplant with increasing dyspnea and falling spirometry. Note the hyperinflation and attenuation of pulmonary vascular markings.

progressing to cachexia, and death. Rapid disease progression was observed despite various therapeutic maneuvers, including augmentation of immunosuppression and appropriate antimicrobial therapy utilized in an attempt to stave off the persistent downward spiral.

It was interesting to note that three patients with early onset OB also developed stenosis at the site of the tracheal anastomosis at 2, 3, and 6 months post-transplant. This latter complication responded to tracheal dilatation and insertion of an endotracheal silastic stent (Figures 6A and 6B), but all three patients experienced relentless progression of OB and died within 10 months of transplant. The association of early aggressive OB and tracheal stenosis suggests a more diffuse airway pathology associated with a generalized bronchomalacia.[28]

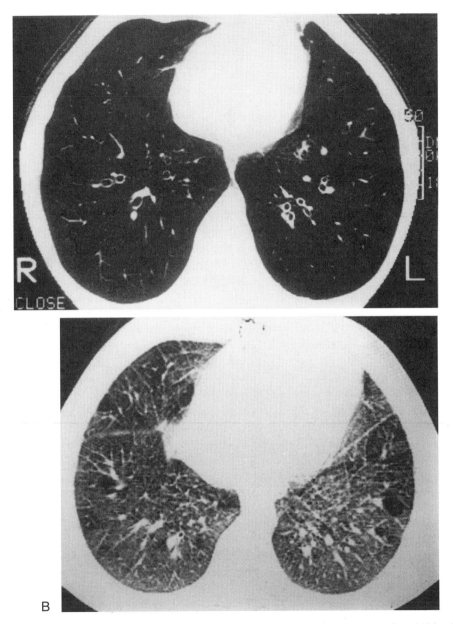

Figures 5A and 5B. High-resolution computed tomography scan appearance of a child with obliterative bronchiolitis. Note bronchial dilatation (**A**) and ground glass opacification which may precede the clinical onset of obliterative bronchiolitis (**B**).

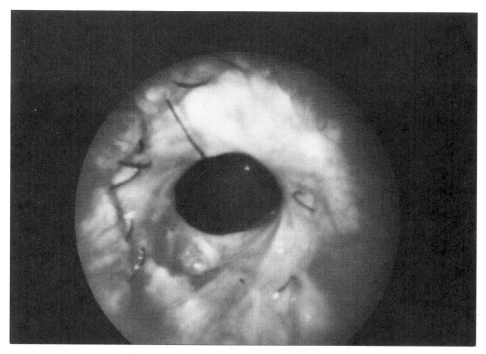

Figure 6A. Bronchoscopic appearance of tracheal anastomotic stenosis in a pediatric heart-lung transplant recipient.

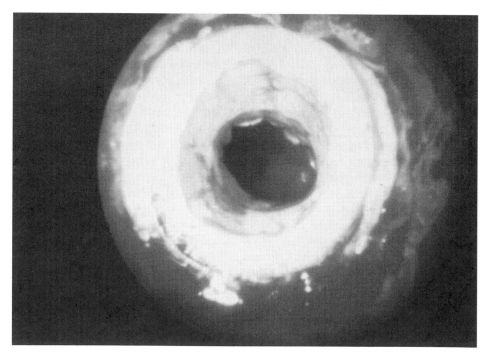

Figure 6B. Appearance following tracheal dilatation and insertion of a silastic stent. Despite this local therapy, the patient developed rapidly progressive obliterative bronchiolitis and died within 10 months of transplant.

Treatment

Therapeutic options available to combat OB are limited. Once fibroproliferation becomes established, it is difficult to halt the process and even more difficult to reverse any fibrosis which has occurred. The main treatment form utilized has been augmentation of immunosuppression with the intention of abrogating any ongoing immunologically related pulmonary damage. This has usually involved increasing steroid therapy which has previously shown initial success.[29] However, by further immunosuppressing the lung transplant recipient, the risk of infective complications is increased, possibly accentuating the lung damage and further progression of the disease. Currently, there appears to be a trend to boost immunosuppression when the development of OB is initially suspected, with subsequent reduction in the level of immunosuppression to the original baseline maintenance dose to avoid further infective events.

Obviously, all pulmonary infections must be aggressively and adequately treated with the appropriate antimicrobials, both before and after the onset of OB. Anti-infective treatment should be guided by clinical assessment, including the regular use of bronchoscopy, bronchoalveolar lavage (BAL), and transbronchial biopsy.[30]

In addition, general measures to maintain the patient in an optimal clinical state should be instituted. These include maintenance of adequate nutritional intake, use of bronchodilators as required, regular aerobic exercise to maintain muscle strength, and the provision of psychosocial support for both the child and family. This last measure is particularly important in ensuring adherence to the therapeutic regimen. With disease progression, associated with increasing dyspnea and hypoxia, oxygen therapy will be required and it is important to organize home as well as portable oxygen therapy to be available to maximize patient mobility.

The only cure for established OB is retransplantation with a single lung, bilateral lungs, or combined heart-lung block. Results of retransplantation for OB in adult lung transplant recipients have been inferior to those for primary lung transplantation.[31] Experience in the pediatric arena is more limited, but results of pediatric heart-lung retransplantation also appear poor (Figure 7).

Accordingly, the issue of retransplantation raises an ethical dilemma, that is should a precious donor organ be used to perform a procedure in a patient who has an inferior outcome, particularly when considering the greater than 50% attrition rate in those children waiting for their first lung transplant.[32] Therefore, depending upon the transplant center's approach to retransplantation, management of the terminally ill lung transplant recipient with OB needs to be adjusted accordingly, i.e., whether to bridge with intensive care therapy and ventilation to retransplantation, or to provide dignified terminal care. This may be less of a dilemma in a setting of plentiful donor organs, e.g., xenografts (see below).

Research Strategies

Despite an increasing experience with both adult and pediatric lung transplantation, there has been a relative void in the understanding of the pathophysiologic processes leading to OB. As a consequence, little progress has been made in the methods of prevention and treatment of this condition. One of the major obstacles to im-

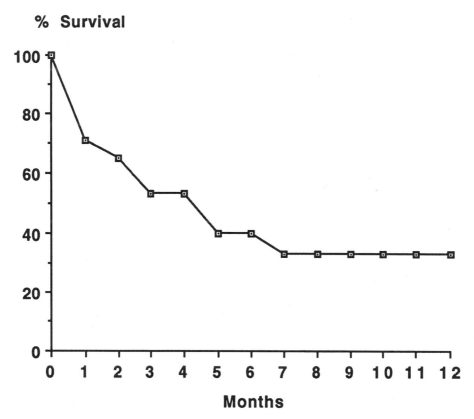

Figure 7. Actuarial survival over the first 12 months after heart-lung retransplantation. (Reproduced with permission from Kaye MP: Pediatric thoracic transplantation—world experience. *J Heart Lung Transplant* 12:S344-S350, 1993.)

proved understanding has been the difficulty in developing an adequate experimental model of OB to employ as a template for examining the pathophysiology and evaluating new therapies. Models which have been developed include those using viruses as the injurious agent. Winter et al used parainfluenza virus type 1[33] while Yagyu et al used CMV in rats to induce OB.[34] In addition, adenovirus-induced OB was developed in young dogs by Castleman et al.[35] Charcoal has also been used to induce lung injury and OB in rats by Shennib and colleagues.[36]

However, if it is to be believed that OB is consequent upon an immunologically derived injury, then an allograft model would seem more appropriate. Hertz et al developed a heterotropic murine transplanted airway model using MHC matched and mismatched donor-recipient pairs.[37] With this model, they found that airway fibroproliferation was reduced by the administration of CsA in a dose-dependent fashion. More recently, Al-Dossari and colleagues have induced OB in miniature swine using whole-lung allografts with suboptimal immunosuppression.[38] All of the above models have yielded further insight into the pathophysiology of OB and may be utilized to try new therapies. For example, Cao et al, using the heterotropic airway model, have shown exciting results with the administration of rapamycin in abrogating the fibroproliferative response.[39]

In the clinical arena, research strategies have been mainly directed toward the (early) detection of OB. These have included the identification of growth factors (platelet-derived growth factor, fibroblast growth factor, transforming growth factor) from BAL samples.[40] Also utilizing BAL, the analysis of the cellular profile, as well as the identification of activation markers of alveolar-derived cells, may be of assistance in unravelling the pathophysiology.[41,42]

Clinical therapeutic research strategies have revolved around maximizing immunosuppression and more recently the use of topical immunosuppression. Inhaled steroids are currently often prescribed for the treatment of established OB, while prophylactic aerosilized steroids are under trial following transplant in high-risk patients. The Pittsburgh group has also recently reported their experience with inhaled CsA, again in adult recipients, which has also shown promise.[43]

The technique of using living-related lung transplant donors, pioneered by Vaughan Starnes et al in California, may not only have an impact on the scarcity of donor organs, but as there is (usually) greater MHC matching between donor and recipient and, therefore, possibly less rejection, may also influence the incidence of OB.[44]

Genetic manipulation of the allograft is also being evaluated in an attempt to reduce the host rejection response and decrease the risk of OB development. Xeno transplantation is becoming more of a clinical possibility with the success in the production of a transgenic pig which expresses human cell surface molecules which inactivate human complement.[45] In addition, a recent report has detailed the experience of transplanting a transgenic pig's heart into a baboon with prolonged survival of the xenograft.[46] The clinical use of genetically engineered xenografts may possibly provide protection against the longer term development of OB in addition to providing a more reliable donor organ source.

Conclusion

OB remains one of the major obstacles to the long-term success of pediatric (and adult) lung transplantation. It appears to be secondary to an immunologically mediated lung injury, although the etiology may be multifactorial. Pathologically, the end result is marked fibrosis of the smaller airways, leading to an obstructive lung defect often associated with recurrent infections consequent upon the development of a central bronchiectasis. Medical therapy, usually comprising augmentation of immunosuppression, has not been effective in either preventing or treating OB and the only cure remains retransplantation which has inferior results. A greater understanding of the pathophysiology is being made possible following the development of experimental models of OB which will also enable the appraisal of various new therapies. Genetic and transgenic techniques may, in the future, aid in the prevention of OB, as well as widen the available donor pool.

References

1. Burke CM, Glanville AL, Theodore J, Robin ED: Lung immunogenicity, rejection, and obliterative bronchiolitis. *Chest* 92:547–549, 1987.

2. Whitehead B, Rees P, Sorensen K, et al: Incidence of obliterative bronchiolitis after heart-lung transplantation in children. *J Heart Lung Transplant* 12:903–908, 1993.
3. Yousem SA, Berry GJ, Brunt EM, et al: A working formulation for the standardization of nomenclature in the diagnosis of heart and lung rejection: lung rejection study group. *J Heart Transplant* 9:593–601, 1990.
4. Yousem SA, Burke CM, Billingham ME: Pathologic pulmonary alterations in long-term human heart-lung transplantation. *Hum Pathol* 16:911–923, 1985.
5. Hardy KA, Schidlow DB, Zaeri N: Obliterative bronchiolitis in children. *Chest* 93:460–466, 1988.
6. Chamberlain D, Maurer J, Chaparro C, Idolor L: Evaluation of transbronchial lung biopsy specimens in the diagnosis of bronchiolitis obliterans after lung transplantation. *J Heart Lung Transplant* 13:963–971, 1994.
7. Cooper JD, Billingham M, Egan T, et al: A working formulation for the standardization of nomenclature and for clinical staging of chronic dysfunction in lung allografts. *J Heart Lung Transplant* 12:713–716, 1993.
8. Scott JP, Higenbottam TW, Sharples L, et al: Risk factors for obliterative bronchiolitis in heart-lung transplant recipients. *Transplantation* 51:813–817, 1991.
9. Yousem SA, Dauber J, Keenan R, et al: Does histologic acute rejection in lung allografts predict the development of bronchiolitis obliterans? *Transplantation* 52:306–309, 1991.
10. Keenan RJ, Lega ME, Dummer JS, et al: Cytomegalovirus serologic status and post operative infection correlated with risk of developing chronic rejection after pulmonary transplantation. *Transplantation* 51:433–438, 1991.
11. Tilney NL, Whitley WD, Diamond JR, et al: Chronic rejection—an undefined conundrum. *Transplantation* 52:389–398, 1991.
12. Taylor TM, Rose ML, Yacoub M: Expression of class I and II MHC antigens in normal and transplanted human lungs. *Transplant Proc* 21:451, 1989.
13. Sly PD, Soto-Quiros, Landau LI, et al: Factors predisposing to abnormal pulmonary function after adenovirus type 7 pneumonia. *Arch Dis Child* 59:935–939, 1984.
14. Milne DS, Gascoigne AD, Ashcroft T, et al: Organising pneumonia following pulmonary transplantation and the development of obliterative bronchiolitis. *Transplantation* 57:1757–1762, 1994.
15. Reid KR, McKenzie FN, Menkis AH, et al: Importance of chronic aspiration in recipients of heart-lung transplants. *Lancet* 336:206–208, 1990.
16. Korsch BM, Fine RN, Negrete VF: Noncompliance in children with renal transplants. *Pediatrics* 61:872–876, 1978.
17. Dunn J, Golden D, Van Buren CT, et al: Causes of graft loss beyond two years in the cyclosporine era. *Transplantation* 49:349–353, 1990.
18. Serrano-Ikkos E, Whitehead B, Lask B: Cystic fibrosis: nonadherence after transplantation. *Pediatr Pulmonol* 9(suppl):274, 1993.
19. Wallwork J: Risk factors for chronic rejection in heart and lungs—why do hearts and lungs rot? *Clin Transplant* 8:341–344, 1994.
20. Burke CM, Theodore J, Baldwin JC, et al: Twenty-eight cases of human heart-lung transplantation. *Lancet* 1:517–519, 1986.
21. Radley-Smith RC, Burke M, Pomerance A, Yacoub MH: Graft vessel disease and obliterative bronchiolitis after heart lung transplantation in children. *Transplant Proc* 27:2017–2018, 1995.
22. Metras D, Shennib H, Kreitmann B, et al: Double-lung transplantation in children: a report of 20 cases. *Ann Thorac Surg* 55:352–357, 1993.
23. Spray TL, Mallory GB, Canter CB, Huddleston CB: Pediatric lung transplantation: indications, techniques, and early results. *J Thorac Cardiovasc Surg* 107:990–1000, 1994.
24. Theodore J, Starnes VA, Lewiston NJ: Obliterative bronchiolitis. *Clin Chest Med* II:309–321, 1990.
25. Skeens JL, Fuhrman CR, Yousem SA: Bronchiolitis obliterans in heart-lung transplantation patients: radiologic findings in eleven patients. *AJR* 153:253–256, 1989.
26. Lentz D, Bergin CJ, Berry GJ, et al: Diagnosis of bronchiolitis obliterans in heart-lung transplantation patients: importance of bronchial dilatation on CT. *AJR* 159:463–467, 1992.

27. Scadeng M, Dicks-Mireaux C, Flower CDR, Whitehead B: High resolution CT in the detection of obliterative bronchiolitis in paediatric heart-lung transplantation. *AJR* 1995. (Submitted.)

28. Novick RJ, Ahmad D, Menkes AH, et al: The importance of acquired diffuse bronchomalacia in heart-lung transplant recipients with obliterative bronchiolitis. *J Thorac Cardiovasc Surg* 101:643–648, 1991.

29. Glanville AR, Baldwin JC, Burke CM, et al: Obliterative bronchiolitis after heart-lung transplantation: apparent arrest by augmented immunosuppression. *Ann Intern Med* 107:300–304, 1987.

30. Whitehead B, Scott JP, Helms P, et al: Technique and use of transbronchial biopsy in children and adolescents. *Pediatr Pulmonol* 12:240–246, 1992.

31. Novick RJ, Andreassian B, Schafers H-J, et al: Pulmonary retransplantation for obliterative bronchiolitis: intermediate-term results of a North American-European series. *J Thorac Cardiovasc Surg* 107:755–763, 1994.

32. Whitehead BF, de Leval MR: Paediatric lung transplantation: the agony and the ecstasy. *Thorax* 49:437–439, 1994.

33. Winter JB, Gouw AS, Groen M, Wildevuur C, Prop J: Respiratory viral infections aggravate airway damage caused by chronic rejection in rat lung allografts. *Transplantation* 57:418–422, 1994.

34. Yagyu K, Van Breda Vriesman BJC, Duijvestijn AM, et al: Reactivation of cytomegalovirus with acute rejection and cytomegalovirus infection with obliterative bronchiolitis in rat-lung allografts. *Transplant Proc* 25:1152–1154, 1993.

35. Castleman WL: Bronchiolitis obliterans and pneumonia induced in young dogs by experimental adenovirus infection. *Am J Pathol* 119:495–504, 1985.

36. Shennib H, Serrick C, Corris P, Giaid A: Development of a nonallogeneic animal model of obliterative bronchiolitis. *J Heart Lung Transplant* 14:S44, 1995.

37. Hertz MI, Jessurun J, King MB, Sarik SK, Murray JJ: Reproduction of the obliterative bronchiolitis lesion after heterotopic transplantation of mouse airway. Am J Pathol 142:1945–1951, 1993.

38. Al-Dossari GA, Kshettry VR, Jessurun J, Bolman RM III: Experimental large-animal model of obliterative bronchiolitis after lung transplantation. Ann Thorac Surg 58:34–40, 1994.

39. Cao W, Mohacsi P, Pratt R, Morris RE: Effects of rapamycin on growth factor-stimulated vascular smooth muscle cell DNA synthesis: inhibition of bFGF and PDGF action and antagonism of rapamycin by FK 506. *Transplantation* 1995. (In press.)

40. Al-Dossari GA, Jessurun J, Bolman RM III, et al: Pathogenesis of obliterative bronchiolitis. *Transplantation* 59:143–145, 1995.

41. Haslam PL, Whitehead BF, Hughes DA, et al: BAL neutrophil counts but not lymphocyte profiles are associated with chronic deterioration in lung function in children after heart/lung transplantation. *Am J Resp Crit Care Med* 151:A121, 1995.

42. Haslam PL, Whitehead BF, Hughes DA, et al: Changes in the BAL macrophage population reflecting early-stage instability in children after lung transplantation. *Am J Resp Crit Care Med* 151:A257, 1995.

43. Iacono A, Keenan R, Zeevi A, et al: Aerosilized cyclosporine improves acute allograft rejection refractory to conventional immunosuppression. *Am J Resp Crit Care Med* 151:A258, 1995.

44. Starnes VA, Barr ML, Cohen RG: Lobar transplantation: indications, technique, and outcome. *J Thorac Cardiovasc Surg* 108:403–411, 1994.

45. Rosengard AM, Cary NRB, Langford GA, et al: Tissue expression of human complement inhibitor, decay-accelerating factor in transgenic pigs. *Transplantation* 59:1325–1333, 1995.

46. McCurry KR, Kooyman DL, Alvarado CG, et al: Human complement regulatory proteins protect swine-to-primate cardiac xenografts from humoral injury. *Nature Med* 1:423–427, 1995.

Chapter 19

Pulmonary Retransplantation

Ko Bando, MD; Bartley P. Griffith, MD

During the last decade, isolated lung transplantation has become an established treatment for selected patients with end-stage pulmonary disease.[1,2] As with any transplant procedure, some grafts fail and these recipients become potential candidates for retransplantation. At the University of Pittsburgh, between January 1989 and May 1994, 119 single lung transplantation (SLT) and 106 bilateral lung transplantation (BLT) procedures were performed in 210 patients; 13 recipients required retransplantation. This chapter documents our experience with pulmonary retransplantation and discusses the indication, technique, and postoperative management of pulmonary retransplantation, as well as the feasibility and risks associated with this procedure.

Indications for Pulmonary Retransplantation (Table 1)

Between January 1, 1989, and May 1, 1994, 210 patients underwent isolated lung transplantation and 42 (21%) of these recipients were activated for retransplantation because of primary graft failure (n = 16), obliterative bronchiolitis (OB)(n = 17), post-transplant lymphoproliferative disease (PTLD) (n = 2), refractory acute rejection and OB (n = 4), or ischemic airway injury (n = 3). Five recipients were later removed from the list for retransplantation because their graft dysfunction resolved; 23 recipients died before a suitable donor was found, 1 recipient has become too ill to be retransplanted, 1 recipient is still waiting for a donor, and 13 recipients (31%) underwent pulmonary retransplantation.

Donor Lung Preservation

Criteria for selection of a donor included: a clear chest radiograph; a PaO_2 greater than 350 mm Hg on an FiO_2 of 1.0, or a PaO_2 greater than 100 mm Hg on an FiO_2 of 0.4;

From: Franco KL (ed). *Pediatric Cardiopulmonary Transplantation*. Armonk, NY: Futura Publishing Company, Inc.; © 1997.

Table 1.

Indication for Pulmonary Retransplantation at University of Pittsburgh

Indication	Activated	ReTX	No. of Patients died before TX	Recovered	Withdrew
CR	17	6	9	1	1
Primary graft failure	16	4	8	4	0
AR/CR	4	1	3	0	0
PTLD	2	2	0	0	0
Airway ischemia	3	0	3	0	0
TOTAL	42	13	23	5	1

CR = chronic rejection; AR = acute rejection; PTLD = post-transplant lymphoproliferative disease.

negative HIV antibody titer; minimal sputum production; and no evidence of aspiration as detected by bronchoscopy. However, for the second lung transplant, we were willing to accept a donor with more marginal oxygenation (PaO_2 = 280 to 350 mm Hg on FiO_2 of 1.0) or less than clear chest radiograph. After heparinization with 300 u/kg, prostaglandin E_1 at a dose of 50 ng/kg was infused into the superior vena cava of the donor. The main pulmonary artery was cannulated and University of Wisconsin (UW) or Euro-Collins (EC) solution was infused at approximately 800 mL/min with a mechanical pump for a total infusion of 100 mL/kg.[3] The lungs were expanded with 100% oxygen and stapled two cartilaginous rings above the carina.[4] The harvested lungs were immersed in 4°C UW or EC solution. The preservation solution was washed out from the lung via the left atrial anastomosis with a wasted blood flush immediately before reperfusion. This preservation technique was applied to both the original and second lung transplants.

Operative Technique

SLT[5] or BLT[6] was performed as previously described with the following modifications. We stapled the pulmonary artery, ligated the pulmonary veins, and performed the bronchial anastomosis first. We used a continuous monofilament suture for the membranous wall of the bronchus, followed by interrupted telescopic sutures for the cartilaginous portion.[7] No omental wrapping of the airway anastomosis was performed. Cardiopulmonary bypass (CPB) was required if pharmacologically unmanageable hypoxemia or hemodynamic instability occurred.[8]

Extracorporeal Membrane Oxygenation

Three recipients required support on extracorporeal membrane oxygenation (ECMO) as a bridge to redo lung transplant. The indications for ECMO were marginal oxygenation with a PaO_2 less than 100 mm Hg on an FiO_2 of 1.0 for more than 8 hours, and diffuse opacification of the lungs by chest radiograph.[9] These recipients were placed on venoarterial ECMO by the cannula placed into the right atrium and the ascending aorta via a reopened or new sternotomy incision. Extracorporeal flow was maintained with a centrifugal pump (Biomedicus, St. Paul, MN) at approximately 80% of the cardiac output by the pulsatile counter observed in the systemic arterial pressure tracing. Anticoagulation was maintained with a continuous infusion of heparin that was titrated to keep the whole-blood activated clotting time between 180 and 220 seconds. Platelets were administered when platelet count was less than $100,000/mm^3$. The risks of barotrauma and oxygen toxicity to the lungs were minimized by using minimal ventilatory assistance with a respiratory rate of 6 to 12 per minute, positive end-expiratory pressure (PEEP) of 5 to 8 cm H_2O, and an FiO_2 of 0.28 to 0.4. Minimal anxiolytic and narcotic medications were used during ECMO in order to adequately assess neurologic function. Prophylactic vancomycin was administered to prevent *Staphylococcus aureus* infection, and specific antibiotics were employed if positive blood cultures were identified.

Retransplantation Technique

Preservation and operative techniques were the same as for the original transplant except that 6 of 13 recipients (46%) required CPB because of preretransplant support on ECMO, unstable hemodynamics during the retransplant procedure, or poor oxygenation at the time of retransplantation. Removal of the original lung(s) was sometimes technically difficult because of adhesions and parenchymal consolidation. Maximal attention was taken to minimize air leaks from the invariably inflated lung. It was also important to identify and protect the phrenic and, when possible, recurrent laryngeal nerves.

Postoperative Care and Immunosuppressive Protocol

Immunosuppressive therapy after the initial and second transplants included cyclosporine (CsA), azathioprine, and low dose corticosteroids. Immediately before the first, but not the second, transplantation, azathioprine (4 mg/kg) and methylprednisolone (5 mg/kg) were administered intravenously. CsA was begun by continuous infusion as soon as the recipient was hemodynamically stable, usually 6 to 8 hours after transplantation. The dose was titrated to maintain a whole blood level by the Abbott TDx method of 700 to 1000 ng/dL for the first month after transplantation, followed by a reduction to 500 to 700 ng/dL thereafter. After the second lung transplant, CsA was initiated later at 16 to 72 hours after transplantation, and at a lower dose to maintain a blood level of 500 to 700 ng/dL in an attempt to avoid infection and minimize renal dysfunction. Following the initial procedure, the dose of azathioprine was titrated to maintain a white blood cell count of about 5000 mm^3. After retransplantation, azathioprine was withheld until immediately prior to discharge to minimize the risk of infection. Two recipients received rabbit antithymocyte globulin (RATG) intramuscularly at a dose of 1.5 mg/kg/d for 5 days after the first transplant. No recipients received RATG after the second transplant. Corticosteroids (prednisone or methylprednisolone 10 to 15 mg/d) were begun when more than one episode of grade II acute rejection occurred after the first or second pulmonary transplantation.

The results of microbiologic cultures obtained from the airways of the donor and recipient at the time of each transplant were used to institute antibiotic treatment.[10] Blood, urine, and sputum cultures were performed as clinically indicated. Bronchoscopy with bronchoalveolar lavage (BAL) and transbronchial lung biopsy (TBBx) were performed every 2 weeks during the initial hospital stay after the first and second transplants, every 3 months during the first year post-transplant, every 4 months during the second year post-transplant, twice a year thereafter, and whenever infection or rejection was suspected.

Definition and Treatment of Complications

Acute allograft rejection (AR) was defined histologically[10] or clinically by new or increased radiographic infiltrates in the absence of infection, volume overload, or the adult respiratory distress syndrome (ARDS). Methylprednisolone 1000 mg/d for 3 days was used to treat the first and sometimes the second episode of acute rejection. RATG was administered at a dose of 1.5 mg/kg/d for 5 days for the third and sometimes for the second episode of acute rejection. Bacterial pneumonia was defined histologically or clinically by symptoms, new or increased radiographic infiltrates, gram stain, and culture results of sputum or BAL fluid, and was treated by appropriate antibiotics for at least 2 full weeks. ARDS was defined histologically by diffuse alveolar damage (DAD) (Figure 1), or clinically by radiographic infiltrates in the absence of volume overload, infection, or rejection. ARDS/DAD was treated by minimizing the potential for oxygen toxicity, by maintaining an arterial oxygen hemoglobin saturation around 90%, minimizing the risk of infection by omitting corticosteroids and azathioprine, and by maintaining a lower CsA blood level at around 500 ng/dL. Chronic rejection (CR) was defined as histologic OB[10] (Figure 2) and was treated with RATG at a dose of 1.5 mg/kg/d for 5 days or methylprednisolone 1000 mg/d for 3 days. PTLD was defined by histologic criteria[11] (Figure 3) and was treated by lowering the CsA level to 100 to 300

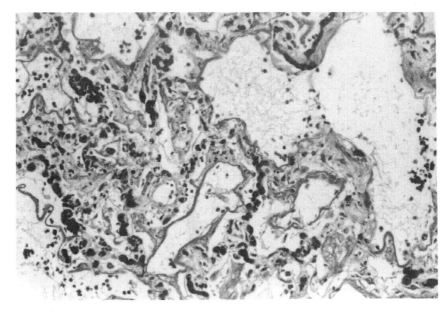

Figure 1. Diffuse alveolar damage. Eosinophilic hyaline membranes with airspace edema form the early histologic manifestation of the adult respiratory distress syndrome.

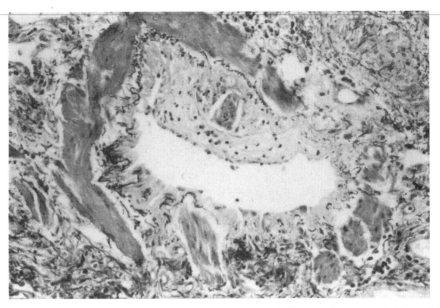

Figure 2. Obliterative bronchiolitis. An eccentric plaque of fibrous tissue partially occludes the lumen of this terminal bronchiole.

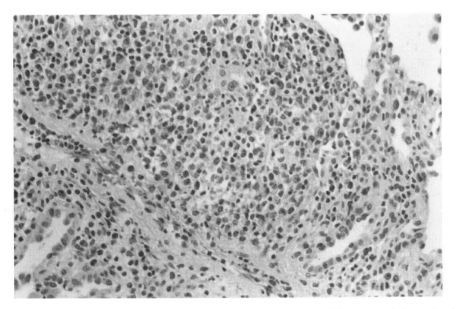

Figure 3. Post-transplant lymphoproliferative disorder. Consolidative nodules of polymorphous lymphoid cells characterize post-transplant lymphoproliferations.

ng/mL and by discontinuing azathioprine and corticosteroids. In the absence of infection, early airway ischemia was defined by the presence of cyanosis and inflammation in the airways of the allograft closest to the anastomosis. Late ischemia evolved into stenosis or bronchomalacia at and below the anastomosis.

Results

The Original Transplant

There were no significant differences in age, gender, or underlying diseases between recipients who did and those who did not require retransplantation. Two graft failures involved recipients with septic lung disease. CPB was required for three patients be-

Table 2.

Outcome of First Lung Transplantation

Recipient #	Complications	Etiology of graft failure	Life of 1st TX	Ventilator/inotrope support	Duration of EMCO
114	ARDS,DAD	Primary graft failure	3	yes/yes	36 hrs
120	ARDS,DAD	Primary graft failure	14	yes/yes	6 days
131	PTLD,AR	PTLD—>AR	184	yes/no	—
152	ARDS,DAD,HSV pneumonitis	Primary graft failure	18	yes/yes	8 days
174	DAD,ARDS,AR PTLD,Klebsiella pneumonia	PTLD	102	yes/yes	—
183	Airway ischemia, ARDS, Enteroacter pneumonia	Primary graft failure	45	yes/yes	—
204	Airway ischemia, PTLD,CR	PTLD—>CR	402	yes/no	—
214	*P. aeruginosa* pneumonia, AR,CR	CR + P. aeruginosa pneumonia	369	yes/yes	—
226	PTLD	PTLD	92	yes/yes	—
254	DAD,CR,AR	CR	561	no/no	—
319	PTLD, bronchomalacia CR,AR	PTLD—>CR	717	no/no	—
334	CMV syndrome, CR,AR	CR	631	no/no	—
342	Legionella pneumonia, CR,AR	CR	3075	no/no	—

ECMO = extracorporeal membrane oxygenation; ARDS = acute respiratory distress syndrome; DAD = diffuse alveolar damage; AR = acute rejection; CR = chronic rejection; PTLD = post-transplant lymphoproliferative disease.

cause of intraoperative hypoxemia, hemodynamic instability, and the nature of the procedure (heart-lung transplantation [HLT]). This rate of CPB was similar to that for our entire series of lung transplant procedures. The ischemic time, preservation technique, or combination of recipient/donor (cytomegalovirus [CMV]) seropositivity were similar between recipients who did and those who did not require retransplantation. There were no instances of transplantation across ABO (Rh) incompatibility.

Outcome of First Lung Transplant (Table 2)

There were no major intraoperative complications after initial lung transplants. ARDS/DAD was the cause of acute graft failure in four recipients and was due to herpes simplex virus (HSV) pneumonitis (one), acute rejection (one), and unknown (two). PTLD was the cause associated with graft failure in five patients. Overwhelming infiltration and destruction of the allograft was the indication for retransplant in two (Figure 4), while treatment of PTLD with reduced immunosuppression resulted in the loss of the three other allografts (one AR, two CR) (Figure 5). AR or CR with resultant allograft failure subsequently occurred in two patients, but there was no

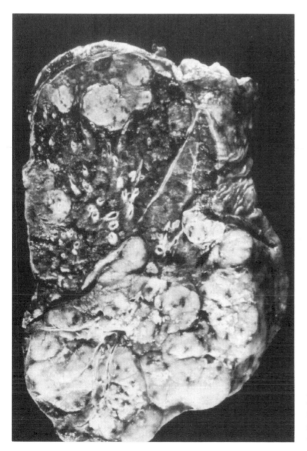

Figure 4. Post-transplant lymphoproliferative disorder. Gross photograph demonstrating fleshy, confluent tumor nodules distorting the lung parenchyma.

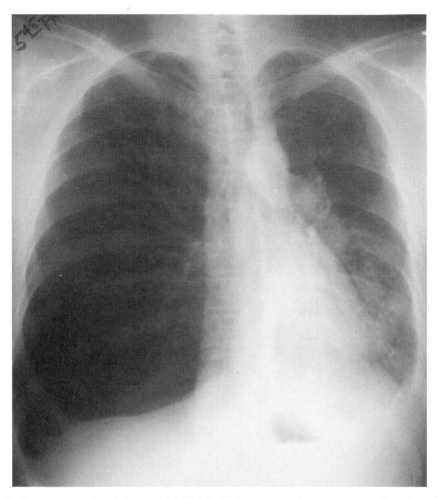

Figure 5. Chest x-ray of recipient #131 (Table 2) demonstrating post-transplant lymphoproliferative disorder involving the left hilum.

PTLD recurrence post-transplant. CR was the primary cause of graft failure in four patients and required retransplantation between 369 and 3075 days, postoperatively (Figure 6).

Nine of 13 recipients (69%) were critically ill and required ventilator or inotropic support by the time of retransplantation, and three recipients required ECMO for up to 8 days to support oxygenation as a bridge to retransplantation (Figure 7).

Outcome of Redo Lung Transplant (Table 3)

Seven of 13 recipients are surviving between 240 and 1440 days and developed ARDS/DAD between 1 and 13 days after retransplantation; this was related to the

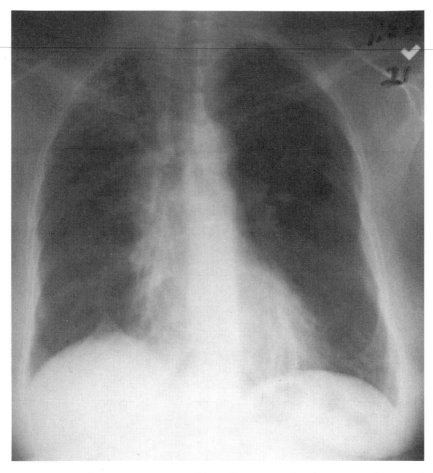

Figure 6. Chest x-ray of recipient #254 (Table 2) demonstrating hyperaeration consistent with obliterative bronchiolitis of left lung.

development of infection of the allograft in four recipients. Four recipients eventually recovered, but only after prolonged periods (5 to 7 weeks) of assisted ventilation. All but three retransplant recipients who survived more than 1 week experienced pneumonia, bronchitis, or sepsis due to bacteria or fungus after the second transplant; three recipients died primarily because of infection and multisystem organ failure. Bleeding related to adhesions from the first lung transplant and to anticoagulation required by CPB was a major concern as a potential complication with retransplantation. We did encounter severe adhesions between the lung allograft and the chest wall in two recipients which resulted in massive bleeding, coagulopathy, and death. Although a mean of 10 units of blood and platelet transfusions were required during and after the retransplant procedure among the other 11 recipients, hemostasis was maintained, and no patients required a return to the operating room for surgical management.

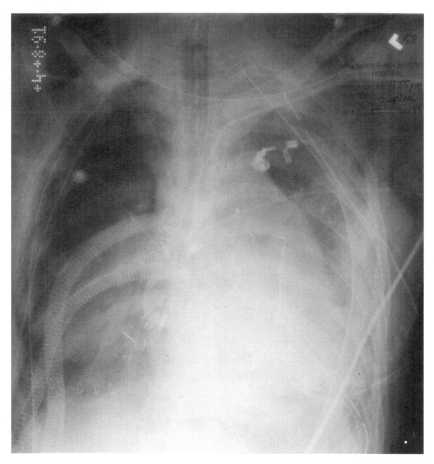

Figure 7. Chest x-ray of recipient #120 (Table 2) demonstrating near bilateral opacification associated with the diffuse alveolar damage from preservation injury. Patient is on extracorporeal membrane oxygenation.

Functional Recovery and Current Status of Retransplanted Patients

All but one survivor have achieved NYHA class I functional state (Table 3). Two recipients have returned to gainful employment, and another has returned to school on a full-time basis. Pulmonary function after the second transplant reveals a moderate restrictive defect, but with a slow improvement in the forced vital capacity (FVC) and forced expiratory volume (FEV_1) up to 24 months post-transplant. Only one recipient requires supplemental oxygen.

Discussion

During the past decade, lung transplantation has become the accepted treatment for selected patients with end-stage pulmonary, parenchymal, or vascular disease, pri-

Table 3.

Outcome of Redo Lung Transplantation

Recipient #	Complications	Outcome (days)	NYHA Class
114	ARDS,DAD, sepsis, secondary abscess at right PV anastomosis	Died (22)	—
120	Airway ischemia, ARDS,DAD, pneumonia, AR,CR	Alive(>1440)	I
131	Airway ischemia, DAD, left bronchial stenosis, CR	Alive(>1260)	I
152	ARDS, sepsis, multiple pulmonary emboli	Died(26)	—
174	ARDS,DAD, sepsis, Klebsiella pneumonia	Alive(>1050)	I
183	CMV pneumonia	Alive(>990)	I
204	ARDS,DAD, A. flavus infection	Died(25)	—
214	Cardiac arrest, interstitial lung hemorrhage	Died(1)	—
226	Cardiac arrest, massive chest wall bleeding	Died(3)	—
254	Anastomotic stenosis, ARDS,CR	Alive(>690)	I
319	DAD,ARDS,CR	Died(51)	—
334	AR,DAD	Alive(>270)	III
342	None	Alive(>240)	I

ARDS = acute respiratory distress syndrome; DAD = diffuse alveolar damage; PV = pulmonary vein; AR = acute rejection; CR = chronic rejection

marily because postoperative morbidity and mortality have declined.[12] However, despite these improvements, the 1-year survival is still only 68% and the 5-year survival is only 45%.[13] This indicates that a significant number of allografts fail. Of the many recipients with failing allografts, only a few are considered to be acceptable candidates for retransplantation, and fewer yet have survived long enough to receive a second allograft. In our experience, only 13 of 44 recipients (30%) who developed poor allograft function due to CR (n = 6), primary graft failure (n = 4), PTLD (n = 2), and combined CR and AR (n = 1) (Table 2) have been retransplanted. Our success with retransplantation was 54%, which is lower than our success rate for first time lung transplantation. The important observation here, however, is that all but one survivor (six of seven, 86%) have achieved a functional outcome equal to that of first time recipients.

ECMO as a bridge to retransplantation or infection in the first allograft was associated with a negative outcome. Of the six recipients with infection in the allograft at the time of retransplantation, three died after the second transplant. Of the three recipients on ECMO prior to retransplantation, two died after the second transplant. Of the six recipients with a negative outcome, all but one recipient had either infection in the allograft or a need for ECMO preretransplant. No retransplant recipient was septic or in a state of multisystem organ failure at the time of retransplantation. Thus, in our limited experience, the optimum candidate for retransplantation should have neither infection in the allograft nor such severe allograft failure that ECMO is required. Although two of the three recipients on pretransplant ECMO died after the second transplant, one recipient survived despite infection in the allograft at the time of retransplantation and despite being on ECMO for 6 days.

Despite treatment with reduced immunosuppression, PTLD was the direct or indirect cause of graft failure in four patients. In one recipient, the PTLD did not remit with reduced levels of immunosuppression. After treatment with alpha interferon, the PTLD did remit, but severe AR developed and this led to allograft failure. In another recipient, the PTLD did remit with reduced levels of immunosuppression, but CR later developed and this led to graft failure. These recipients were retransplanted and one recipient has no evidence of PTLD more than 36 months after retransplantation. Although disseminated PTLD is a contraindication for retransplantation, selected patients with PTLD localized to the lungs can be treated by retransplantation if conventional medical therapy is unsuccessful.

Recipients with late allograft dysfunction secondary to CR may also be suitable candidates for lung retransplantation, although the likelihood of redeveloping CR after pulmonary retransplantation is not known.[14,15] A recent survey conducted by Novick and associates on a 34 multicenter experience indicated that CR does not appear to recur in a more accelerated manner after retransplantation.[16] In our series, CR was the most common indication for retransplantation (6 of 13). Three recipients have survived with no evidence of recurrent CR up to 8 to 23 months postretransplant. In another recipient, the original transplant procedure was a BLT and the retransplant procedure was an SLT. The patient died 25 days after retransplantation from a disseminated aspergillus flavus infection that originated in the "native" lung with the CR. Adams and associates from Harefield reported a similar experience in redo SLT for patients with CR after initial HLT.[15] Based on these experiences, BLT is preferred when possible. Thus far, only one recipient has developed CR after retransplantation.

The risk of infection in retransplant recipients was markedly increased compared to first time recipients.[17,18] Infection is increased due to pretransplant immunosuppressive infection in the diseased allograft and the native lung, and requires ICU care and associated ventilation.[15] In our series, 8 of 13 (62%) recipients experienced pneumonia or sepsis, and 3 of 6 deaths were due to infection. Since perioperative infection was the most significant complication after retransplantation (62% retransplant versus 29% original transplant), this procedure probably should not be performed if infection is poorly controlled.

ARDS was the second most common complication after retransplantation (7 of 13), and the risk of this complication was much higher as compared to the first transplant (54% versus 26%). Increased risk of this complication was probably due to the severe degree of illness in these candidates and our willingness to accept marginal donors. Nevertheless, all but two recipients with ARDS recovered with conventional therapy.

We conclude that pulmonary retransplantation can be successfully performed with reasonable hope for extended high-quality survival; perioperative infection and severe allograft failure are the major risk factors associated with a poor outcome following lung retransplantation; short-term ECMO support may be successfully applied as a bridge to pulmonary retransplantation; and PTLD localized to the lungs and resistant to treatment with reduced immunosuppression can be successfully treated by retransplantation. Future efforts in this area should be directed toward determining the optimum candidate for this procedure.

References

1. The Toronto Lung Transplant Group: Unilateral lung transplantation for pulmonary fibrosis. *N Engl J Med* 314:1140–1145, 1986.
2. Egan TM, Kaiser LR, Cooper JD: Lung transplantation. *Curr Probl Surg* 26(10):673–752, 1989.
3. Griffith BP, Zenati M: The pulmonary donor. *Clin Chest Med* 11(2):217–225, 1990.
4. Weder W, Harper B, Shimokawa S, et al: Influence of intraalveolar oxygen concentration on lung preservation in a rabbit model. *J Thorac Cardiovasc Surg* 101:1037–1043, 1991.
5. Calhoon JH, Grover FL, Gibbons WJ, et al: Single lung transplantation: alternative indications and technique. *J Thorac Cardiovasc Surg* 101:816–825, 1991.
6. Cooper JD, Pearson FG, Patterson GA, et al: Technique for successful lung transplantation in humans. *J Thorac Cardiovasc Surg* 93:182–198, 1987.
7. Pasque MK, Cooper JD, Goldman B, et al: Improved technique for bilateral lung transplantation: rational and initial clinical experience. *Ann Thorac Surg* 49:785–791, 1990.
8. Aeba R, Griffith BP, Kormos RL, et al: Effect of cardiopulmonary bypass on early graft dysfunctioning clinical lung transplantation. *Ann Thorac Surg* 57:715–722, 1994.
9. Dowling RD, Zenati M, Yousem SA, et al: Donor-transmitted pneumonia in experimental lung allografts: successful prevention with donor antibiotic therapy. *J Thorac Cardiovasc Surg* 103:767–772, 1992.
10. Yousem SA, Berry GJ, Brunt EM, et al: A working formulation for the standardization of nomenclature in the diagnosis of heart and lung rejection. Lung Rejection Study Group. *J Heart Lung Transplant* 9(6):593–601, 1990.
11. Yousem SA, Randhawa P, Locker J, et al: Post-transplant lymphoproliferative disorders in heart-lung transplant recipients: primary presentation in the allograft. *Hum Pathol* 20:361–369, 1989.
12. Shapiro RS, Chauvenet A, McGuire W, et al: Treatment of B-cell lymphoproliferative syndrome with interferon alpha and intravenous gamma globulin. *N Engl J Med* 318:1334, 1988.
13. Bando K, Paradis IL, Komatsu K, et al: Analysis of time-dependent risks for infection, rejection, and death after pulmonary transplantation. *J Thorac Cardiovasc Surg* 109:49–59, 1995.
14. Hosenpud JD, Novick RJ, Breen TJ, Daily OP: The Registry of the International Society for Heart and Lung Transplantation: eleventh official report—1994. *J Heart Lung Transplant* 13:561–570, 1994.
15. Adams DH, Cochrane AD, Khaghani A, Smith JD, Yacoub MH: Retransplantation in heart-lung recipients with obliterative bronchiolitis. *J Thorac Cardiovasc Surg* 107:450–459, 1994.
16. Novick RJ, Schafers HJ, et al: Recurrence of obliterative bronchiolitis and determinants of outcome in 139 pulmonary retransplants recipients. Presented at the 75th Annual Meeting of the American Association for Thoracic Surgery, April 23–26, Boston, MA.
17. Novick RJ, Kaye MP, Patterson GA, Klepetko W, Menkis AH, McKenzie FN: Redo lung transplantation: a North American-European experience. *J Heart Lung Transplant* 12:5–16, 1993.
18. Baumgartner WA: Retransplantation of the heart. In: Baumgartner WA, Reitz BA, Achuff SC (eds). *Heart and Heart-Lung Transplantation*. Philadelphia: WB Sanders, Co.; 279–283, 1990.

Chapter 20

Pediatric Lung Transplantation:

Report of the St. Louis International Registry Results

Thomas L. Spray, MD; Mary S. Pohl, RN, BSN

Although the majority of lung transplants performed during the development of clinical lung transplantation were in adult patients, progressive improvement of the techniques and results in adults have resulted in the application of lung transplantation to the pediatric patient population. Children represent a distinctly different group as compared to adults when considered for lung transplantation, as they have different forms of end-stage pulmonary vascular disease and different types of fibrotic pulmonary disease.[1] In spite of these differences between pediatric and adult lung transplantation, the number of pediatric pulmonary transplants gradually increased worldwide and the short-term results suggest that pulmonary transplantation will become more widely used as a treatment for end-stage pulmonary or cardiovascular disease in children.

Analysis of the data collected by the St. Louis International Lung Transplant Registry and reported in September of 1995 shows a total of 4366 pulmonary transplants performed worldwide.[2] The majority of these transplant procedures were performed in the United States, although a significant number were done in England, France, Canada, and Germany (Figure 1). Single lung transplants (SLT) accounted for 2600 of the 4366 transplants (60% of the total); the remaining transplants were by the en-bloc double (242) or bilateral sequential (1515) technique (Table 1).

Analysis of the diagnosis for which transplantation was performed is shown in Figure 2. The majority of transplants reported to the Lung Transplant Registry have been performed in patients with chronic obstructive pulmonary disease (COPD), idiopathic pulmonary fibrosis, or emphysema of the alpha-1 antitrypsin variety. A smaller, but significant proportion of transplants (662 of the total) were performed in patients with cystic fibrosis (CF). The remaining diagnoses, including Eisenmenger's syndrome and primary pulmonary hypertension, represent a relatively smaller proportion of patients

From: Franco KL (ed). *Pediatric Cardiopulmonary Transplantation.* Armonk, NY: Futura Publishing Company, Inc.; © 1997.

Table 1.

**St. Louis International Lung Transplant Registry
September 1995 Report
Indications for Transplantation (Excludes En-bloc doubles)**

Diagnosis	*n*	*Single Lung (n=2600)*	*Bilateral Lung (n=1515)*
COPD	1284	1055	229
A-1 Emphysema	489	337	152
Cystic Fibrosis	601	2	599
PPH/Eisenmengers	426	239	187
IPF	685	614	71
Other	630	353	277

COPD=Chronic obstructive pulmonary disease; A-1 = alpha–1 antitrypain; PPH = primary pulmonary hypertension; IPF = idiopathic pulmonary fibrosis.

in the total group. As noted in Table 1, the majority of transplants for the diagnosis of CF were performed by the bilateral sequential technique, and patients in this group represent almost one-half of all the bilateral sequential lung transplants (BSLTs) that have been recorded.

Clinical activity in transplantation has progressively increased, such that in 1992, 795 transplants were reported to the International Lung Transplant Registry, 930 in 1993, and 913 in 1994 (Figure 3). In 1994, 488 SLTs, 390 BSLTs, and 32 en-bloc double procedures were performed. Projection of the data in the 1995 group (Figure 4) would suggest that as greater experience has been obtained, the number of double lung transplants has increased, while the number of SLTs has decreased.

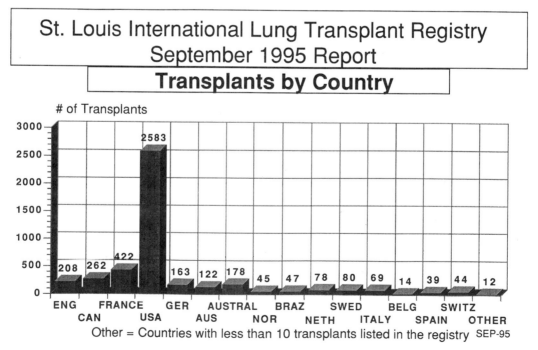

Figure 1.

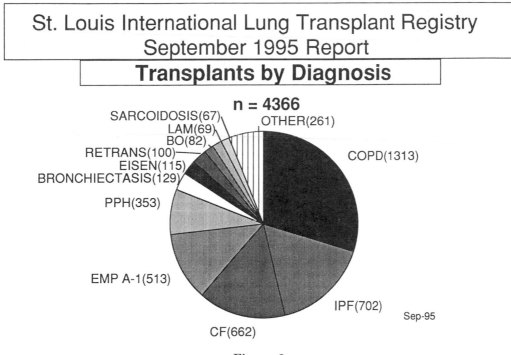

Figure 2.

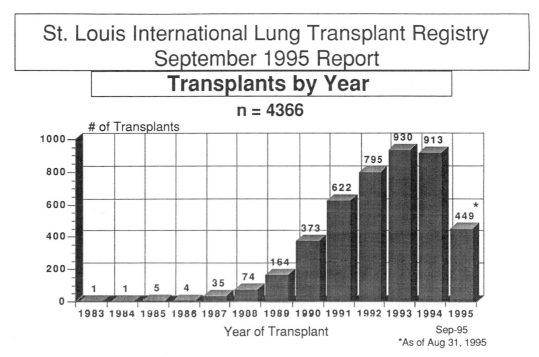

Figure 3.

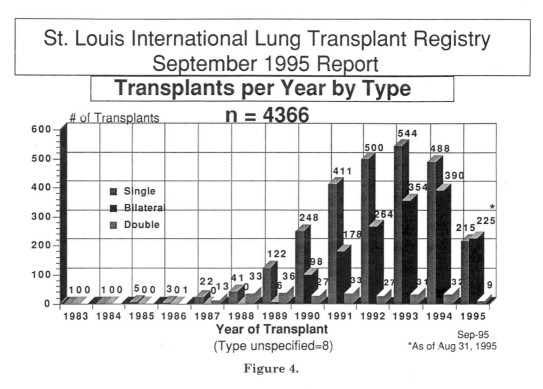

Figure 4.

Pediatric Lung Transplantation

Figure 5 shows the age distribution of the 4366 transplants performed and reported to the Lung Transplant Registry by September of 1995. The majority of patients have been over 21 years of age, with only 330 patients transplanted at less than 20 years of age. In addition, only 76 patients under 10 years of age were transplanted. This data confirms the fact that pediatric lung transplantation is relatively unusual, but that the numbers are gradually increasing. A breakdown of the transplants in patients less than 16 years of age (Table 2) shows that the majority of transplants have been BSLTs, with fewer en-bloc double lung transplants and SLTs. Analysis in Table 3 of the breakdown of diagnoses in the pediatric patients shows that the majority of children transplanted to date have CF; almost half of the total group (87 of 187 patients) had this diagnosis. A relatively smaller proportion of patients had a pretransplant diagnosis of pulmonary hypertension or pulmonary fibrosis, and only a few patients were transplanted for Eisenmenger's syndrome or were retransplanted. Thus, the pediatric patients who have undergone transplantation have a disease spectrum requiring transplantation that is more similar to that seen in heart-lung transplantation (HLT) than that seen in adult lung transplantation. Emphysema and alpha-1 antitrypsin deficiency are virtually nonexistent in children who require transplantation, and idiopathic pulmonary fibrosis is rarely severe enough to require transplantation in childhood. Thus, the majority of pediatric patients who come to lung transplantation will have rare fibrotic lung disease, CF with progressive pulmonary dysfunction, complications of repaired or unrepaired congenital heart disease, or primary pulmonary hypertension.

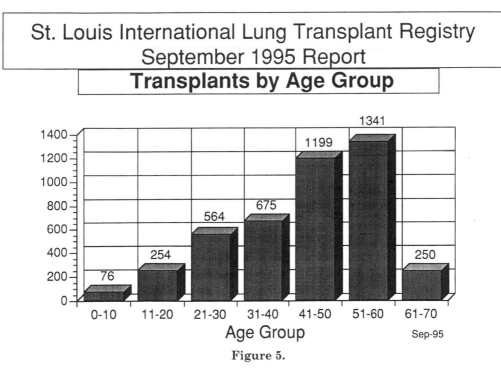

Figure 5.

Analysis of the 771 early (within 90 days post-transplant) deaths of recipients after lung transplantation reported to the Lung Transplant Registry shows that the majority were caused by sepsis (27%) and primary organ failure (12%). A few instances of death from airway dehiscence (5%), rejection (5%), or hemorrhage (7%) were noted. These data confirm the risks associated with sepsis in immunosuppressed patients, especially in patients who have colonization of the lungs prior to transplant. Although early deaths were likely due to sepsis or primary organ failure, late deaths (after 90 days post-transplant) were often (27%) caused by obliterative bronchiolitis (OB) and rejection, with sepsis becoming the second most common identifiable cause of late death (25%). This data reflects the known concerns about the development of OB in

Table 2.

St. Louis International Lung Transplant Registry
September 1995 Report
Pediatric Transplants (0–16 Years)
Age in Years

Group	0–5 (n=39)	6–10 (n=37)	11–16 (n=111)	Total (n=187)
Single	7	6	21	34
Bilateral	31	28	76	135
Double	1	3	13	17
Unknown	0	0	1	1

Table 3.

St. Louis International Lung Transplant Registry
September 1995 Report
Pediatric Transplants (0–16 Years)
Age in Years

Diagnosis	*0–5* *(n=39)*	*6–10* *(n=37)*	*11–16* *(n=111)*	*Total* *(n=187)*
CF	2	18	67	87
IPF	2	1	9	12
PPH	12	4	14	30
EISEN	2	1	5	8
OB	1	5	3	9
RETRAN	0	3	5	8
OTHER	20	5	8	33

lung transplant patients, and reflects the relatively high incidence of chronic rejection which is not adequately managed by current immunosuppressive regimens.

Actuarial Survival

The overall analysis of actuarial survival of the 3113 patients on whom data was collected by the Lung Transplant Registry is demonstrated in Figure 6. The 1-year survival rate was 71%, with a 3-year survival rate of 57%. When comparison is made based on transplant type, rather than overall survival (Figure 7), the SLTs and BSLTs have a virtually identical 1-year survival rate, but BSLTs have a slightly better survival at 2 and 3 years, while en-bloc double lung transplants have a significantly lower survival rate. In addition, when comparison is made on the basis of diagnosis for which transplantation was performed (Figure 8), emphysema patients are noted to have a higher (69%) 2-year survival rate than patients with CF (63%), pulmonary hypertension (58%), or pulmonary fibrosis (56%).

Analysis of pediatric transplants reported through September 1995 (Figure 9) shows a small number of patients for whom data is available at 1 and 2 years. Survival of 67% in a total group of 180 pediatric transplants at 1 year, 58% at 2 years, and 54% at 3 years was reported.

It has been suggested that double lung transplantation is a better procedure for patients with pulmonary hypertension and Eisenmenger's syndrome than SLT and cardiac repair.[3] Analysis of the data presented to the International Lung Transplant Registry at 2 years suggests a slight difference between these two techniques, with a 55% to 62% survival at 2 years in both groups (Figure 10). Most of the difference, however, is in early mortality, with a slightly better early survival in double lung recipients. This difference perhaps reflects the better early hemodynamic stability with double lung transplants versus SLTs for pulmonary hypertension. In addition, SLT and BSLT results for patients with alpha-1 emphysema and COPD at 1, 2, 3, and 4 years are similar (Figure 11). Longer follow-up may be necessary to define a survival difference between these two procedures, as is reflected in the emerging significant survival differences between SLT and double lung transplants at 2 years and greater, as OB be-

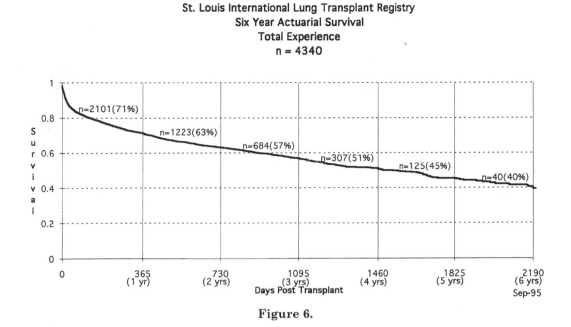

Figure 6.

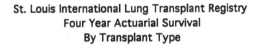

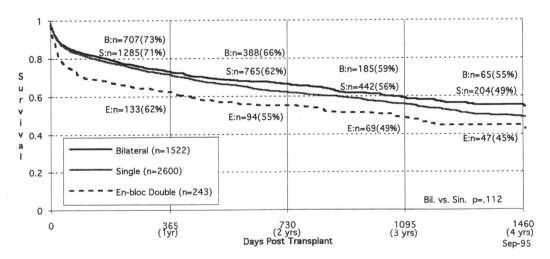

Figure 7.

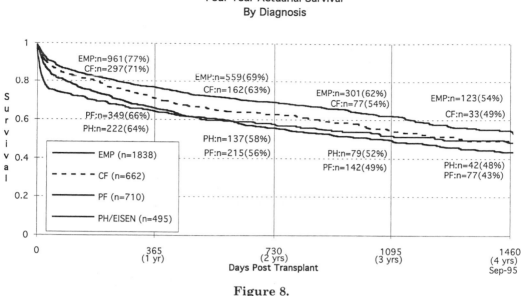

Figure 8.

differences between SLT and double lung transplants at 2 years and greater, as OB becomes a more common cause of late mortality.

The requirement for cytomegalovirus (CMV) matching between donor and recipient has not been supported by data from the Lung Transplant Registry. Analysis of the donor and recipient CMV status, and the long-term results at 3 and 4 years in the total group of reported patients as seen in Figure 12 shows a similar survival with all CMV matches.

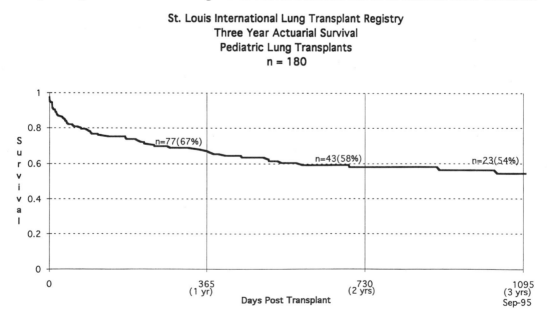

Figure 9.

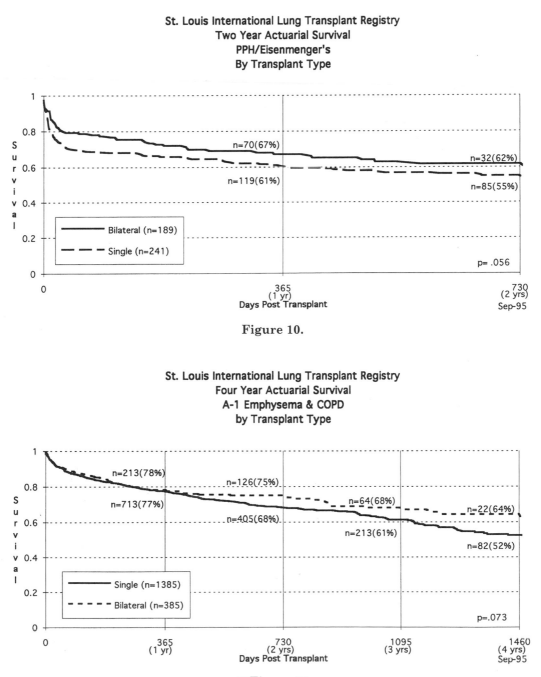

St. Louis International Lung Transplant Registry
Two Year Actuarial Survival
PPH/Eisenmenger's
By Transplant Type

n=70(67%)

n=32(62%)

n=119(61%)

n=85(55%)

Bilateral (n=189)

Single (n=241)

p= .056

0

365
(1 yr)
Days Post Transplant

730
(2 yrs)
Sep-95

Figure 10.

St. Louis International Lung Transplant Registry
Four Year Actuarial Survival
A-1 Emphysema & COPD
by Transplant Type

n=213(78%)

n=126(75%)

n=713(77%)

n=64(68%)

n=22(64%)

n=405(68%)

n=213(61%)

n=82(52%)

Single (n=1385)

Bilateral (n=385)

p=.073

0

365
(1 yr)

730
(2 yrs)
Days Post Transplant

1095
(3 yrs)

1460
(4 yrs)
Sep-95

00Figure 11.

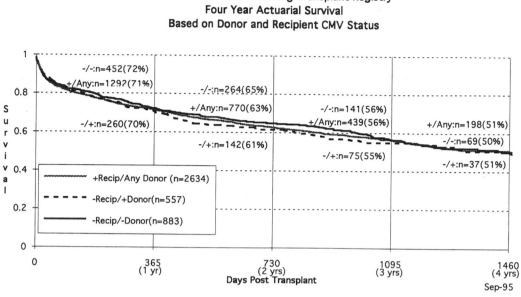

Figure 12.

A group in which the reported results are particularly poor are those patients who have undergone retransplantation of lungs. Ninety-nine such patients have been reported to the International Lung Transplant Registry in the September 1995 report with a very significant early mortality of approximately 40% and a 1-year survival of only 48%. The early steep slope of the actuarial survival curve in this group reflects problems with sepsis and early graft failure in patients who undergo retransplantation after increases in immunosuppressive therapy in hopes of improving pulmonary function in patients with OB.[4] In addition, retransplantation of a patient who develops acute graft failure after initial lung transplant has been associated with very poor results due to the high incidence of sepsis.

Conclusions

Analysis of the data collected from over 94 international lung transplant centers by the St. Louis International Lung Transplant Registry has provided invaluable data regarding the expected outcome after lung transplantation. While long-term follow-up is not available on the majority of recipients, continued monitoring and the reporting of results will hopefully shed light on the relative advantages of SLT versus double lung transplantation for certain pulmonary conditions and the effects of development of OB on the late functional results. Although a significant early mortality remains after lung transplantation, the actuarial survival after successful transplantation appears to be satisfactory, with a significantly good late functional result in those patients who do not develop OB.

Pediatric lung recipients represent a relatively small proportion of cases that have been reported to the International Lung Transplant Registry. The markedly different distribution of clinical diseases for which pediatric lung transplantation is performed as compared to adults make direct comparison between the patient populations difficult. Therefore, continued reporting of pediatric lung recipients to registries such as the International Lung Transplant Registry may provide sufficient numbers to be able to compare the results of this therapy to reported results of HLT in children.

References

1. Spray TL, Huddleston CB: Pediatric lung transplantation. *Chest Surg Clin North Am* 3:123–143, 1993.
2. St. Louis International Lung Transplant Registry, Suite 3108 Queeny Tower, 4989 Barnes Hospital Plaza, St. Louis, MO 63110. September 1995 Summary.
3. Trinkle JK: Discussion of Pasque MK, Kaiser LR, Dresler CM, Trulock E, Triantafillow AN, Cooper JD: Single lung transplantation for pulmonary hypertension. *J Thorac Cardiovasc Surg* 103:475–482, 1992.
4. Miller JD, Patterson GA: Retransplantation following isolated lung transplantation. *Semin Cardiovasc Surg* 4:122–125, 1992.

Index